Practical Clinical Hematology
Interpretations and Techniques

STANFORD SERIES ON METHODS AND TECHNIQUES
IN THE CLINICAL LABORATORY

Edited by Paul L. Wolf, M.D.
Director of Clinical Laboratory
Clinical Pathology and School of Medical Technology,
Stanford University Medical Center,
Stanford, California

METHODS AND TECHNIQUES IN CLINICAL CHEMISTRY
by Paul L. Wolf, Dorothy Williams,
Tashiko Tsudaka, and Leticia Acosta

PRACTICAL CLINICAL ENZYMOLOGY: TECHNIQUES
AND INTERPRETATIONS
by Paul L. Wolf and Dorothy Williams
AND BIOCHEMICAL PROFILING
by Elisabeth Von der Muehll and Paul L. Wolf

PRACTICAL CLINICAL HEMATOLOGY: INTERPRETATIONS
AND TECHNIQUES
by Paul L. Wolf, Patricia Ferguson, Irma Torquati
Mills, Elisabeth Von der Muehll, and Mary Thompson

PLANNED FOR SERIES:

COMPUTER METHODS AND TECHNIQUES IN CLINICAL MEDICINE
by Herbert Ludwig, Ph.D.

METHODS, TECHNIQUES, AND INTERPRETATIONS OF
BLOOD TRANSFUSION
by Paul L. Wolf, Betsy Hafleigh, and
Gabriel Korn

PRACTICAL CLINICAL MICROBIOLOGY AND MYCOLOGY:
TECHNIQUES AND INTERPRETATIONS
by Paul L. Wolf, Betty Russell, and
Adrienne Shimoda

Practical Clinical Hematology Interpretations and Techniques

Paul L. Wolf, M.D.
Director of Clinical Laboratory
Clinical Pathology and
School of Medical Technology
Associate Professor of Pathology

Patricia Ferguson, M.T. (ASCP)
Chief Technologist
Clinical Hematology Laboratory

Irma Torquati Mills, M.T. (ASCP)
Supervisor Morphologic Hematology
Clinical Hematology Laboratory

Elisabeth Von der Muehll, M.T. (ASCP)
Supervisor
School of Medical Technology

Mary Thompson, M.T.
Supervisor Coagulation Laboratory
Clinical Hematology Laboratory

Stanford University Medical Center
Stanford, California

A Wiley Biomedical-Health Publication

JOHN WILEY & SONS

New York   London   Sydney   Toronto

LIBRARY OF CONGRESS CATALOGING IN PUBLICATION DATA:

Main entry under title:

Clinical hematology procedures.

    (Stanford series on methods and techniques in the
clinical laboratory)
    "A Wiley-Biomedical-Health publication."
    1. Hematology--Technique. I. Wolf, Paul L.
II. Series. DNLM: 1. Blood chemical analysis--
Laboratory manuals. 2. Hematology--Laboratory manuals.
Qy25 C641 1973
RB145.C53   616.07'561   73-7968
ISBN 0-471-95910-3

Printed in the United States of America

10 9 8 7 6 5 4 3 2 1

Dedication

To all of our devoted teachers and especially to the
residents, medical students, and medical technology students
from whom we receive continual inspiration and knowledge.

Preface

This book is intended as a review and reference text book for Clinical Pathologists and Medical Technologists who are concerned with daily problems in diagnostic Clinical Hematology. We have cited a majority of the past and current technical information relevant to the determination of common Clinical Laboratory Hematology procedures and their diagnostic interpretation. A great proliferation of knowledge has occurred in the last fifteen years in this field. The emphasis of this book is on the practical aspects of Clinical Hematology with a tendency to refer to only a minimal amount of esoteric clinically irrelevant information. We have attempted to cover each Clinical Hematologic determination performed in the Stanford Clinical Laboratory completely from a technical and clinical viewpoint. The book is organized such that, the hematologic and chemical determinations are listed alphabetically to enable the reader to quickly obtain the needed information. All of the important diagnostic tests pertaining to Hematology and Coagulation are included in this book.

We thus hope that this book will provide the necessary current knowledge required by Clinical Pathologists, Medical Technologists, and Medical Technology Students for optimal care of their patients.

The Authors gratefully acknowledge the cooperation of Ruth Coleman, M.T. (ASCP), Frances MacMillan, M.T. (ASCP), Wilma Mesa, M.T. (ASCP), Charles Blankenship, M.T. (ASCP), Cheryl Haiflich, M.T. (ASCP), Karen Claridge, M.T. (ASCP), Karen Hudon, M.T. (ASCP), and others of our technical staff for their valuable contribution in compiling information and helping to revise these techniques. We also wish to thank for their technical expertise, Mr. Donald E. Morris, for the excellent technical drawings, and Mr. Leonard Winograd, for the excellent photography.

We also gratefully acknowledge the excellent secretarial work of Miss Elisabeth Von der Muehll, M.T. (ASCP), Supervisor School of Medical Technology, and Miss Charlotte Farber, who typed and edited the entire manuscript.

THE AUTHORS

Contents

Contents (Continued):

Contents (Continued):

Contents (Continued):

Contents (Continued):

xiii

Contents (Continued):

Contents (Continued):

Contents (Continued):

Contents (Continued):

Contents (Continued):

Practical Clinical Hematology
Interpretations and Techniques

ACID SERUM TEST
FOR
PAROXYSMAL NOCTURNAL HEMOGLOBINURIA (PNH)

PRINCIPLE: The hemolytic anemia PNH is characterized by the red blood cells of PNH being especially sensitive to hemolysis when the serum is acidified.

SPECIMEN: 10 ml. defibrinated blood.

REAGENTS AND EQUIPMENT:

1. Erlenmeyer Flask, 50 ml.

2. Glass Beads, 3 to 4 mm. in diameter, 10

3. Normal Saline, 0.85% NaCl

4. Centrifuge

5. Waterbath or Heat Block, 37°C.

6. Waterbath or Heart Block, 56°C.

7. Hydrochloric Acid, 0.2 N.

PROCEDURE:

1. Defibrinate 10 ml. of blood in a 50 ml. Erlenmeyer flask with 10 glass beads.

2. Centrifuge blood in a test tube for 10 minutes.

3. Wash red blood cells with 0.85% saline three times.

4. Prepare a 50% red blood suspension in saline.

5. Prepare control red blood cells in similar manner.

6. Number seven test tubes sequentially 1 through 7 and place them in a waterbath at 37°C.

7. Place 0.5 ml. of normal control serum in test tubes 3, 4, and 5, and 0.5 ml. of the patient's test serum in test tubes 1, 2, 6, and 7.

1

Acid Serum Test for PNH (Continued):

8. Immerse test tube 3 in a 56°C. waterbath or heat block for 30 minutes. Return test tube 3 to the 37°C. waterbath.

9. To test tubes 2, 3, 5, and 7 add 0.05 ml. of 0.2 N. Hydrochloric acid.

10. Add 1 drop of normal control red blood cell suspension to test tubes 6 and 7, and 1 drop of patient's test red blood cells to test tubes 1 through 5.

11. All of the test tubes should be incubated at 37°C. for 1 hour.

12. Centrifuge the test tubes for 5 minutes at 1000 rpm and observe them for hemolysis.

Test Tube	Serum	HC1	Red Blood Cells	Hemolysis
1	P*	-	P	None
2	P	+	P	Yes
3	C**(56°C.)	+	P	None
4	C	-	P	None
5	C	+	P	Yes
6	P	-	C	None
7	P	+	C	None

*   P = Patient Test
** C = Normal Control

NORMAL VALUES: Negative Test

REFERENCES:

1. Ham, T. H.: "Studies on Destruction of Erythrocytes". Arch. Int. Med. 64:1271, 1939.

2. Dacie, J. V. and Lewis, S. M.: PRACTICAL HEMATOLOGY, Grune and Stratton, New York, pg. 180, 1968.

INTERPRETATION:

A diagnosis of PNH is suggested if hemolysis occurs in Test Tubes 2 and 5.

False positive Test with hemolysis may be seen in hereditary spherocytic anemia. Spherocytes may undergo hemolysis in Test Tubes 2, 3,

Acid Serum Test for PNH (Continued):

and 5. Since PNH red blood cells require complement for hemolysis, there will be no hemolysis of PNH red blood cells in Test Tube 3, in contrast to hemolysis of spherocytic red blood cells at 56°C.

If hemolysis occurs in Test Tubes 2 and 7, but not in Test Tube 5, a warm hemolysin antibody may be present in the patient's serum.

ALPHA-HYDROXYBUTYRATE DEHYDROGENASE
(α-HBD)

PRINCIPLE: Advantage is taken of the clinical differentiation of the serum lactic dehydrogenase (LDH) isoenzymes. It has been shown that the faster moving isoenzymes reduce α-ketobutyrate while the slower moving ones show negligible activity. Damage to heart muscle, altered erythropoiesis and extreme damage to other tissue could lead to increased HBD activity.

The HBD measurement in relation to total LDH becomes of great value in the measurement of the "heart" fractions of LDH isoenzymes.

This test has the advantage of being performed quite rapidly and simply.

The following reaction takes place:

$$\alpha\text{-oxobutyrate} + NADH_2 \underset{}{\overset{HBD}{\rightleftharpoons}} \alpha\text{-hydroxybutyrate} + NAD$$

SPECIMEN: A pipetable 100 microliters (0.10 ml.) of serum, free from hemolysis, is required. This specimen is stable for several days at room temperature or 4°C.

REAGENTS AND EQUIPMENT:

(Biochemica Kit TC-HD, Cat. No. 15953 THAD for 60 Determinations)

Bottle No. 1 0.05 M. Phosphate Buffer, pH 7.4
Bottle No. 2 0.004 M. NADH
Bottle No. 3 0.10 M. alpha-oxobutyrate

1. Dissolve contents of Bottle No. 1 in 200 ml. deionized water.

2. Dissolve contents of Bottle No. 2 in 2.5 ml. deionized water.

   Mix these reagents together in a brown glass bottle. This makes Solution 1. (Stable four weeks at 4°C.)

3. Dissolve the contents of Bottle No. 3 in 6.5 ml. of deionized water. This makes Solution 2. (Stable three months at 4°C.)

   Do not mix the two solutions.

4

Alpha-hydroxybutyrate Dehydrogenase (Continued):

4. <u>DBG or Gilford 300 N Spectrophotometer</u>
An instrument with temperatured controlled cuvette well and recorder should be used.

5. <u>Eppendorf Pipette</u>
Use a 100 microliter Eppendorf pipette for dispensing serum sample.

PROCEDURE:

Place into a 10 mm. square cuvette:

1. 3.1 mol of Solution 1.

2. 0.10 ml. (100 microliters) of serum.

Mix and place into a 30°C. waterbath for approximately 15 minutes.

3. Add 0.10 ml. (100 microliters) of Solution 2. Mix. Place cuvette in cuvette well and record Absorbance change for two minutes of linearity.

4. CALCULATIONS:

Based on $\Delta A/1$ minute and a light path of 1.0 cm.

(ϵ NADH at 340 nm. = 6.22 Liter/Mole x cm.)7

$$\frac{\Delta A}{\epsilon x d} \times 10^6 \times \frac{TV}{SV} \times \frac{1}{Time} = \text{I.U./L. or mU/ml.}$$

$$\Delta A \times \frac{1}{6.22 \times 10^3 \times 1} \times 10^6 \times \frac{3.3}{0.1} \times \frac{1}{1} = \text{mU/ml.}$$

$$\Delta A \times F = \text{mU/ml.}$$

$$F = 5305$$

NORMAL VALUES: Up to 168 mU/ml. at 30°C.

6

Alpha-hydroxybutyrate Dehydrogenase (Continued):

REFERENCES:

1. Rosalki, S. B. and Wilkinson, J. H.: Nature, 188:1110, 1960.

2. Rosalki, S. B.: British Heart Journal, 25:795, 1963.

3. Preston, J. A., Batsakis, J. G., and Briere, R. O.: Amer. J. Clin. Path., 41:237, 1964.

INTERPRETATION:

The value of determining alpha-hydroxybutyrate dehydrogenase is that this enzyme corresponds to LDH-one which is from a myocardial source. Myocardial damage results in liberation of this enzyme and elevation in the serum. Hemolytic anemia and metastatic malignant melanoma will result in an elevated serum alpha-hydroxybutyrate dehydrogenase. The enzyme is present in the erythrocyte and the malignant melanoma cells.

When myocardial damage is present, LDH-one or alpha-hydroxybutyrate dehydrogenase will be increased in the serum. At times the total LDH will be normal, but the former isoenzymes will always be increased. It is more difficult to perform an electrophoresis to ascertain the level of LDH-one. In addition the determination of heat stable LDH requires more time than the determination of alpha-hydroxybutyrate dehydrogenase. Heat stable LDH corresponds to LDH-one and alpha-hydroxybutyrate dehydrogenase. It is determined by ascertaining the amount of LDH remaining after total serum LDH is heated in a water-bath at 60°C. for 30 minutes. Heat stable LDH originates from myocardial cell mitochondria and the erythrocyte. Heat labile LDH is derived from the liver and skeletal muscle. Thus, a rapid method to ascertain the presence of myocardial necrosis is the determination of alpha-hydroxybutyrate dehydrogenase. It is more rapid and simpler than the determination of LDH-one by electrophoresis or heat stability.

AUTOHEMOLYSIS TEST FOR HEMOLYTIC ANEMIA

PRINCIPLE: Normal cells undergo a small amount of hemolysis when incubated. Blood from patients with Dacie Type I Hemolytic Anemia (G-6-PD) deficiency) have increased incubated autohemolysis which corrects to some extent upon the addition of glucose or ATP. In Dacie Type II (Pyruvic Kinase deficiency), the autohemolysis is increased greatly and corrects toward normal only with ATP. Dacie III (Triosphosphate Isomerase deficiency) corrects completely with ATP or glucose. Hereditary spherocytosis has greatly increased autohemolysis and like Type I corrects toward normal with glucose or ATP.

SPECIMEN: 25 ml. of blood. On infants it is possible to use 10 to 15 ml. of blood; however, there won't be enough sample for duplicates.

EQUIPMENT AND REAGENTS:

1. Sterile 20 or 30 ml. siliconized or plastic syringe

2. 19 Gauge thin-walled needle

3. Sterile 125 ml. Erlenmeyer Flask
   Containing 25 glass beads about 4.0 mm. in diameter.

4. Sterile 5.0 ml. Screw-topped Vials

5. Sterile Dextrose, 50%
   Dilute 1:5 with sterile water just prior to use.

6. ATP, 0.4 M., Disodium Salt (M.W. 623.2)
   Use 2.5180 gm. per 10 ml. of water, pH to 7.0 with NaOH before diluting to volume. Freeze in 1.0 ml. aliquots. Stable indefinately.

7. 37°C. Waterbath

8. Sahli Hemoglobin Pipettes (0.02 ml.)

9. Drabkin's Solution

10. Centrifuge Tubes

11. Sterile Tuberculin Syringe and Needle (2)

12. 0.2 ml. Pipettes

Autohemolysis Test (Continued):

13. <u>Spectrophotometer, Coleman Jr.</u>
    Set wavelength at 540 nm.

PROCEDURE: All Steps must be kept Sterile. Always run a Normal Contr(

A. Part 1. <u>Initial Autohemolysis</u>
    1. Draw 25 ml. of blood or 10 to 15 ml. of blood on infants.

    2. Place all of sample in the sterile Erlenmeyer flask and
       defibrinate gently until there is no longer any sound of
       the glass beads swirling in the flask (5 - 15 minutes).
       Continue defibrinating sample for another 5 minutes. In
       defibrinating a smaller volume, use few glass beads or
       about 1 bead per ml. blood as in the case of infants.

    3. Pour 2.0 ml. whole blood into each of 6 sterile vials.

    4. Into 2 vials put 0.1 ml. 10% glucose using the tuberculin
       syringe (0.05 ml. glucose/ml. blood). Mix.

    5. Into 2 other vials put 0.1 ml. 0.4 M. ATP using a tuberculin
       syringe (0.05 ml. ATP/ml. blood). Mix.

    6. The remaining 2 vials are incubated with nothing added.

    7. Incubate all vials for 48 hours in the 37°C. waterbath.

    8. Measure initial autohemolysis.

B. Part II. <u>Autohemolysis</u>
            This is done on an initial sample the day the test is
            started and on the six incubated samples 48 hours later.

    1. Mix blood well by <u>gentle</u> inversion.

    2. Pipette 0.02 ml. whole blood into 5.0 ml. Drabkin's solution.

    3. Take 2 micro-hematocrits from each sample.

    4. Centrifuge remaining blood and remove serum.

    5. Pipette 0.2 ml. serum into 5.0 ml. Drabkin's solution and
       let sit 10 minutes.

Autohemolysis Test (Continued):

6. Read hemoglobins on Coleman Jr. Spectrophotometer at 540 nm.

7. Centrifuge and read hematocrits.

CALCULATIONS:

$$\frac{\text{O.D. Serum} \quad x \quad \dfrac{100 - \text{Hct.}}{100}}{\text{O.D. Whole Blood} \quad x \quad 10} \quad x \quad 100 = \frac{\text{O.D. Serum} \quad x \quad (100 - \text{HCT})}{\text{O.D. Whole Blood} \quad x \quad 10}$$

$$= \text{Percent (\%) Autohemolysis}$$

NOTES AND PRECAUTIONS:

1. Always read Optical Density and use O.D. in calculations.

2. If excessive hemolysis has taken place, use 0.02 ml. serum instead of 0.2 ml. Calculations then become:

$$\frac{\text{O.D. Plasma} \quad x \quad (100 - \text{Hct.})}{\text{O.D. Whole Blood}} = \% \text{ Autohemolysis}$$

3. If duplicates don't check, there has probably been some contamination.

4. It is almost impossible to run an autohemolysis on sickle cell blood because cells clump together due to decreased oxygen tension and are difficult to resuspend after 48 hours incubation.

NORMAL VALUES:

	Initial	Incubated	10% Glucose	0.4 M ATP
Normal	0-0.94%	0.2-2.7%	0-2.2%	0.5-2.3%
Dacie I	Normal	3-5%	Normal	Normal
Dacie II		12-16%	12-16%	Normal
Hereditary Spherocytosis		12-15%	3-5%	3-5%

REFERENCE: Selwyn, J. and Dacie, J.: "Autohemolysis and Other Changes Resulting from the Incubation In Vitro of Red Cells from Patients with Congenital Hemolytic Anemia". Blood 9:414, 1954.

Autohemolysis Test (Continued):

INTERPRETATION:

The value of this test is to assess hereditary spherocytosis. It was at one time valuable in the diagnosis of nonspherocytic congenital hemolytic anemia, but now that specific enzyme analyses are available, this test is not as important.

Hereditary spherocytosis has a greatly increased autohemolysis with the absence of added glucose. The hemolysis is corrected by adding glucose.

The congenital nonspherocytic hemolytic anemias which exhibit moderate autohemolysis, 3 to 5 percent, which is corrected by glucose are the Type I. The Type II have prominent autohemolysis, 12 to 16 percent, not corrected by the addition of glucose, but are corrected by the addition of ATP.

AUTOMATED BLOOD COUNTS
(Model S Coulter)

PRINCIPLE: The Model S Coulter uses the Coulter counting principle for WBC, RBC, and MCV. Hemoglobin is converted to cyanmethemoglobin and measured by a photocell. The PCV, MCH, and MCHC are calculated. In the diluter, blood is aspirated, automatically diluted, mixed, lyzed, and sensed. From the analyzer unit, signals in the form of voltages representing values are applied to the electronic circuits located in the power supply. The signals are converted from voltage information to digital data for use by the printer (or computer), where a numerical printout takes place.

EQUIPMENT AND REAGENTS:

1. Model S Coulter

2. Isoton

3. S Lysing Agent

4. Printout Cards

5. Isoterge

6. 4-C Control

7. Pipettes, 44.7 lambda

8. Pipettes, 10 ml.

PROCEDURE:

1. Introduce aspirator tip into tube of well-mixed blood.

2. Press "touch control bar". Do not remove blood until the red light appears above the "touch control bar".

3. Remove the blood, and wipe the aspirator with a Kimwipe or gauze.

4. Insert a card into the printer until the red light on the printer is activated. Label card with patient's name and number.

Automated Blood Counts - Model S Coulter (Continued):

5. The next specimen may be aspirated when the green light appears above the "touch control bar".

6. Fingersticks may be introduced by switching from "whole blood" to "224:1 dilution".

COMMENTS:

1. If WBC is 20,000 or more, repeat the following count.

2. If WBC is 30,000 or more (incl. 99.9), repeat entire CBC manually, and repeat the following count.

3. If WBC is 3,000 or less, repeat the count, using second value.

4. If WBC is 1,000 or less, run the count two times in succession and use the last count.

5. If PCV is 50 percent or more, repeat the following count if it is low (under 20).

6. Make sure the correct amount of lysing reagent is dispensed, approximately 1.0 ml.

7. Keep a close watch on isoton and lysing reagent levels.

ROUTINE CARE:

Blood must not be left in the aspirator tubing for more than 2 minutes. Isoton must be aspirated (press "aspirator priming" button on control panel) through the sandwich (valve) if the machine is to be stopped momentarily. (There is no need to prime the machine if it is not cycled with isoton). If the pause is for 20 minutes or more, cycle with isoton and the blood should be removed from the L-1A card by aspirating isoterge through the aspirator tip. The machine can be left with isoterge in the L-1A card, and the pneumatic power supply off, but the electronic power supply should be left on.

CLEANING:

A. Daily
1. Drain aperture bath.

2. Empty apertures by lifting out of baths, turning upside down, and pressing "count button".

Automated Blood Counts - Model S Coulter (Continued):

3. Fill WBC bath with bleach twice and drain into waste chamber.

4. Soak WBC apertures in 50% bleach and 50% isoton for 5 minutes, pushing count and clear buttons alternately for a few times (5-6). At the same time, soak RBC apertures in isoterge. Allow to soak for a few minutes. Do not let apertures fill completely up with bleach.

5. Drain both baths, and allow to soak in isoterge for 20 to 30 minutes. Use count and clear buttons again.

6. Drain baths, and rinse with isoton a few times.

7. Empty apertures as in Step 2.

8. Fill baths with isoton with "rinse button" and press "count" button until lines to the vacuum isolator jar are clear of bubbles.

9. Clean L-1A card with 50% bleach/isoton.

10. Cycle isoton through system until clear of bleach and isoterge.

11. Check bubbles rates while cycling isoton.

B. Weekly
1. Soak both RBC and WBC apertures in 50% bleach and 50% isoton for 5 minutes.

2. Turn off valve on R-1 card and remove valve. Unscrew black screw in front of valve, and remove. The middle section is carefully removed and placed in isoterge to soak for 20 minutes. Do not scratch, scrub, or drop valve. Use only Kimwipes. Rinse with isoton, and replace with the sides wet with isoton. The screw should not be put on too tight.

3. Remove diluting chambers, lysing chamber, and aperture baths - one side at a time. Wash in Haemo-Sol and bleach. Rinse with water and then isoton. Dry with Kimwipes.

4. Clean air filter on pump with water.

5. Check pressure gauges, especially the 5 PSI. Correct positions are marked with orange crayon.

Automated Blood Counts - Model S Coulter (Continued):

CALIBRATION:

1. Run isoton through the complete cycle, and check the bubble and drain rates throughout the diluting system. There should not be excessive bubbling or backing up in the system. Excessive bubbling into the counting baths will give erroneous results. Adjustments are made with the knobs on the cards on the sides of the diluter unit.

2. Run about 3 or 4 blood samples through the instrument. Check bubble rates.

3. Check background count by cycling isoton and getting a printout on a card (RBC no higher than 0.2; WBC no higher than 0.4).

4. Run 3 to 4 specimens 3 or 5 times to check for duplication.

5. Run 4-C through twice (4-C must be mixed carefully and well; it must be at room temperature). Save card with second set of values Values should be within 2 SD of values given. Record on quality control sheets. Return to refrigerator and repeat in p.m.

6. Run daily controls.* They must also be at room temperature. Record on log sheet.
   * Controls are pulled in afternoon from normal out-patients (OB-GYN, Emergency Room, Employee Health, etc.) Make sure there are 5 controls and correct values on log sheet.

NOTE ON 4-C CONTROL:

1. If 4-C does not correspond with values on sheet, run controls before becoming alarmed.

2. Check quality control sheets to see if values have been consistently high or low for that Lot Number. Notify someone if there is a trend.

3. Make sure machine is calculating correctly by using slide rule or wheel, using values printed out.

4. If 4-C is really bad, get a new bottle (using old to prime). The dilution could be off, due to an aspiration after improper mixing.

Automated Blood Counts - Model S Coulter (Continued):

NORMAL VALUES: WBC   5,000 - 10,000/cu. mm.
                    RBC   3.50 - 5.50 million/cu. mm.
                    Hgb.   12.5 - 16.0 gm./cu. mm.
                    PCV   Corresponds with MCV and RBC
                    MCV   82   - 95 cu. mm.

                    These values should agree with 2 SD of values obtained on previous day, with the exception of WBC due to protein build-up on apertures.

REFERENCE: COULTER COUNTER MODEL S MANUAL.

MODEL S TROUBLE-SHOOTING GUIDE
(INTERPRETATION)

RBC IS ERRATIC:

1. Insure external electrode is in bath.

2. Remove and clean Blood Sampling Valve.

3. The RBC aspirator (located inside WBC Mixing Chamber B-1) should be just below the entrance hole from the WBC Mixing Chamber A-1. It must not touch the sides of the B-1 chamber, and the bevel should be facing away from the hole.

4. Are there air bubbles in the blood line behind the Blood Sampling Valve?

5. Is the Blood Sampling Valve leaking from the side?

6. Is the flow rate into the RBC Mixing Chamber (A-2) too turbulent?

7. Is the RBC sample hitting the rubber cap on the A-2 Chamber and causing carry-over?

8. The Diluent Dispenser should dispense approximately 10 ml. of isoton each stroke. Check to see that there are no air bubbles in Diluent Dispenser.

9. Is the RBC sample flowing into the bath with too much turbulence?

10. Is the instrument background count normal? (RBC no higher than .02; WBC no higher than .4.)

Automated Blood Counts - Model S Coulter (Continued):

11. Clean and wash the RBC Mixing Chambers and rubber caps.

12. Check Mercury Manometer. Make sure the Indicating Fluid level is stable. When the instrument is counting, the level should not vary more than ¼".

WBC IS ERRATIC:

1. Check to see if RBC and Hgb. are also erratic. If they are, check for RBC erratic problem.

2. Check the mixing rate in the A-1 to B-1 and Lyse Chambers.

3. Check the flow rate into the WBC bath.

4. Make sure the sample is not splashing the rubber cap on the A-1 Chamber and causing carry-over.

5. Check background count with and without lysing reagent. Maximum background count for white side is .4 with lysing reagent and lower value without lysing reagent. Insure there are no bubbles in lyse dispensed into C-1 Chamber.

6. Grass on pattern is sign of defective lyse reagent.

MCV IS ERRATIC (always high or too low):

1. Insure RBC's are not voting out.

2. Clean apertures.

3. Clean the mixing chambers.

4. Clean the sampling valve.

5. Inspect tygon tubing in blood and diluent lines for foggy appearance.

6. The RBC background count should be low (.02 maximum printout).

PCV IS ERRATIC OR WRONG:

1. Make sure the RBC and MCV are not erratic.

2. Check calculations of machine. The PCV depends on the RBC and MCV.

Automated Blood Counts - Model S Coulter (Continued):

HEMOGLOBIN IS ERRATIC:

1. Is the Hgb. lamp burned out or does the face appear black? If so, change the Hgb. lamp.

2. Insure that WBC bath drains completely.

MCH OR MCHC WRONG OR ERRATIC:

Check calculations.

THE BATHS WILL NOT EMPTY:

1. Check the pinch valve between the baths and the "T" which leads to the Waste Chamber.

2. Is the tubing leading from the bath through the pinch valve to the "T" pinched?

3. Do you have at least 15 inches of vacuum at the Pneumatic Supply? Is the tubing from the Pneumatic Supply plugged? Pinch off vacuum line from Pneumatic Supply, and observe the vacuum gauge. If needle increases more than 4", this will indicate a possible vacuum leak in the Diluter Unit.

4. Check the Waste Chamber for leaks and associated check valves.

5. Check fitting at bottom of bath to insure it is clear from any foreign matter.

THE BATHS WILL NOT FILL:

Check with an experienced technologist who has been to Coulter School.

THE WASTE CHAMBER WILL NOT EMPTY:

1. Remove and check the Waste Chamber thoroughly for damage. Rinse the Waste Chamber with isoterge and reinstall.

2. Insure Waste "T" is not plugged. Run pipe cleaner through.

Automated Blood Counts - Model S Coulter (Continued):

BUBBLE TRAP IS DRAINING:

1. Check level of isoton.

2. Check the fittings on the "T" above the normally open pinch valve (next to the diluent dispenser). They should be tight.

3. Insure that the fittings on the Bubble Trap are not loose.

4. The tubing passing through the normally open pinch valve may have a crack. Replace it if necessary.

A PARAMETER IS PRINTING 999:

1. If the parameter is the WBC, check the lyse reagent supply. Cycle the instrument to see if 1.0 ml. of lyse reagent is dispensed into Lysing Chamber C-1.

2. Observe the C-1 Chamber, and insure the RBC's are lysed.

MISCELLANEOUS:

1. If there are any questions, ask an experienced techologist who has been trained in the Coulter system to assistance.

2. Do not change any voltages.

3. Do not change any parameters on the Timing/Generator Card (otherwise known as the Idiot Card).

REFERENCE: MODEL S TROUBLESHOOTING GUIDE.

BASOPHIL COUNT

PRINCIPLE: This is a procedure to determine the absolute basophil count, especially in patients with myeloproliferative disease, chronic inflammation, immunological disease and ulcerative colitis. Basophils stain a bright red color with neutral red, supravital stain.

SPECIMEN: 0.05 ml. heparinized blood.

REAGENTS:

1. Neutral Red, Supravital Red Stain Solution
   Prepare the stain by dissolving 6.0 mg. of neutral red in 50 ml. of buffer solution at pH 5.4. The solution is stable for 7 days.

2. Saponin Solution, 4.0%

3. Formaldehyde, 40%

PROCEDURE:

1. Prepare neutral red supravital dye and saponin solution by mixing 1.0 ml. of neutral red dye and 0.25 ml. of 4% Saponin solution buffered at pH 5.4.

2. Prepare buffered 40% formaldehyde solution by mixing 0.5 ml. formaldehyde with 3.5 ml. of pH 5.4 buffer.

3. Mix 0.05 ml. heparinized venous blood with 0.4 ml. neutral red-Saponin solution and 0.05 ml. buffered formaldehyde in a polyethylene tube.

4. Load 4 chambers of an eosinophil counting chamber.

5. Allow to stand approximately 10 minutes on moistened filter paper in a covered Petri dish.

6. Count basophils with the high dry objective.

7. CALCULATION:

   Total Number Basophils in all ten (10) 1 x 1 mm. squares in each of four chambers x 1.25 = Absolute Basophil Count/cu. ml. peripheral blood.

19

Basophil Count (Continued):

NORMAL VALUES: 20 - 50 Basophils per cu. ml. blood.

REFERENCE: Shelley, W. B. and Parnes, H. M.: "Technique of the
Absolute Basophil Count". J. Amer. Med. Assoc. 192:368.
1965.

INTERPRETATION:

Elevations of the basophil count occur most commonly in the myeloproliferative syndrome, especially myelogenous leukemia and polycythemia vera. Increased peripheral blood basophils are found in the
diseases of hypersensitivity, including drug reactions and the collagen vascular diseases. Other causes for basophilia are ulcerative
colitis, myxedema, urticaria pigmentosa, and systemic mast cell
disease.

BLEEDING TIME (BORCHGREVINK METHOD)

PRINCIPLE: A prolonged bleeding time generally means either that the subject has reduced platelet numbers or defective platelet function.

EQUIPMENT:

1. Sphygmomanometer

2. Sterile Bleeding Time Gauges

3. Filter paper

4. Stopwatch

PROCEDURE:

1. Apply blood pressure cuff and inflate to 40 mm. of mercury.

2. Clean the volar surface of the forearm with alcohol.

3. Using Bleeding Time Gauge, make three cuts approximately 1 mm. deep and 10 mm. in length. Start stopwatch at this point.

4. Absorb with filter paper, the drops of blood every 30 seconds being careful not to touch the wound.

5. The bleeding time is finished when the spots on the filter paper are no longer red. In many patients there will be an oozing of a blood-tinged fluid from the wound after the free flow of blood has ceased and the size of the drop has significantly decreased. At the first sign of this, the test is considered finished.

6. The test is stopped at 25 minutes and reported as greater than 25 minutes.

NORMAL VALUES: 3 - 12 minutes

REFERENCES:

1. Johnson and Greenwalt: COAGULATION AND TRANSFUSION IN CLINICAL MEDICINE, Little, Brown, and Co., Boston, pp. 12-15, 1965.

Bleeding Time (Borchgrevink Method) (Continued):

2. Borchgrevink, C. F., and Waaler, B. A.:   Acta Med. Scand.
   162:361, 1958.

INTERPRETATION:

The Bleeding Time is prolonged when severe thrombocytopenia is present
(below 25,000 cu. mm.) or when platelet function is abnormal with a
normal platelet count.   Abnormal platelet function may be hereditary,
such as in von Willebrand's disease or may be acquired, such as in
uremia or excessive utilization of drugs such as aspirin.

DUKE'S BLEEDING TIME

PRINCIPLE: Capillary bleeding time measures vascular and platelet factors in hemostasis.

EQUIPMENT:

1. Glass slide

2. Bard-Parker blade No. 11.

3. Stopwatch

4. Filter paper

PROCEDURE:

1. Cleanse the ear lobe with 70 percent alcohol and dry.

2. Place a clean slide behind the lobe.

3. Puncture through the lobe quickly so that the tip of the blade strikes the glass slide.

4. When the first drop of blood appears, start the stopwatch.

5. Absorb the blood on filter paper every 30 seconds, taking care not to touch the wound.

6. Record the time the bleeding stops.

SPECIMEN: This test cannot be used in infants since the ear lobe is too thin for an adequate puncture.

NORMAL VALUES: 1 - 3 minutes

REFERENCE: Miale, John B.: LABORATORY MEDICINE HEMATOLOGY, 3rd Ed., C. V. Mosby Co., St. Louis, pg. 1192, 1967.

INTERPRETATION:

The Bleeding Time is prolonged when severe thrombocytopenia is present (below 25,000 cu. mm.) or when platelet function is abnormal, with a

23

Bleeding Time (Duke's Method) (Continued):

normal platelet count. Abnormal platelet function may be hereditary, such as in von Willebrand's disease or may be acquired, such as in uremia or excessive utilization of drugs such as aspirin.

BLEEDING TIME
(Ivy's Method)

PRINCIPLE: A prolonged bleeding time generally means either that
the subject has reduced platelet numbers or that the platelets present
in the circulation, although normal in number, are pathological in
function.

EQUIPMENT:

1. Sphygmomanometer

2. Bard-Parker Blade No. 11

3. Filter Paper, Whatman No. 11

4. Stopwatch

PROCEDURE:

1. Apply blood pressure cuff and inflate to 40 mm. of mercury.

2. Clean the volar surface of the forearm with alcohol.

3. Make an incision 2.0 mm. deep and 2.0 mm. long with the Bard-
    Parker blade 3 fingerbreadths below the fold of the antecubital
    fossa. Start the stopwatch at this point.

4. Absorb with filter paper, the drops of blood every 30 seconds
    being careful not to touch the wound.

5. The bleeding time is finished when the spots on the filter paper
    are no longer red. In many patients there will be an oozing of a
    blood-tinged fluid from the wound after the free flow of blood has
    ceased and the size of the drop has significantly decreased. At
    the first sign of this, the test is considered finished.

6. The test is stopped at 25 minutes and reported as greater than
    25 minutes.

NORMAL VALUES: 1 - 7 Minutes

REFERENCE: Roskam, J.: ARREST OF BLEEDING, Charles C. Thomas,
             Springfield, Ill., 1954.

Bleeding Time (Ivy's Method) (Continued):

INTERPRETATION:

The Bleeding Time is prolonged when severe thrombocytopenia is present (below 25,000 cu. mm.) or when platelet function is abnormal, with a normal platelet count. Abnormal platelet function may be hereditary, such as in von Willebrand's disease or may be acquired, such as in uremia or excessive utilization of drugs such as aspirin.

BENCE-JONES PROTEIN
(Heat Test)

PRINCIPLE: Bence-Jones protein precipitates at 56°C. which differentiates the Bence-Jones proteins from other fractions of human serum proteins. It is soluble at 100°C., and thus characteristically at this temperature the precipitate and therefore, the turbidity of the test solution disappears. Cooling to 56°C. reprecipitates the protein. Control of pH is one of the important parameters of the qualitative heat test and optimal precipitation occurs at a pH range of 4.6 to 5.4.

REAGENTS:

1. Acetic Acid, 2.0 M.

2. Sodium Acetate, 2.0 M.
   Dilute 136.1 gm. sodium acetate to 500 ml. with distilled water.

3. Buffer Solution, 2.0 M., pH 4.9
   Mix 140 ml. of the 2.0 M. acetic acid and 260 ml. of the 2.0 M. sodium acetate. Check with pH meter.

PROCEDURE:

1. To 4.0 ml. of a centrifuged urine sample, add 1.0 ml. of 2.0 M. acetate buffer.

2. Heat buffered sample in a 56°C. waterbath for 15 minutes.

3. Precipitation is an indication that Bence-Jones proteins may be present.

4. Heat the sample for 3 minutes at 100°C. and observe the specimen while it is in the boiling bath.

5. A decrease in the amount of precipitate confirms results.

NORMAL VALUES: Report positive Bence-Jones protein if the precipitate at 56°C. disappears at 100°C. and reappears upon cooling.

REFERENCE: Snapper, I. and Ores, R. O.: Jour. Amer. Med. Assoc. 173:1137, 1960.

Bence-Jones Protein - Heat Test (Continued):

INTERPRETATION:

Bence-Jones protein represents a light chain immunoglobulin which is present in the blood and urine of patients with multiple myeloma and rarely in other conditions, such as systemic amyloidosis, neoplastic lymphoproliferative diseases, such as lymphoma and chronic infections, e.g. tuberculosis.

BENCE-JONES PROTEIN
(Para-Toluene Sulfonic Acid Procedure)

PRINCIPLE: This procedure is a rapid chemical method to detect the presence of light chain immunoglobulins in the urine of patients with multiple myeloma or other conditions in which Bence-Jones protein is present.

SPECIMEN: 2.0 ml. of urine

REAGENTS:

1. Glacial Acetic Acid

2. Para-Toluene Sulfonic Acid Reagent,
   Prepare the para-toluene sulfonic acid by adding 12 gm. of para-toluene sulfonic acid to 100 ml. of glacial acetic acid.

PROCEDURE:

1. Place 2.0 ml. of urine to a test tube and add 1.0 ml. of the para-toluene sulfonic acid to the urine by carefully permitting it to run down the side of the test tube.

2. Gently mix and permit it to stand at room temperature for five minutes.

3. Observe for a precipitate within five minutes. If a precipitate forms, the test is positive for Bence-Jones protein.

REFERENCE: Cohen, E., Raducha, J. J.:   Amer. J. Clin. Path., 37:660, 1962.

INTERPRETATION:

Bence-Jones protein represents a light chain immunoglobulin which is present in the blood and urine of patients with multiple myeloma and rarely in other conditions, such as systemic amyloidosis, neoplastic lymphoproliferative diseases, such as lymphoma and chronic infections, e.g. tuberculosis.

BONE MARROW ASPIRATES

PRINCIPLE: Bone marrow smears exhibit spicules and a small amount of
blood.

SPECIMEN: Bone marrow aspirate and peripheral blood smears.

EQUIPMENT AND REAGENTS:

A Bone Marrow Tray containing:
1. 20 gauge needles (2)

2. Alcohol Preps, Gauze

3. 20 cc. Plastic Syringes (2)

4. Petri Dish

5. Bouin's Solution

6. Glass Slides

7. WBC or Pasteur Pipettes

8. EDTA (Sequester - Sol in Refrigerator)

9. Micro - Lance

PROCEDURE:

1. Preparing syringe for aspirate
    A small amount of sterile EDTA is drawn into 20 cc. plastic
    syringe using sterile technique. Then EDTA is expressed leaving
    0.25 ml. which is sufficient for 2.0 to 2.5 ml. of aspirate.

2. Smear Procedure
    a). (Preferable) Aspirate is placed immediately in Petri dish
         and spicules transferred to a slide with pipette.

    b). If marrow is rich in spicules, smears may be made directly
         from syringe. Mix contents of syringe well and place drop
         on slide, draining excess blood off with gauze. Make about
         one dozen smears and stain four.

30

Bone Marrow Aspirates (Continued):

c). Make three or four peripheral smears and stain in regular Wright's and Giemsa.

3. Preparation of Pathology Specimen
a). Place remainder of aspirate in approximately 20 ml. Bouin's solution for one hour.

b). Filter fixed aspirate through nylon stocking, washing excess tissue away with saline.

c). Place remaining washed spicules on lens paper, close tightly and return to Bouin's solution.

4. Staining Procedure

AIR DRY

Absolute Methanol
230 ml.
30 seconds

Tap water
230 ml.
Rinse

Wright's Stain (Filtered)

2 minutes

Giemsa (Filtered)
10 ml.
Buffer
230 ml. 6 to 8 minutes

Tap water
230 ml.
Wright's Stain (Filtered)
8.0 ml.   6 to 8 minutes

Tap water
230 ml.
Rinse

5. Number of Smears
Finished preparation includes 3 bone marrow smears, 3 peripheral blood smears, and 1 iron stained slide.

COMMENT ON STAINING PROCEDURE:

Failure to get satisfactory results most frequently due to incorrect reaction of staining fluid. Reaction of staining solution most affected by pH and oxidation of methanol to formic acid. This requires changing stain often, twice a week or more.

32

Bone Marrow Aspirates (Continued):

REFERENCES:

1. Davidsohn & Wells: TODD-SANFORD CLINICAL DIAGNOSIS BY LAB-
   ORATORY METHODS, 13th. Ed., W. B. Saunders Co., Phil., pgs.
   112-114; 146-150, 1965.

2. Miale, John B.: LABORATORY MEDICINE HEMATOLOGY, 4th. Ed.,
   C. V. Mosby Co., St. Louis, pg. 1208-1209, 1972.

INTERPRETATION:

The indications for aspirating bone marrow and preparing smears for
interpretation are numerous. A few of the important indications are:

1. Assessment of anemia
2. Assessment of leukemia
3. Assessment of leukopenia
4. Assessment of thrombocytopenia
5. Identification of bone marrow parasites
6. Diagnosis of lipid storage disease
7. Follow-up of therapy of anemia and leukemia
8. Assessment of hypoplasia or aplasia
9. Assessment of plasmacytic disorders
10. Assessment of metastatic cancer

TOTAL BILIRUBIN
(Spectrophotometric Method)

PRINCIPLE: The yellow color of serum or plasma is due in part to bilirubin. This fact is the basis for the icterus index test. The icterus index is an imprecise and relatively nonspecific test; however, the simplicity of the test and its potential utility have led to numerous refinements and applications. The test described here is the direct spectrophotometric determination of total bilirubin. As a refinement of the icterus index, precision in this test has been achieved by the use of an ultramicrodilutor, a buffered diluent, and a spectrophotometer. Specificity has been improved by making corrections for hemoglobin and turbidity. This is accomplished by substracting the absorbance at 551 nm. from the absorbance at 461 nm. The latter wavelength is the peak for bilirubin; whereas, absorbance due to hemoglobin and turbidity is practically the same at these two wavelengths; by subtracting the absorbance at 551 nm. from the absorbance at 461 nm., any absorbance due to hemoglobin and turbidity is effectively cancelled out of the final answer. Thus, this method is a very simple, rapid, precise, ultramicro determination for bilirubin. The lack of specificity inherent in the method does not detract from its utility, particularly when it is restricted to its intended uses of monitoring neonatal jaundice and estimating bilirubin levels in adults.

SPECIMEN: 20 microliters of serum or plasma. Specimen should be processed as soon as possible or stored in a light-tight container at refrigerator temperature until assayed.

REAGENTS AND EQUIPMENT:

1. Citrate Buffer, 5% (W/V)
   Weigh out 50 gm. of Reagent Grade Sodium Citrate into a one liter volumetric flask. Dilute to volume with deionized water, pH = 8.8.

2. Ultramicro dilutor
   Set up to dilute 20 microliters of specimen with 1 0 ml. of sodium citrate.

3. Gilford Spectrophotometer 300N
   Instrument should be fitted with a microaspiration cuvette.

4. Calibration Standard
   An elevated Bilirubin Control with an Assay of around 20 mg%. Always check the assay, which varies with different lot numbers.

Total Bilirubin (Continued):

Several dilutions are made to give bilirubin concentrations of 2.0, 5.0, 7.0 15, and 20 mg%.

PROCEDURE:

1. Standardization. A calibration curve is made by diluting 20 microliters of each of the diluted standards with 1.0 ml. of sodium citrate. Set the machine to 0.000 absorbance at 551 nm. with a blank containing citrate buffer. Take the reading of the buffer at 461 nm. Take the absorbance readings of the standards at 461 nm. and 551 nm. Calculate the true absorbance of the bilirubin standards. Plot absorbance versus concentration on regular graph paper.

   A = (A of test at 461 nm.) — (A of Blank at 461 nm.) —

   (A of test at 551 nm.)

   The A of Blank at 551 nm. was preset to zero.

2. Using the dilutor, dilute 20 microliters of serum (Test) with 1.0 ml. of sodium citrate.
   Blank - Sodium Citrate
   Controls - Abnormal Control and Elevated Bilirubin Control.

3. Using the blank, set the machine to 0.000 absorbance at 551 nm. Take another reading at 461 nm.

4. Read the Test at 461 nm. and 551 nm.
   Calculate the bilirubin absorbance and refer to the curve.

NOTES:

1. Indirect sunlight lowers bilirubin values drastically. After standing for ½ hour under the influence of indirect sunlight, the values are lowered by an average of 7% of the original concentration.

2. The 5% sodium citrate maintains the pH of the solution, making absorbance readings more stable. To keep the effects of light on bilirubin to the minimum, read test very soon after each dilution.

NORMAL VALUES: Adults   - less than 0.8 mg%.
                Children - 0.1 to 0.7 mg%.
                Infants   - 5.0 mg%.

Total Bilirubin (Continued):

REFERENCES:

1. Henry, R. J., Golub, O. J., Berkman, S., and Segalove, M.: Am. J. Clin. Path., 23:841, 1953.

2. Chiamori, N., Henry, R. J., and Golub, O. J.: Clin. Chim. Acta, 6:1, 1961.

3. Gambino: MANUAL ON BILIRUBIN ASSAY, ASCP, 1968.

INTERPRETATION:

The three main causes for jaundice are hemolytic, hepatic and obstructive. The main reason for elevation of the non-conjugated bilirubin is hemolytic anemia. Conjugated bilirubin may rise in hemolysis if the liver is competent.

Other Etiologies for an elevated non-conjugated bilirubin are:

1. Presence of a large hematoma
2. Hemorrhagic pulmonary infarction
3. Utilization of a large number of blood bank units of blood in blood transfusions which are not fresh
4. Absence of liver glucuronyl transferase (Crigler-Najjar Syndrome)
5. Deficiency of liver glucuronyl transferase (Gilberts Syndrome)

There are many causes for liver disease responsible for a hepatic type of jaundice. Patients who have hepatic disease have elevation of conjugated and non-conjugated bilirubin. If the hepatic disease is due to infiltrative etiologies such as are seen in primary or metastatic cancer to the liver, granulomata, lymphoma, or chole-stasis secondary to drugs, the conjugated bilirubin will be more elevated than the unconjugated bilirubin. Patients who have ob-structive jaundice usually have an increased conjugated bilirubin. If liver disease develops after obstructive jaundice due to carcin-oma of the head of the pancreas, choledocholithiasis, carcinoma of the bile ducts or sclerosing cholangitis, the unconjugated bilirubin will also become elevated. Patients with the Dubin-Johnson Syndrome also have an elevated conjugated bilirubin.

SERUM BILIRUBIN, DIRECT REACTING
(Ultramicro Method)

PRINCIPLE: Lathe and Ruthven have shown that a sharp distinction between the diazo coupling rate of conjugated and unconjugated bilirubin may only be achieved under the following conditions:

1. a low pH
2. a low concentration of diazotized sulfanilic acid

These two conditions are satisfied by the method presented, the reagents being optimal for the measurement of direct reacting bilirubin. Since standards of conjugated bilirubin are unavailable at the current time, the method must be standardized against a total bilirubin determination which uses the same reagents.

SPECIMEN: 40 microliters of unhemolyzed serum or plasma. Hemolysis will significantly lower the bilirubin result. For accurate results, specimen should be separated from cells as soon as possible, and stored in a light-tight container at refrigerator temperatures until assayed. Determination should be performed as soon as possible The instability of bilirubin when exposed to light and room temperature cannot be overemphasized.

REAGENTS AND EQUIPMENT:

1. Sulfanilic Acid, 0.2%
   Place 2.0 gm. of sulfanilic acid into a 1.0 liter volumetric flask, and bring to volume with 0.04 N. HCl. Stable indefinitely at room temperature.

2. HCl, 0.04 N.

3. Sodium Nitrite, Stock Solution, 5.0%
   Dissolve 12.5 gm. $NaNO_2$ in deionized water, and bring to volume in a 250 ml. volumetric flask. Store in dark bottle at refrigerator temperatures; reagent is labile at room temperature and when exposed to light.

4. Sodium Nitrate, Working Solution, 0.1%
   Place 2.0 ml. of the stock $NaNO_2$ into a 100 ml. volumetric flask, and bring to volume with deionized water. Prepare fresh solution weekly, and store in a dark bottle at refrigerator temperatures. Use fresh aliquots of this reagent with each set of determinations.

36

Serum Bilirubin, Direct Reading (Continued):

5. Brij.-Water, approximately 0.1%
   Add 1.0 ml. Brij.-35 to 1000 ml. deionized water.

6. Methanol, absolute
   This reagent is only required for standardization.

7. Ultramicro Dilutor
   500 microliter flush syringe set to deliver 350 microliters of sulfanilic acid reagent.

   100 microliter sample syringe set to take up 20 microliters of specimen.

8. Gilford Spectrophotometer 300 N
   Instrument should be fitted with a microaspiration cuvette.

COMMENTS ON PROCEDURE:

1. The presence of hemoglobin in the sample will significantly affect the accuracy of the diazo reaction. While the exact mechanism is unknown, hemolysis interferes with the coupling reaction resulting in a loss of azobilirubin, which is proportional to the amount of hemoglobin present. It has also been suggested that hemolysis interferes with the final reading of azobilirubin values, due to the increased rate of conversion of hemoglobin to methemoglobin as a result of the presence of nitrite in the test solution and its absence in the blank.

   Increased amounts of protein will proportionally decrease the amount of azobilirubin formed; this has been proposed as a partial explanation for the effect of hemolysis.

2. The instability of bilirubin when exposed to light and room temperature cannot be over emphasized.

3. When performing the direct bilirubin determination, timing of the readings is critical to reproducible results, particularly when the specimen has an elevated value.

4. Specimens with a direct bilirubin value greater than 20 mg%. must be repeated on dilution. Dilute with saline.

5. Standardization of the azobilirubin absorption values must be achieved by carrying the direct bilirubin procedure on to a

Serum Bilirubin, Direct Reading (Continued):

total bilirubin content. The addition of methanol will dilute
the direct test volume in half; one must keep this in mind when
assigning bilirubin values to the absorbance units.

6. Standardization

A. A series of specimens or control sera, or standards of known
   total bilirubin concentration (ranging in value up to 20 mg%.)
   are used.

Total Bilirubin Determination

B. Perform steps #1 through #4 of the direct bilirubin procedure
   on the above samples.

C. After a five minute time period, add 0.7 ml. of methanol to
   each tube, and vortex well. Allow five minutes of color
   development.

D. Determine absorbance value of specimen, and specimen blank
   against water at 540 nm. using the Gilford microaspiration
   cuvette.

E. Subtract absorbance value of specimen blank from that of the
   specimen.

F. Plot mg%. against absorbance on linear graph paper. From
   this curve, prepare a calibration chart for direct bilirubin.
   The absorbance values for a given mg%. should be multiplied
   by 2 to account for the difference in dilution between the
   direct and total methods.

PROCEDURE:

1. Prepare two microcentrifuge tubes or A.A. cups for each specimen
   to be analyzed. One tube is for sample color development, and
   one is reserved for the sample blank.

2. Using the ultramicrodilutor, draw up 20 microliters of freshly
   aliquoted 0.1% sodium nitrite, and flush this with 350 microliters of sulfanilic acid. Deliver into the color development
   tube, and vortex or mix thoroughly.

Serum Bilirubin, Direct Reading (Continued):

3. Take up 20 microliters of serum, and flush with 350 microliters
   of sulfanilic acid into the sample blank tube; dilute with an
   additional 350 microliters of sulfanilic acid. Vortex or mix
   thoroughly.

4. Take up a second 20 microliters of serum and flush into the tube
   with diazotized sulfanilic acid. Vortex and start timer.

5. At exactly one minute, determine absorbance of the azobilirubin
   against a Brij.-water blank at 540 nm. using the Gilford microaspiration cuvette. Determine the absorbance of the specimen
   blank against Brij.-water.

6. Subtract absorbance of specimen blank from absorbance of specimen. Determine the mg%. direct reacting bilirubin from the
   calibration chart. Repeat values greater than 20 mg%. on dilution with saline.

NORMAL VALUES: Less than 0.1 mg%.

REFERENCES:

1. Lathe, R. and Ruthven, C.: "Factors Affecting the Rate of
   Coupling of Bilirubin and Conjugated Bilirubin in the van
   den Bergh Reaction", J. Clin. Path., 11:155, 1958.

2. Jacobs, Henry, R., Segalove, M.: "Studies on the Determination of Bile Pigments", Clin. Chem., 10:433, 1964.

3. Amatuzio, D.: "The Rate of Coupling of Diazotized Sulfanilic
   Acid with Bilirubin", Archives of Biochemistry and Biophysics,
   86:77, 1960.

4. Meites, S. and Hogg, C.: "Studies on the Use of the van den
   Bergh Reagent for Determination of Serum Bilirubin", Clin.
   Chem., 5:470, 1959.

5. Gambino: MANUAL ON BILIRUBIN ASSAY, ASCP, 1968.

INTERPRETATION:

Refer to Interpretation section under Total Bilirubin - Spectrophotometric Method on page 35.

CHOLINESTERASE

PRINCIPLE: In most of the quantitative methods, the enzymatic hydrolysis of an organic ester of choline under controlled conditions of
sample size, substrate concentration, time, temperature, pH, ionic
strength, and various salt concentrations results in the liberation
of a choline salt and an organic acid. In this method, acetylthiocholine is used as a substrate; giving off hydrolysis products of
thiocholine and acetic acid. The thiocholine is further reacted with
dithiobisnitrobenzoic acid which gives off a colored product with
maximum absorbance at 405 nm.

Acetylthiocholine $\xrightarrow{\text{Cholinesterase}}$ Thiocholine + Acetic Acid

Thiocholine (Sulfhydryl Group) + Dithiobisnitrobenzoic Acid

$\xrightarrow{\hspace{2cm}}$ Color

The product formed is proportional to the concentration of the enzyme.
Cholinesterase is an enzyme found in the tissues of all animals and
formed in the liver. When this enzyme is low, acetylcholine accumulates, resulting in the continuous stimulation of the parasympathetic
system with undesirable symptoms. Cholinesterase activity is another
diagnostic test for liver disease. It is very useful in detecting
poisoning by organic phosphate insecticides or some drugs as in
anesthesia.

SPECIMEN: 0.02 ml. of fresh, unhemolyzed serum is required. Plasma
should not be used. Samples are stable for several days at 4°C. and
for weeks in the freezer.

REAGENTS AND EQUIPMENT: (Biochemica Test Combination Colorimetric
                         Method, Cat. No. 15984 TCAB).

1. Buffer (Bottle No. 1)
   0.05 M. Phosphate Buffer, pH 7.2, and 0.00025 M. Dithiobisnitrobenzoic acid.

2. Substrate
   0.156 M. Acetylthiocholine Iodide.

3. Spectrophotometer
   A. Gilford 300N, 405 nm.
   This instrument is used when analyzing one sample at a time.

Cholinesterase (Continued):

The change in absorbance per minute is read from the Data
Lister printout. The linearity of the reaction is visually
monitored on the strip chart recorder. The instrument is
used with the thermocuvette set at 25°C.

B. Gilford 222, 405 nm.
This instrument is used when analyzing four samples at a time.
Temperature control is maintained by means of a 25°C. circulating waterbath. Rate of reaction is determined from the
strip chart recorder set for 0.200 A. full scale and run at
one inch per minute.

COMMENTS:

1. Reconstituted solutions are stable for six weeks at 4°C.

2. All specimens with optical density differences greater than
   0.200/30 seconds should be diluted with physiological saline.

3. The amount of non-enzymatic hydrolysis of acetylthiocholine which
   may occur during the test should be determined for each new pack.
   This can be done by running it with deionized water in place of
   serum. The resulting optical density difference/30 seconds
   should be deducted from the optical density difference of each
   test result.

PROCEDURE:

1. Using pyrex cuvettes (10 mm. light path, 10 mm. wide), pipette
   3.00 ml. of buffer xolution, 0.02 ml. of serum and 0.10 ml. of
   acetylthiocholine iodide.

2. Dilute three more specimens in the same manner.

3. Place four specimens in the cuvette chamber of the Gilford 222.

4. Set the baseline of specimen No. 1 with the slit, and No.'s 2,
   3, and 4 with the OFF-SET knobs. Switch to "AUTO" and scan all
   four channels.

5. Scan immediately, and record 2 minutes of linear reaction time
   at 405 nm. Determine $\Delta A/30$ seconds from the recorder chart.

6. CALCULATIONS:

Cholinesterase (Continued):

$$I.U. = \frac{\Delta A/30 \text{ Sec.}}{\varepsilon xd} \times 10^6 \times \frac{TV}{SV} \times \frac{1}{Time}$$

ε = Molar Extinction Coefficient of the product at 405 nm.
  = 13.3×10^3 Liter/Mole x cm.
d = Diameter of the cuvette in cm.
  = 1.0 cm.
TV = Total Volume
  = 3.12 ml.
SV = Sample Volume
  = 0.02 ml.
T = Time
  = 0.5 minutes

10^6 converts Moles/Liter into micromoles/liter
    1.0 I.U./Liter = 1 mU/ml.

$$I.U. = \frac{\Delta A/30 \text{ Sec.}}{13.3 \times 10^3} \times 10^6 \times \frac{3.12}{0.02} \times \frac{1}{0.5}$$

$$= \Delta A/30 \text{ Sec.} \times 23400$$

$$\Delta A/30 \text{ Sec.} \times 23400 = mU/ml. \text{ of serum}$$

Report results in I.U. at 25°C.

NORMAL VALUES: Normal Values compiled by BMC at 25°C.:
                1900 - 3800 mU/ml. of serum.

REFERENCES:

1. Bergmeyer, H. U.: METHODS OF ENZYMATIC ANALYSIS, 2nd. Ed.,
   Academic Press, New York, pg. 771, 1965.

2. STANDARD METHODS OF CLINICAL CHEMISTRY, Vol. 3, pg. 93 - 98,
   1961.

3. STANDARD METHODS OF CLINICAL CHEMISTRY, Vol. 4, pg. 47 - 56,
   1963.

Cholinesterase (Continued):

INTERPRETATION:

The red blood cell cholinesterase is a reflection of the cholinesterase of the central nervous system. It is preferable to measure the red blood cell enzyme than serum pseudocholinesterase to evaluate organic phosphate poisoning. Enzyme activity may be decreased to approximately 40 percent of the initial red blood cell level before clinical symptoms appear in an acute exposure to an organic phosphate insecticide. Prolonged low level exposure to a toxic insecticide may not result in illness until the enzyme decreases to 25 percent of pre-exposure levels.

SERUM OR PLASMA CHOLINESTERASE
(Acholest Test Paper)

PRINCIPLE: Cholinesterase, an enzyme found in the tissues of all animals, formed in the liver, hydrolyzes acetylcholine to choline and acetic acid.

Acetylcholine ⟶ Choline + Acetic Acid

Acetylcholine stimulates the nerve impulses in the parasympathetic nervous system. When cholinesterase is low, acetylcholine accumulates, resulting in continuous stimulation of the parasympathetic system with undesirable symptoms.

The ACHOLEST TEST PAPER is a rapid, simplified screening test for the determination of plasma or serum cholinesterase. The kit consists of a test strip impregnated with a special substrate and a control strip (comparative color strip). The time required to reach the endpoint with the control strip is a measure of cholinesterase activity, described as "increased", "normal", "suspicious", or "decreased".

Cholinesterase activity is another diagnostic test for liver disease. It is very useful in detecting poisoning by organic phosphate insecticides or some drugs as in anesthesia.

SPECIMEN: 0.1 ml. of non-hemolyzed plasma or serum is required. Samples are stable for several days at 4°C. and for weeks in the freezer.

REAGENTS AND EQUIPMENT:

1. ACHOLEST, cholinesterase Test Paper
   Bottle I.

2. Comparative Color Strip
   Bottle II.

3. Clean Slides

4. 0.05 ml. Wiretrol Disposable Pipettes

5. Stopwatch

6. Tweezers

44

Serum or Plasma Cholinesterase (Continued):

The whole kit (for 30 determinations) is available and supplied by E. Fougera and Co., New York).

PROCEDURE:

1. Using Wiretrol disposable pipettes, pipette 0.05 ml. of plasma or serum on each of two clean slides. Label one slide "Test" and the other one "Control".

2. Cut the "Test" Strip and the "Control" Strip in half.

3. Using tweezers, place the Test Strip and Control Strip on the respective slides.

4. Cover with clean slides to ensure complate saturation of the paper.

5. Set the stopwatch. The Test Paper turns green, gradually developing into a yellowish color, which is the color of the Control Paper.

6. Cholinesterase activity is measured by the time required for the Test Paper to reach the color of the Control Paper.

7. From the moment of contact of the serum or plasma and Test Paper, to the point where the comparative tone of color has been reached, the following time values have been established:

Minutes	Activity of Plasma or Serum Cholinesterase
Below 5	"Increased"
5 - 20	"Normal"
20 - 30	"Suspicious"
30 and Longer	"Decreased"

NORMAL VALUES: 5 - 20 Minutes

REFERENCES:

1. STANDARD METHODS OF CLINICAL CHEMISTRY, 3:93-98, Academic Press, 1961.

2. STANDARD METHODS OF CLINICAL CHEMISTRY, 4:47-56, Academic Press, 1963.

Serum or Plasma Cholinesterase (Continued):

INTERPRETATION:

A rapid test to qualitatively determine the plasma level of cholinesterase. The test paper known as Acholest Test Paper is utilized
as a simple screening method for plasma cholinesterase. Determination of this enzyme is important in suspected decrease due to
poisoning by organic phosphate insecticides. Enzyme levels also
are low in hepatic disease due to various causes. If succinyl choline is utilized before surgery in patients with hepatic disease
when there are low enzyme levels, patients may suffer undesirable
"overdose" type effects. Thus, the determination of plasma cholinesterase may be extremely useful in the surgical patient. The lab
kit consists of a test strip impregnated with a special substrate
and a control strip. The time required to reach the endpoint with
the control strip is a measure of cholinesterase activity which is
reported as normal or decreased. The plasma cholinesterase acts on
the substrate to liberate choline and acetic acid. The acetic acid
changes the color of the test strip containing an acid base indicator.

TITRATION OF CIRCULATING ANTICOAGULANT

PRINCIPLE: The semiquantitation of the titer of a circulating anti-coagulant is determined by diluting the patient's plasma and measuring the prolongation of the activated partial thromboplastin time.

SPECIMEN: 1.0 ml. of citrated plasma.

REAGENTS AND EQUIPMENT:

1. Aluminum Hydroxide

2. Ice Waterbath

3. Fibrometer

4. Stopwatch

5. Verify Normal
   Reconstitute with 0.5 ml. distilled water. Do not shake. Let stand at room temperature 20 minutes before mixing. Then mix and put in ice waterbath. May be reconstituted and frozen in advance to save time.

6. Platelin
   Reconstitute with 2.5 ml. distilled water. Shake well. Incubate at 37°C. for 8 minutes before using. DO NOT USE after 30 minutes. Values will become too short.

7. $CaCl_2$, 0.025 M.
   Prewarm to 37°C.

8. HCl, 0.1 N.

9. Acid Citrate
   2 Parts 0.1 M. citric acid to 3 parts 0.1 M. Na_3 citrate.

PROCEDURE:

1. Add 0.03 ml. of aluminum hydroxide to absorb 1.0 ml. of patient's citrated plasma.

2. Incubate 3 minutes and then centrifuge.

47

Titration of Circulating Anticoagulant (Continued):

3. Next dilute the absorbed plasma in plastic test tubes serially to 50%, 25%, 12.5%, and 6.25% with citrated saline.

4. Mix 0.1 ml. normal citrated plasma and 0.1 ml. absorbed test plasma dilution in a 10 x 75 mm. test tube.

5. Incubate 10 minutes at 37°C. and put into ice waterbath.

6. Mix platelin well with 0.2 ml. pipette to resuspend the Celite. Blow 0.1 cc. into first cup. Add 0.1 ml. plasma (with gun off) and start stopwatch.

7. Mix thoroughly by shaking fibrometer cup. Return to fibrometer.

8. At about 4.5 minutes mix cup again by shaking, and position for probe.

9. At exactly 5 minutes, with gun on, add 0.1 ml. of 0.025 $CaCl_2$.

10. Run in duplicate.

NORMAL VALUES: No Circulating Anticoagulant should be Present.

REFERENCE: Hardesty, R. M. and Ingram, C. I. C.: BLEEDING DISORDERS INVESTIGATION AND MANAGEMENT, Blackwell Scientific Pub., Oxford, pg. 315, 1965.

INTERPRETATION:

Each plasma dilution should be run in triplicate. The dilutions of the patient's plasma should be compared with a control containing 0.1 ml. citrated saline instead of absorbed test plasma. The semi-quantitative titer of the circulating anticoagulant corresponds to the dilution of patient plasma which prolongs the Control PTT.

WHOLE BLOOD EUGLOBULIN CLOT LYSIS

PRINCIPLE: To assay the fibrinolytic activity of circulating blood by measuring the fibrinolytic activity of the euglobulin fraction.

SPECIMEN: 9.0 ml. of patient's blood added to 1.0 ml. of 3.8% sodium citrate. Run a normal control along with patient. Mix both tubes gently by inversion.

REAGENTS AND EQUIPMENT:

1. Sodium Citrate, 3.8%

2. Acetic Acid, 1.0%

3. Epsilon-amino Caproic Acid (EACA), 2.8 x 10^{-3} M. (M.W. 117)

4. Thrombin, 2 NIH Units/0.2 ml.
   Thrombin lyophilyzed for fibrinogen contains 10 NIH Units/Vial. Reconstitute with 1.0 ml. of saline. Thrombin made up just before use.

5. Saline-Phosphate Buffer
   Saline 0.07 M. - Phosphate 0.06 M., pH 7.5
   NaCl   4.092 gm.
   Na$_2$HPO$_4$ 7.156 gm.
   KH$_2$PO$_4$ 1.306 gm.
   Merthiolate 10 mg.
   Dissolve in approximately 900 ml. of distilled water. Adjust to pH 7.5 and dilute to 1 liter.

COMMENTS ON PROCEDURE:

1. The Euglobulin fraction is precipitated when ionic strength is decreased to 0.008 at pH 5.2 to 5.9.

2. The precipitate contains activator and/or plasmin from plasma and red blood cell stroma, plasminogen, and fibrinogen.

3. The major fibrinolytic inhibitors are either labile at a pH of 5.2 to 5.9 or remain in the supernatant.

4. Activator and plasmin are quantitatively differentiated when the precipitate is reconstituted by the addition of EACA.

49

Whole Blood Euglobulin Clot Lysis (Continued):

5. Final EACA concentration in reaction is 4×10^{-4} M.

6. The Euglobulin should be precipitated as soon as the blood is drawn to permit measurement of activity before any loss occurs from enzyme lability.

7. Rapidity of clot lysis is dependent upon activity present and fibrinogen content of clot.

8. Low fibrinogen samples are characterized by small precipitate, inadequate co-precipitation of activator and plasmin, and poor clot formation.

9. If low fibrinogen is suspected, run a fibrinogen on a versenated sample.

PROCEDURE:

1. After blood is drawn, immediately add 1.3 ml. of blood to each of two tubes containing 13.5 ml. distilled water to which 0.22 ml. 1% acetic acid has been added.

2. Place tubes in ice bath for 7 minutes.

3. Centrifuge 3000 rpm for 15 minutes at 4°C.

4. Decant supernatant thoroughly.

5. 0.7 ml. Saline-Phosphate Buffer is added to one precipitate of each set.

6. 0.6 ml. Saline-Phosphate Buffer and 0.1 ml. of the 0.0028 M. EACA is added to the second precipitate of each set.

7. Stir to dissolve precipitates.

8. 0.7 ml. reconstituted Euglobulin is placed in a 12 x 75 mm. tube.

9. 2 NIH Units (0.02 ml. of 100 U./ml.) thrombin is added and mixed.

10. Incubate at 37°C.

11. Examine for clot lysis every 15 minutes the first 2 to 3 hours then every half hour up to 5 hours.

Whole Blood Euglobulin Clot Lysis (Continued):

NORMAL VALUES: Normal Whole Blood Euglobulin Clot Lysis requires
at least 2 hours.
Normal Euglobulin Clot Lysis with Epsilon amino
caproic acid requires about 4 hours for lysis to
occur.

REFERENCE: Tocantins, L. M.: BLOOD COAGULATION, HEMORRHAGE, AND
THROMBOSIS, 2nd. Ed., pg. 465, 1964.

INTERPRETATION:

If clot lysis is inhibited by Epsilon amino caproic acid, the fibrinolysis is assumed to be due to the presence of a fibrinolytic activator in the blood. If clot lysis occurs uninhibited by Epsilon
amino caproic acid, it is due primarily to plasmin. Fibrinolysis
occurs rarely as a consequence of severe brain injury, cardiovascular,
pulmonary, or pancreatic surgery.

CLOT RETRACTION

PRINCIPLE: Normally the blood clot separates from the wall of the tube and expresses serum. This is observed after one hour and is usually complete in 4 hours. Generally, clot retraction is a useful index of platelet activity.

SPECIMEN: Whole venous blood.

EQUIPMENT:

1. Syringe

2. Plain Glass Tube with Stopper

3. Waterbath, 37°C.

PROCEDURE:

1. Draw blood with a syringe. Place 5 to 7 ml. in plain glass tube (a red top Vacutainer may be used).

2. Place tube in waterbath and note time blood clots.

3. Two hours later examine for clot retraction and report retraction as follows:

0 - No serum extruded.
1 + 5 - 10% serum extruded.
2 + 10 - 20% serum extruded.
3 + 20 - 35% serum extruded.
4 + 35 - 50% extruded.

4. Read in 24 hours for retraction and clot lysis.

REFERENCE: Miale, John B.: LABORATORY MEDICINE HEMATOLOGY 4th Ed., C. V. Mosby Co., St. Louis, pg. 1268, 1972.

INTERPRETATION:

A clot will retract poorly if there is severe thrombocytopenia or poor platelet function as is found in von Willebrand's disease, uremia, or excessive utilization of drugs as aspirin. In vivo, it

Clot Retraction (Continued):

is normal for a thrombus to retract if normal platelet activity is present, since a smaller thrombus is tougher and serves as a better clot. This in vivo retraction thus occurs in vitro if normal platelet activity is present.

DRAWING BLOOD FOR CLOTTING STUDIES

Blood for clotting studies must be free from tissue thromboplastin which initiates clotting. Blood must be obtained by a clean stick, and the first five ml. of blood that enter the syringe discarded (or used for other tests).

Fill the PTT tube first, and mix without delay. Mix well but gently since hemolysis alters PTT values. Never add blood through a vacutainer stopper with a syringe needle. This frequently causes hemolysis.

9 parts of blood must be anticoagulated by 1 part of trisodium citrate or acid citrate. Therefore, blood must be added to the designated line on the PTT tubes (5 ml. or 2.5 ml.) Prothrombin in tubes should have 4.5 ml. blood added, or filled to about three-quarters of an inch from the top. (Special tubes for newborns will be furnished on request).

Patients with PCV's of greater than 70% should be drawn in special tubes, which have less anticoagulant because the plasma volume is so small.

PTT's should be sent to the lab promptly. Thrombin times should not be frozen. Separate the plasma, stopper, and refrigerate. Fibrinogens should not be frozen.

LEE-WHITE CLOTTING TIME

PRINCIPLE: The clotting time of whole blood is a procedure which
tests the composite action of all plasma factors acting simultaneously. The time required for the blood to clot is a function of the
combined factors favoring coagulation on one hand as opposed to the
combined factors inhibiting coagulation on the other.

EQUIPMENT:

1. Thermos bottle

2. 12 x 75 mm. tubes

3. Glass syringe

4. Stopwatch

COMMENTS ON PROCEDURE: The venous clotting time is the one done in
this laboratory. The capillary clotting time, because of the intro-
duction of tissue thromboplastin masks a defect in intrinsic thromboplastin formation.

PROCEDURE:

1. Place three tubes, 12 x 75 mm. in a 37°C. incubator or in a
    thermos with 37°C. water.

2. With a non-traumatic venipuncture, draw into a glass syringe
    approximately 4 to 5 cc. of blood. Start stopwatch as the blood
    enters the syringe. If there is difficulty in the venipuncture,
    a few cc. should be drawn in the syringe and a second syringe used
    to draw the blood for testing as there will be tissue thrombo-
    plastin in the first syringe. Do not use a syringe larger than
    20 cc. when drawing a clotting time.

3. Measuring from the syringe without the needle, place 1 cc. of
    blood in each of the three tubes.

4. At 3 minutes and at 30 second intervals thereafter, tilt all
    three tubes to approximately a 45° angle.

5. When the blood ceases to run, tilt to a 90° angle, but do not

Lee-White Clotting Time (Continued):

invert completely, and when the blood ceases to run at 90°, the test is completed.

6. The clotting time is not stopped until the blood has clotted. After 20 minutes, however, the tubes can be tilted every 5 minutes rather than every 30 seconds and reported to the nearest 5 minutes.

7. Average clotting time of the three tubes and report out average to nearest one-half minute. The three tubes should be within 2 minutes of each other.

NORMAL RANGE: 5 - 15 minutes.

REFERENCE: Miale, John B.: LABORATORY MEDICINE HEMATOLOGY 4th. Ed., C. V. Mosby Co., St. Louis, pg. 1267, 1972.

INTERPRETATION:

The Lee-White Clotting Time is prolonged primarily in diseases associated with deficiencies of the intrinsic system, such as extreme deficiencies of Factors XII, XI, IX, VIII. The Lee-White Clotting Time has also been utilized to follow the course of Heparin Anticoagulant Therap

There has been general agreement for some time that the Lee-White Coagulation Time has poor reproducibility and is extremely time consuming. Its lack of sensitivity makes it useless as a screening test.

Several new tests can be used to monitor heparin therapy that have proved much more satisfactory. These include the Activated Clotting Time, Recalcification Time, and the Activated Partial Thromboplastin Time. The Whole Blood Activated Partial Thromboplastin is a substitute for the Lee-White.

The Partial Thromboplastin Time, especially performed on the Fibrometer, is more accurate than the Lee-White Clotting Time because it eliminates variations in surface activation, phospholipid release from platelets, temperature, and endpoint detection. For monitoring heparin therapy, whole blood is preferable to plasma, because platelets have anti-heparin activity which should affect the determination.

The Whole Blood PTT has a reproducibility of $\pm$ 2% at normal levels and $\pm$ 3% at therapeutic levels. Reproducibility of Lee-Whites is $\pm$ 30%.

COLD AGGLUTININ TEST

PRINCIPLE: The serum of most normal individuals has an antibody-like substance that will cause the agglutination of Group O human erythrocytes at temperatures between 0° and 5°C. This type of substance has been termed "Cold Agglutinin". The agglutination is reversible, since erythrocytes clumped by cold agglutinins disperse when warmed to 37°C. This is a good method for detecting true cold agglutination. The titer may be elevated after a disease process.

SPECIMEN: Draw 10 ml. patient's blood and let 5.0 ml. clot at 37°C., and the remaining 5.0 ml. defibrinate. Blood should not be refrigerated after the specimen is drawn since the antibody will be absorbed upon the surface of the red cell, resulting in a false negative reaction. It is recommended that, as a precaution, blood be warmed to 37°C. before separating the serum from the clot, to elute any agglutinin which might be absorbed onto the cells. Inactivation of the serum is not necessary.

REAGENTS:

1. 2.0% Suspension of Human "O" Red Cells or Patient's Own Cells
    Suspension is in 0.85% NaCl. The cells should not be over 5 to 6 days old, from blood which is either defibrinated or anticoagulated with EDTA, citrate or oxalate. A fresh cell suspension should be prepared daily; wash the cells three times in saline, followed by centrifugation for 5 to 10 minutes at 1500 rpm. The final or fourth wash is followed by 10 minute centrifugation at 1500 rpm to pack the cells.

2. Normal Saline, 0.85% NaCl

COMMENTS ON PROCEDURE:

1. It is absolutely necessary to wash cells with 37°C. saline to remove any agglutinin which may have attached to cell during defibrination or clotting.

2. Reading of the tubes must be done as soon as they are removed from the refrigerator. If many tubes are set up, it might be wise to refrigerate all tubes not being read to prevent the warming to room temperature from dispersing the agglutination.

Cold Agglutinin Test (Continued):

3. The tubes are read by gentle shaking sufficient to disperse the red cells into solution. Vigorous shaking will result in lower titers and an increase of negative agglutination.

4. Serum may be stored, preferably frozen.

5. Group O cells may be used if patient cells are not available; however, the titer might be a bit different.

6. Generally, the higher the titer, the higher the thermal amplitude.

PROCEDURE:

1. After blood has been drawn separate the clot at 37°C.

2. Wash cells 4 times in normal saline packing the cells after the 4th wash.

3. Make doubling dilutions of patient's serum in saline; i.e. 0.2 ml. saline + 0.2 ml. serum.

4. Set up one control tube of saline; i.e. 0.2 ml.

5. Make a 2.0% suspension of patient's cells in saline or use human "0" red cells.

6. Add one volume of cells to each serum-saline tube EXCEPT the last one (this can then be used to continue titer if necessary) and one volume of 2.0% cells to saline control; i.e. if 0.2 ml. volume used, add 0.2 ml. 2.0% cells.

7. Shake rack to mix well.

8. Refrigerate 4°C. 20 to 24 hours.

9. Centrifuge quickly and lightly and read immediately BEFORE tubes warm up.

NORMAL VALUES: Normal titers up to 1:64.
Report the highest positive dilution.

REFERENCE: Cartwright, G.: DIAGNOSTIC LABORATORY HEMATOLOGY 4th. Ed., Williams & Wilkins, Baltimore, pgs. 274-275, 1965.

Cold Agglutinin Test (Continued):

INTERPRETATION:

Cold agglutinins and hemolysins are associated with benign and malignant lymphoproliferative diseases. Their presence may result in severe hemolytic anemia. A false elevation of MCV may occur with a cold agglutinin since doublets or triplets of red blood cells may be processed by the Coulter S and render false elevations of the MCV. Cold agglutinins and hemolysins are found in Mycoplasma pneumonia, infectious mononucleosis, Waldenstrom's macroglobulinemia, various lymphomas, such as Hodgkin's disease, and lymphocytic lymphoma, and autoimmune disease such as systemic lupus erythematosus.

PLASMA CRYOFIBRINOGEN

PRINCIPLE: To demonstrate the presence of a fibrinogen in plasma which precipitates between 0°C. and 4°C. The precipitation is reversible on warming to 37°C.

SPECIMEN: 2.0 ml. of plasma. Ten ml. of blood should be obtained by vacutainer technique in a violet top tube anticoagulated with EDTA.

PROCEDURE:

1. Using two 12 x 75 mm. tubes, pipette 1.0 ml. of plasma in each tube.

2. Appropriately label tubes with patient's name, date, and hospital number.

3. Cork both tubes, and place one in the refrigerator and keep the other tube at room temperature.

4. Read both tubes 24 hours later.

5. To read: Compare Room Temperature Control tube with refrigerated tube for discrete white particles or gel formation.

NORMAL VALUES: Negative Test

CONFIRMATION OF POSITIVE TEST:

Incubate both tubes at 37°C. for 30 minutes. If the precipitate or gel disappears, the test was a true positive.

REFERENCES:

1. Ealbfleisch, J. M. and Bird, R. M.: New England Jour. Med., 263:881, 1960.

2. Korst, D. R., Kratochvil, C. H.: Blood, 10:445, 1955.

3. Smith, S and Arkin, C.: "Cryofibrinogenemia". Am. J. Clin. Path. 58:524, 1972.

Plasma Cryofibrinogen (Continued):

INTERPRETATION:

Cryofibrinogens are complexes of fibrinogen which precipitate at $4^{\circ}C$. Cryofibrinogenemia occurs in a variety of clinical conditions, especially carcinoma, multiple myeloma, acute and chronic leukemia, pregnancy, and utilization of oral contraceptives. An association with diabetes mellitus has also been demonstrated.

The association of cryofibrinogenemia and cancer is not clear. Alpha$_1$ and alpha$_2$ macroglobulins are elevated with the presence of cryofibrinogenemia resulting in recurrent thromboembolism, since these proteins inhibit plasmin. Hyperfibrinogenemia is also usually found.

CRYOGLOBULIN TEST

PRINCIPLE: Cryoglobulin is an abnormal globulin characterized by spontaneous but reversible gelation or precipitation on cooling. It occurs most often in multiple myeloma and cryoglobulinemia. It may also be related to abnormalities in the immune process.

SPECIMEN: 2.0 ml. serum.

PROCEDURE:

1. Using two 12 x 75 mm. tubes, pipette 1.0 ml. of serum in each tube.

2. Appropriately label tubes with patient's name, date and hospital number.

3. Cork both tubes, and place one in the refrigerator and keep the other tube at room temperature.

4. Read both tubes 24 hours later.

5. To read: Compare Room Temperature Control tube with refrigerated tube for discrete white particles or gel formation.

NORMAL VALUES: Negative Test.

CONFIRMATION OF POSITIVE TEST:

Incubate both tubes at 37°C. for 30 minutes. If the precipitate or gel disappears, the test was a true positive.

REFERENCE: Henry, J. B.: CLINICAL CHEMISTRY: PRINCIPLES AND TECHNIQUES, Hoeber, pg. 241 - 242, 1965.

INTERPRETATION:

Cryoglobulins are globulins that precipitate irreversibly on cooling. Most cases of cryoglobulinemia are associated with multiple myeloma or Waldenstrom's Macroglobulinemia. It may also be found in other conditions such as rheumatoid arthritis, other collagen diseases, sarcoidosis and cirrhosis. The globulin may be a 7S Gamma G, a 19S Gamma M or a mixture of both. Symptoms of the condition are purpura, petechiae, and Raynaud's Phenomenon with painful blanching of the extremities on exposure to cold.

Cryoglobulin Test (Continued):

Many cryoglobulins, especially the mixed immunoglobulins may only precipitate if exposed to a temperature of 0 to 4°C. for 12 to 24 hours. Cryoprecipitation depends on the formation of weak, noncovalent bonds between Gamma globulin molecules at low temperatures. It can be prevented by pH changes, ion concentration or addition of urea. Abnormal globulins in rheumatoid Factor type cryoglobulinemia resemble Classic RF. They are Gamma M immunoglobulins with specificity for Fc fragment of a Gamma G Globulin.

DONATH-LANDSTEINER TEST
FOR
PAROXYSMAL COLD HEMOGLOBINURIA

PRINCIPLE: This procedure is performed to detect the hemolysin which is associated with paroxysmal cold hemoglobinuria. The hemolysin attaches to the red blood cells in the cold and causes hemolysis at 37°C.

SPECIMEN: 10 ml. of the patient's blood is collected in a warm syringe. The blood is transferred to a centrifuge tube in a waterbath at 37°C. and the blood is permitted to clot. Centrifuge at 2000 rpm for 10 minutes. Transfer the serum to a test tube immersed in a waterbath at 37°C. Separate the red cells and wash 3 times with warm saline. Make a 50% suspension of cells in saline. Repeat the procedure with normal ABO compatible blood.

REAGENTS AND EQUIPMENT:

1. Small test tubes

2. Incubators or Heat Blocks, 37°C. and 56°C.

3. Centrifuge

PROCEDURE:

1. Number 8 small test tubes and place in a waterbath at 37°C.

2. Place 0.5 ml. of the patient's serum in Tubes 1, 3, 4, and 6; 0.5 ml. of the normal serum in Tubes 5, 7, and 8; 0.25 ml. of the patient's serum and 0.25 ml. of normal serum Tube 2.

3. Incubate Tube No. 3 at 56°C. for 30 minutes.

4. After incubation, return it to 37°C.

5. Add 0.05 ml. of the patient's erythrocytes in Tubes 1, 2, 3, 5, 6, and 7.

6. Add 0.05 ml. of normal cells in Tubes 4 and 8, and place Tubes 1 through 5 in an ice bath for 30 minutes.

7. Return them to the 37°C. waterbath and incubate for 1 hour.

64

Donath-Landsteiner Test (Continued):

8. Centrifuge at 1000 rpm for 2 minutes and look for hemolysis in the supernatants.

9. Incubate Tubes 6, 7, and 8 for 1 hour at 37°C.

10. Centrifuge at 1000 rpm for 2 minutes and look for hemolysis in the supernatants.

RESULTS:

Tube	Serum 0.5 ml.	Cells 0.05 ml.	Temperature and Time		Hemolysis
1	P*	P	2°C., ½ Hr.;	37°C. 1 Hr.	Yes
2	P & C**	P	2°C., ½ Hr.;	37°C. 1 Hr.	Yes
3	P (Heated)	P	2°C., ½ Hr.;	37°C. 1 Hr.	No
4	P	C	2°C., ½. Hr.;	37°C. 1 Hr.	Yes
5	C	P	2°C., ½ Hr.;	37°C. 1 Hr.	No
6	P	P	37°C., 1 Hr.		No
7	C	P	37°C., 1 Hr.		No
8	C	C	37°C., 1 Hr.		No

*Patient
**Control

REFERENCE: Hinz, C. F.: "Serological and Physiochemical Characterization of Donath-Landsteiner Antibodies from Six Patients".
Blood 22:600, 1963.

INTERPRETATION AND RESULTS:

The presence of hemolysis only in Tubes No. 1, 2, and 4 is found
with paroxysmal cold hemoglobinuria. The paroxysmal cold hemoglobinuria is a condition which occurs in individuals exposed to cold with
development of hemolysis with hemoglobinuria. The D - L type of condition was recognized by Donath and Landsteiner as a hemolytic anemia
associated with syphilis. The condition now is usually associated
with viral diseases or other conditions related to lymphoprolifera-
tion. The D - L antibody is an IgG immunoglobulin and not an IgM
cold agglutinin. The D - L antibody is an autoantibody which fixes
to red blood cells in the presence of complement at 4°C. - 20°C.
When the red blood cell temperature returns to 37°C., hemolysis occurs.
The antibody has specificity for the normal red cell antigen P in the
syphilitic and viral cases.

CIRCULATING EOSINOPHIL COUNTS

PRINCIPLE: Phloxine is an acid dye which stains the eosinophils a bright pink. The propylene glycol lyses the red cells.

SPECIMEN: EDTA tube or capillary blood.

EQUIPMENT AND REAGENTS:

1. Stock Solution:
   0.1% phloxine B in propylene glycol (Randolph's fluid). This should be kept in the refrigerator when not in use.

2. Working Solution:
   1.0 ml. of Stock phloxine and 2.0 ml. of distilled water. (Made fresh each day.)

3. WBC pipettes $\pm$ 1%

4. Aspirator

5. Hemocytometer and coverslip

PROCEDURE:

1. Draw the blood to the 0.5 mark on the WBC pipette and fill to the 11 line with the diluting fluid. Dilute two pipettes.

2. Let the pipettes stand for 15 minutes.

3. Shake the pipettes for 3 minutes, discard the first 3 drops from each pipette. Fill each chamber of the hemocytometer.

4. Let set for 5 minutes and then count 0.9 cu. mm. on each side of the hemocytometer.

5. Add the two sides together and multiply by 11.1
   $$\frac{\text{Dilution}}{\text{Volume}} \left[\frac{20}{1.8 \text{ cu. mm.}} = 11.1 \right]$$

6. If there are no eosinophils seen, dilute 2 additional pipettes and repeat the count.

NORMAL VALUES: 150 - 300 cu. mm.

66

Circulating Eosinophil Counts (Continued):

REFERENCES:

1. Miale, John B.: LABORATORY MEDICINE HEMATOLOGY 4th. Ed.,
   C. V. Mosby Co., St. Louis, pg. 1204, 1972.

2. Randolph, T. G.: "Enumeration of Eosinophils with a Glycol
   Stain". J. Lab. Clin. Med. 34:1696, 1949.

INTERPRETATION:

A total eosinophil count above 300 cu. mm. may be caused by allergic
disorders, such as bronchial asthma, chronic non-allergic skin disease, parasitic infection, hematologic disorders, such as Hodgkin's
disease, or myeloproliferative diseases, or Addison's disease.
Cushing's syndrome is characterized by eosinopenia as is the utilization of exogenous cortisone or various diseases associated with excess
adrenal cortical function. The purpose of the Thorn Test is to evaluate adrenal cortical function. A total eosinophil count is performed,
25 mg. of ACTH is injected, and a total eosinophil count is performed
again 4 hours later. If adrenal cortical function is normal, the
total eosinophil count will decrease by 50 percent.

ERYTHROCYTE COUNT
(Coulter Counter)

PRINCIPLE: The blood is diluted 1:50,000 in 0.85% saline. This dilution is passed through an orifice 100 microns in diameter. Internal and external electrodes maintain a current in the orifice. As each cell enters the orifice, it changes the resistance and a pulse is generated which is proportional in magnitude to the size of the cell.

EQUIPMENT AND REAGENTS:

1. Coulter Counter

2. Plastic Vials

3. Autodilutor or a 20 lambda pipette (Sahli) and a 10 ml. automatic pipette

4. Isoton or Saline, 0.9%

SPECIMEN: EDTA or capillary blood.

COMMENTS ON PROCEDURE:

Errors may result from dust in the vials. The count should stand at least 15 seconds between the mixing and the actual counting. Too vigorous mixing produces air bubbles which will give an elevated count.

PROCEDURE:

1. Place a vial of saline under the orifice and count. This count should be below 70.

2. Make a 1:500 dilution of blood to saline by placing 20 lambda of blood in 10 ml. of saline. (This may be used later for the WBC.) Using 0.1 ml. of this dilution and 9.9 ml. saline, make a 1:50,000 dilution.

3. The aperture current setting should be on 5. The threshhold setting is determined by calibration. Proper setting will be found taped on the face of the Coulter. When running erythrocyte counts, always reset the Coulter Counter for WBC's when finished.

68

Erythrocyte Count (Continued):

4. Erythrocyte counts must always be corrected. Disregard the last two numbers on the digital counter. Use the numbers left and refer to the correction chart by 10,000 and this will give the erythrocytes/mm^3.

NORMAL VALUES:

Male	4.2 million to	5.4 million/mm^3	
Female	3.6 million to	5.0 million/mm^3	
Newborn	4.8 million to	7.0 million/mm^3	
1 Month	4.1 million to	6.1 million/mm^3	
3 Months	3.7 million to	5.2 million/mm^3	
1 Year	3.9 million to	5.3 million/mm^3	
4 Years	4.1 million to	5.6 million/mm^3	
8 Years	4.4 million to	6.0 million/mm^3	
12 Years	4.5 million to	5.8 million/mm^3	

REFERENCES:

1. Miale, John B.: LABORATORY MEDICINE HEMATOLOGY 4th. Ed., C. V. Mosby Co., St. Louis, pgs. 1201-1202, 1972.

2. Brecker, G.: "Evaluation of Electronic Red Cell Counter". Am. J. Clin. Path. 26:1437-1449, 1956.

3. Freichtmir, T. V.: "Electronic Counting of Erythrocytes". Am. J. Clin. Path. 35:373-377, 1961.

INTERPRETATION:

See Interpretation under Red Blood Cell Indices on page 76.

ERYTHROCYTE COUNTS
(Hematocytometer Method)

PRINCIPLE: Anticoagulated blood is diluted with an isotonic solution. After shaking the pipettes, the dilution is introduced into the hemocytometer and the erythrocytes are then counted. The diluting fluid does not destroy the leukocytes. The dilution is so great that they usually do not interfere with the count.

SPECIMEN: An EDTA tube or fingertip blood.

EQUIPMENT AND REAGENTS:

1. RBC pipettes $\pm$ 1%

2. Aspirator

3. Hemocytometer with Coverslip

4. Hayem's Solution
   Mercuric Chloride, C. P.   1.1 gm.
   Sodium Sulfate, anhydrous, C. P.   4.4 gm.
   Sodium Chloride, C. P.   2.0 gm.
   Distilled water q. s. to   400.0 ml.

                    OR

5. Gower's Solution
   Sodium Sulfate, anhydrous, C. P. 12.5 gm.
   Glacial Acetic Acid   33.3 ml.
   Distilled Water q. s. to   200.0 ml.

6. 0.9% Sodium Chloride
   In cases of autoagglutination

PROCEDURE:

1. Fill a RBC pipette with blood to the 0.5 line then fill with diluting solution to the 101 mark. This gives a 1:200 dilution. Dilute two pipettes.

2. Shake the pipettes for 3 minutes.

3. Discard the first 5 drops from the pipettes.

70

Erythrocyte Counts (Continued):

4. Fill the hemocytometer carefully placing one pipette on each side of the chamber. Let settle for 3 minutes.

5. The center area consisting of 25 small squares is the erythrocyte counting area. Count 5 of these 25 squares. (The four corner squares and the middle square.)

6. The difference between the two counts should be no more than 10%.

7. CALCULATIONS:

$$RBC/mm^3 = Cells \text{ counted} \times 5(1/5 \text{ cm}.^2 \text{ counted}) \times 10 \text{ (Depth)}$$

$$\times 200 \text{ (Dilution)}$$

COMMENTS ON PROCEDURE:

Clumping of the red cells in Hayem's Solution may be due to cold agglutinins, in which case it may be prevented by warming the Hayem's solution before use. It may also be produced by precipitation of globulins by the heavy metals in the diluting fluid (as in multiple myeloma and Kala-azar). In cirrhosis of the liver and atypical pneumonia, cold hemagglutinins may be found. This clumping will usually be avoided with Gower's solution.

NORMAL VALUES: Males   4.2 to 5.4 Million/mm^3
               Females   3.6 to 5.0 Million/mm^3
               Newborns   4.8 to 7.0 Million/mm^3
               1 Month   4.1 to 6.1 Million/mm^3
               3 Months   3.7 to 5.2 Million/mm^3
               1 Year   3.9 to 5.3 Million/mm^3
               4 Years   4.1 to 5.6 Million/mm^3
               8 Years   4.4 to 6.0 Million/mm^3
               12 Years   4.5 to 5.8 Million/mm^3

REFERENCES:

1. Miale, John B.: LABORATORY MEDICINE HEMATOLOGY 4th. Ed., C. V. Mosby Co., St. Louis, pgs. 1198-1200, 1972.

2. Hepler, Opal E.: MANUAL OF CLINICAL LABORATORY METHODS 4th. Ed., Charles C. Thomas, Springfield, Ill., pgs. 34-35, 1968.

INTERPRETATION:

See Interpretation under Red Blood Cell Indices on page 76.

ERYTHROCYTE LIFE
SPAN ^{51}CHROMIUM

PRINCIPLE: Red blood cells rapidly incorporate $Na_2{}^{51}CrO_4$. The radio-activity of the radioactive red blood cells is followed for 2 to 4 weeks and the half-life of the red blood cells is ascertained from the loss of radioactivity from the circulation. The normal $T\frac{1}{2}$ is approximately 30 days.

SPECIMEN: 30 ml. of heparinized blood drawn under sterile conditions.

REAGENTS AND EQUIPMENT:

1. 100 Microcuries of ^{51}Cr

2. Centrifuge

3. Sterile Saline

4. Microhematocrit Centrifuge and Reader

5. Scintillation Counter

PROCEDURE:

1. Incubate 30 ml. of heparinized blood with 100 microcuries of ^{51}Cr in a sterile screw-top tube for 30 minutes.

2. Centrifuge the mixture.

3. Remove the plasma.

4. Reinject the red blood cells into the patient after suspending them in saline.

5. Obtain 10 ml. heparinized blood 1 hour later, every day for a week and every 3 days of the second week.

6. Perform a hematocrit on each sample.

7. Place 2.0 ml. of whole blood and 2.0 ml. of plasma from each sample into separate scintillation counting tubes.

Erythrocyte Life Span ^{51}Chromium (Continued):

8. CALCULATIONS:

The counts are expressed in counts per minute per ml. of whole blood. The hematocrit is needed in calculating the amount of radioactivity present in the plasma of each sample.

NORMAL VALUES:

The results are plotted on logarithm paper using the 1 hour sample as representing 100% activity and each subsequent value a percentage of the 1 hour sample. The patient's heart, liver and spleen should be scanned for radioactivity and the possibility of splenic sequestration of red blood cells should be determined.

REFERENCE: Danon, D., Marikovsky, Y. & Gasko, O.: "^{51}Chromium Uptake as a Function of Red Cell Age". J. Lab. Clin. Med. 67:70, 1966.

INTERPRETATION:

The normal T½ erythrocyte life span is approximately 30 days. Smaller sample volumes may be utilized for counting depending on the sample activity.

PRINCIPLE: The indices give an accurate picture of red blood cell morphology in association with the appearance of the red blood cells on fixed smears.

SPECIMEN: 5.0 ml. of whole blood anticoagulated with EDTA.

REAGENTS AND EQUIPMENT:

I. Erythrocyte Counts (Hemocytometer Method)
    1. RBC pipettes $\pm$ 1%

    2. Aspirator

    3. Hemocytometer with Coverslip

    4. Hayems Solution
        Mercuric Chloride, C.P.   1.0 gm.
        Sodium Sulfate, anhydrous, C.P.   4.4 gm.
        Sodium Chloride, C.P.   2.0 gm.
        Distilled Water to   400.0 ml.
                        OR
    5. Gowers Solution
        Sodium Sulfate, anhydrous, C.P. 12.5 gm.
        Glacial Acetic Acid   33.3 ml.
        Distilled Water to   200.0 ml.

    6. In the case of autoagglutination use 0.9% NaCl.

II. Hemoglobin Determination
    A. Cyanmethemoglobin Method
        1. Coulter Autodilutor

        2. Sahli Pipettes (0.02 ml.)

        3. Drabkin's Reagent
            $NaHCO_3$ 1.0 gm.
            K Cyanide (KCN)   50.0 mg.
            K Ferricyanide $K_3Fe(CN)_6$ 200.0 mg.
            Distilled Water to   1000.0 ml.

        4. Spectrophotometer, 540 nm.

Erythrocyte Indices (Continued):

B. Coulter Hemoglobinometer Method
   1. Coulter Autodilutor

   2. Coulter Hemoglobinometer

   3. Sahli Pipettes (0.02 ml.)

   4. Isoton

   5. Zap-oglobin

   6. Cyanmethemoglobin Standard (Coulter)

III. Hematocrit or PCV (Packed Cell Volume)
   1. Heparinized and/or plain Capillary Tubes (I.D. 1.1-1.2 mm.; length 75 mm.

   2. Micro Hematocrit Centrifuge

   3. Sealer for Capillary Tubes

PROCEDURE:

1. See procedure section of erythrocyte count determination on page 70; of hemoglobin determination on pages 141 and 143; hematocrit determination on page 132.

2. Determine the:
   a). Mean Corpuscular Volume (MCV).
   b). Mean Corpuscular Hemoglobin (MCH)
   c). Mean Corpuscular Hemoglobin Concentration (MCHC).

3. CALCULATIONS:

Mean Corpuscular volume (MCV):

$$MCV = \frac{Hematocrit \times 10}{Erythrocyte\ count,\ millions\ per\ cu.\ mm.}$$

Mean Corpuscular Hemoglobin (MCH):

$$MCH = \frac{Hgb.,\ Gm.\ per\ 100\ ml.\ \times 10}{Erythrocyte\ count,\ millions\ per\ cu.\ mm.}$$

76

Erythrocyte Indices (Continued):

Mean Corpuscular Hemoglobin Concentration (MCHC):

$$MCHC = \frac{Hgb., \; Gm. \; per \; 100 \; ml. \; x \; 100}{Hematocrit}$$

NORMAL VALUES: MCV: 87 $\pm$ 5 cubic microns (cu.μ)
                MCH: 29 $\pm$ 2 micromicrograms ($\gamma \gamma$)
                MCHC: 34 $\pm$ 2%

REFERENCE: Miale, John B.: LABORATORY MEDICINE HEMATOLOGY 4th. Ed.
            C. V. Mosby Co., St. Louis, pgs. 643-646; 1205-1206, 1972.

INTERPRETATION:

An MCV above 92 cμ indicates that the red blood cells are macrocytic
while one below 82 cμ indicates that the red blood cells are microcytic. Borderline results should be interpreted with caution. One
should correlate the MCV with the blood smear morphology. The MCV
is only a mean volume index, and represents the mean of the volume
of red blood cells in the peripheral blood. There may be a wide
variation in the red blood cell size in anemic patients.

The MCH is an expression of the average weight of hemoglobin present
in a red blood cell. High MCH values are found in macrocytic anemias
while low MCH results are found in microcytic anemias.

The MCHC represents the hemoglobin concentration in each red blood
cells. A higher than normal hemoglobin concentration is not possible,
but a lower concentration is found in anemia and indicates a hypochromic state.

NORMAL INDICES

AGE	RBC/MILL. PER CC.	HEMOGLOBIN GMS./100 CC.	PCV (%)	MCV (^{3})	MCH (^{3})	MCHC (%)
First Day	5.1 ± 1.0	19.5 ± 5.0	54.0 ± 10	106	38	36
14-60 Days	4.7 ± 0.9	14.0 ± 3.3	42.0 ± 7.0	90	30	33
1 Year	4.5	11.2	35.0	78	25	32
11-15 Years	4.8	13.4	39.0	82	28	34
Adult Female	4.0 - 4.7	12.2 - 14.1	35.8 - 42.0	83-97	28-32	33-36
Adult Male	4.5 - 5.2	13.6 - 16.1	40.0 - 47.1	83-97	28-32	33-36

REFERENCES:

1. Wintrobe, M.: CLINICAL HEMATOLOGY 6th Ed., Lea & Febiger, Phil., 1967.

2. Adult Blood Donors at Stanford University Hospital Blood Bank.

A Complete Blood Count consists of a PCV, WBC, hemoglobin, differential, and RBC morphology and platelet estimation on smear. The RBC morphology and platelet estimation are done on the first CBC done on patient admission, and only on direct smear not on versenate smear.

The CBC is done on a versenate specimen, a lavendar top Vacutainer tube, or by fingerstick. If it is done by fingerstick, the WBC and hemoglobin are drawn in triplicate and 3 or 4 PCV tubes are filled.

One hundred cells are counted for most differentials; in counts of less than 3,000, only a 50 cell differential is counted and multiplied by 2 to report out in percentage. If the WBC count is 15,000 or greater, a 200 cell differential is done divided by 2 and reported out in percent. When a differential of other than 100 cells is done, it is noted under remarks how many cells were counted. In all abnormal differentials at least 200 cells are counted.

In a CBC, the WBC and PCV are always done in duplicate. The MCHC is calculated, and if it does not fall between 33 - 36%, these tests are repeated unless there is hypochromia on the smear. If only a hemoglobin or PCV is ordered, it is always done in duplicate. When a RBC count is ordered, indices are calculated. The indices should agree with RBC morphology or be repeated. An RBC morphology and platelet estimation are done on all admission work even if only a PCV or hemoglobin is ordered.

ETHANOL GELATION TEST
FOR
DISSEMINATED INTRAVASCULAR COAGULATION

PRINCIPLE: This procedure is a simple, rapid screening procedure to detect the fibrin monomer present in the plasma in dimmeminated intravascular coagulation. Ethanol causes the fibrin monomer to gel.

SPECIMEN: 1 to 5.0 ml. plasma obtained in 0.1 M. buffered citrate. The 0.1 M. buffered citrate may be obtained as special anticoagulant solution (Hyland Laboratories, Los Angeles, California). Plasma drawn into the special buffered citrate has a pH of approximately 7.3.

REAGENTS:

1. <u>0.1 M. Buffered Citrate Solution</u>

2. <u>0.1 N. Sodium Hydroxide</u>

3. <u>Ethanol, 50%</u>

PROCEDURE:

1. Add one drop of 0.1 N. sodium hydroxide to nine drops of buffered citrated plasma.

2. Layer 0.15 ml. of 50% ethanol over this mixture.

3. A distinct line appears at the interface within one minute if the fibrin monomer is present.

NORMAL VALUES: A Negative Test

REFERENCE: Breen, F. A., Jr. and Tullis, J. L.: "Ethanol Gelation: A Rapid Screening Test for Intravascular Coagulation". <u>Ann. Intern. Med.</u>, 69:1197-1206, 1968.

INTERPRETATION:

The main value of the Ethanol Gelation Test is to detect soluble fibrin monomer present in the plasma associated with disseminated intravascular coagulation. A positive test with a decrease in platelets, intrinsic and extrinsic factors, and fibrinogen is suggestive of disseminated intravascular coagulation. A false positive Ethanol Gelation Test may occur in other conditions associated with bleeding

Ethanol Gelation Test (Continued):

and clotting, such as post-operative state, idiopathic thrombocytopenic purpura, bleeding gastrointestinal lesions, menstruation,
phlebothrombosis and pulmonary embolism.

QUANTITATIVE TEST FOR FECAL UROBILINOGEN

PRINCIPLE: Urobilinogen, along with other aldehyde reacting substances found in stools, reacts with Ehrlich's Aldehyde Reagent to produce a red color whose intensity is proportional to the amount of pigment present.

SPECIMEN: A 72 hour stool specimen is collected. Keep under refrigeration. The specimen must weigh at least 100 gm. for an accurate determination. Specimens on newborns may weigh less.

REAGENTS:

1. Ferrous Sulfate

2. NaOH, 10%

3. Sodium Acetate, saturated aqueous solution
   Approximately 1,000 gm. of sodium acetate containing 3 molecules of water of crystallization is added to one liter of distilled water. The mixture is heated to approximately 60°C. When the solution cools there should be a large excess of crystals.

4. Ehrlich's Aldehyde Reagent, Watson's modification
   Dissolve 0.7 gm. of paradimethylaminobenzaldehyde in a mixture of 150 ml. of concentrated HCl and 100 ml. distilled water. The reagent is stable if stored in a brown bottle.

5. Stock Standard
   Dissolve 20 mg. Phenol Red in 100 ml. of 0.05% NaOH.

6. Working Standard
   Dilute Stock Standard 1:100 with 0.05% NaOH to make a 0.2 mg%. solution. This 0.2 mg%. solution is equivalent in color to 0.35 (0.0346) mg%. of urobilinogen. The working standard should have an O.D. of 0.38 at a wavelength of 562 nm. against a water blank when read on a spectrophotometer of high resolution.
   NOTE: Phenol Red, pH 6.8 - 8.4 (Code 2411-C) is made by La Motte Chemical Co., Chestertown, Md.

7. 3-Indoleacetic Acid

Fecal Urobilinogen (Continued):

PROCEDURE:

1. Weigh sample.

2. Place 10 gm. of well mixed sample in a Waring blender. Add 20 gm. of ferrous sulfate.

3. Dilute up to 400 ml. with distilled water (marked on blender).

4. Add 100 ml. of 10% NaOH.

5. Mix and decant into a 1000 ml. flask and set in the dark for one hour or longer. If the supernatant solution is not almost color-less at the end of this period, the reduction may be continued for another hour.

6. Filter. If the reduction is not complete, as occasionally is true when the feces contain large amounts of urobilinogen, a meas-ured portion of the filtrate should be mixed with fresh ferrous sulfate as described above, and after standing another hour, this filtrate is taken for the quantitative procedure.

7. Assemble 6 tubes (3 Blanks and 3 Unknowns).

    PART I   Blank: 2.5 ml. filtrate plus 5 ml. sodium acetate mixed thoroughly. Add 2.5 ml. Ehrlich's reagent.

               Unknown: 2.5 ml. filtrate plus 2.5 ml. Ehrlich's reagent. Mix for 15 seconds. Add 5 ml. sodium acetate solution and mix.
NOTE: Sodium Acetate stops the color reaction of Ehrlich's reagent.

               If color appears in Blank for Part I, substitute "Part IV" for "Part I".

    PART II   Blank: Distilled water.

               Standard: 0.35 mg%. urobilinogen standard that has been kept in a brown bottle. Needed for Calculation of Part I.

    PART III Blank: 2.5 ml. of methanol plus 2.5 ml. Ehrlich's reagent (use stopper in test tube as methanol evapor-ates quickly).

Fecal Urobilinogen (Continued):

> Unknown: 0.1 gm. preweighed 3-Indoleacetic acid plus 2.5 ml. methanol; mix until dissolved. Add 2.5 ml. Ehrlich's reagent. Allow to stand at least 15 minutes before reading.
>
> Read Parts I, II, and III Unknowns against their respective Blanks on the Spectrophotometer at 562 nm.

PART IV   Add 100 mg. ascorbic acid (from capsule) to 10 ml. of filtrate.

> Colored Blank: Mix 6.0 ml. of sodium acetate with 3.0 ml. of Ehrlich's reagent. Add 4.5 ml. of this mixture to 1.5 ml. absorbed filtrate.
>
> Unknown: 1.5 ml. absorbed filtrate plus 1.5 ml. Ehrlich's reagent. Mix well for one minute, then add 3.0 ml. sodium acetate solution and mix thoroughly.
>
> Read the Colored Blank and Unknown against colorless Water Blank at 562 nm. on a Spectrophotometer.
>
> Proceed on Part II and III as above

CALCULATIONS:

Part I.

$$\frac{0.35}{\text{O.D. Standard}} = \frac{X}{\text{O.D. Unknown}}$$

Multiply value of "X" x 200 = Conc. of urobilinogen in mg./100 gm. feces.

Factor of 200 is derived from the following:

$$\frac{50 \text{ Total ml. of Solution (500)}}{10 \text{ (gm. of Stool)}} \text{ x } \frac{\text{Volume of Final Sol. (10 ml.)}}{\text{Volume of Filtrate used (2.5 ml.}}$$

Part III.

Part III is a check on the stability of the Ehrlich's reagent.

$$\frac{\text{O.D. Unknown (Part III)}}{\text{O.D. Standard (Part II)}} = \frac{X}{0.35 \text{ mg\%. (Value of Standard)}}$$

84

Fecal Urobilinogen (Continued):

X should fall between 0.35 ——→ 0.395.

Part IV.

$$0.35 \times \left[\frac{\text{O.D. Unknown} - \text{O.D. Colored Blank}}{\text{O.D. Standard}}\right] \times 200 \text{ mg./100 gm.}$$

$$\frac{\text{Urobilinogen in mg./100 gm. x Wt. of Total Sample}}{100 \text{ x number of days}}$$

= mg. Urobilinogen/24 hours.

Report in mg./100 gm. feces and mg./24 hours

NORMAL VALUES: Normal Range 30 - 200 mg./100 gm. feces
                 Maximum   40 - 280 mg./day

REFERENCES:

1. Henry, Richard B.: CLINICAL CHEMISTRY: PRINCIPLES AND TECHNIQUES, Hoeber, New York, pgs. 611-614, 1964.

2. Davidsohn, I. and Wells, B.: CLINICAL DIAGNOSIS BY LABORATORY METHODS, 13th. Ed., Saunders Co., Phil., pgs. 548-550, 1965.

INTERPRETATION:

The urobilinogen excretion in the stool varies daily in normal individuals. It is important to determine the 24 hour fecal urobilinogen and not a single stool specimen. Too wide a range of normal values exists for a single stool specimen. The daily fecal urobilinogen excretion is a measure of daily hemoglobin destruction. Thus, an elevation of fecal urobilinogen occurs in hemolytic anemia.

A decrease in fecal urobilinogen occurs in anemia other than hemolysis obstructive jaundice from intra-or extrahepatic causes, diarrhea, where there is a reduction in time for bacterial transformation of bilirubin glucuronide and utilization of broad spectrum antibiotics. These decrease colonic Gram-negative bacilli.

FIBRINOGEN
(Semiquantitative)

PRINCIPLE: Thrombin and calcium are added to diluted plasma to convert fibrinogen to fibrin. The time required for the clot to form is inversely proportional to the amount of fibrinogen present.

SPECIMEN: Citrated plasma: 9 parts blood to 1 part 3.8% sodium citrate (EDTA plasma may be used - 7.0 ml. blood to 9.0 mg. of EDTA).

REAGENTS AND EQUIPMENT:

1. Thrombin Stock Solution
   Dilute vials of 5000 units with 0.025 M. Calcium chloride to 1000 units/ml. Aliquot 0.1 ml. amounts in 10 ml. plastic tubes. Store in freezer.

2. Thrombin Working Solution
   10 units/ml. Thaw and dilute as needed 1 tube of stock solution with 9.9 ml. of 0.025 M. Calcium chloride.

3. Imidazole Buffer
   Ingredients include: 6.8 gm. imidazole, 16.7 gm. sodium chloride, 372 ml. 0.1 M. HCl. Dilute to 2 liters and check pH. pH should be 7.35 $\pm$ 0.05.

4. Fibrometer and 0.4 ml. Probe

5. Control - CNP
   Dilute as directed on vial. Stable several days in refrigerator.

SOURCES OF ERROR:

Thrombin is stable in plastic, but rapidly adsorbs out on glass. It must be kept in plastic tubes.

PROCEDURE:

1. Prewarm 0.9 ml. of imidazole buffer to 37°C.

2. Prewarm 0.2 ml. aliquots of thrombin in fibrometer cups.

3. Add 0.1 ml. of plasma to the prewarmed buffer. Mix well.

Fibrinogen (Continued):

4. Add 0.2 ml. of diluted plasma to the thrombin, starting the fibrometer.

5. Read value from Curve Chart.

6. If the clotting time is greater than 18 seconds, repeat, using 0.2 ml. plasma and 0.8 ml. buffer. Read value from curve, and divide by 2. If clotting time is less than 9.5 seconds, repeat using 0.1 ml. plasma and 1.9 ml. buffer. Read value from chart, and multiply by 2.

7. Control is run in same manner as patient's plasma. The time in seconds should fall within 2 S.D. of a previously determined time for that Lot No. of CNP.

CALCULATION:

Except in the presence of a rare antithrombin, fibrinogen may be read from a curve previously prepared from a plasma of known fibrinogen value. This gives a variation of 10% and should be reported as $\pm$ 10% of the value obtained.

The Curve is made with the following dilutions of plasma in imidazole buffer:

80%	0.40 ml. plasma	0.10 ml. buffer
70%	0.35 ml. plasma	0.15 ml. buffer
60%	0.30 ml. plasma	0.20 ml. buffer
50%	0.25 ml. plasma	0.25 ml. buffer
40%	0.25 ml. of 80% dil.	0.25 ml. buffer
30%	0.25 ml. of 60% dil.	0.25 ml. buffer
20%	0.25 ml. of 40% dil.	0.25 ml. buffer

The dilutions are treated as whole plasma in the test. Clotting times are plotted against mg%. on Log 2 Cycle Graph Paper.

REFERENCES:

1. Clauss, A.: "Gerinnungsphysiologische Schnellmethode zur Bestimmung des Fibrinogens", Acta Haemat., 17:237 - 246, 1957.

2. Morse, Edward: "Automated Fibrinogen Determination", Am. J. Clin. Path., 55:671 - 676, 1971.

Fibrinogen (Continued):

The following is typical of the Calibration Curves used in our Laboratory and is given here only as an example of the scope of the range used. Each laboratory must set up their own curves each and every time reagents and Lot Numbers are changed.

FIBRINOGEN
(EDTA or Sodium Citrate)

Seconds	Mg%.	Seconds	Mg%.	Seconds	Mg%.
9.2	400 ± 10%	12.2	264 ± 10%	15.2	191 ± 10%
9.3	394 ± 10%	12.3	261 ± 10%	15.3	189 ± 10%
9.4	388 ± 10%	12.4	258 ± 10%	15.4	187 ± 10%
9.5	382 ± 10%	12.5	255 ± 10%	15.5	185 ± 10%
9.6	376 ± 10%	12.6	252 ± 10%	15.6	184 ± 10%
9.7	370 ± 10%	12.7	249 ± 10%	15.7	183 ± 10%
9.8	365 ± 10%	12.8	246 ± 10%	15.8	182 ± 10%
9.9	360 ± 10%	12.9	243 ± 10%	15.9	181 ± 10%
10.0	355 ± 10%	13.0	240 ± 10%	16.0	180 ± 10%
10.1	350 ± 10%	13.1	237 ± 10%	16.1	178 ± 10%
10.2	345 ± 10%	13.2	234 ± 10%	16.2	176 ± 10%
10.3	340 ± 10%	13.3	231 ± 10%	16.3	174 ± 10%
10.4	335 ± 10%	13.4	228 ± 10%	16.4	172 ± 10%
10.5	330 ± 10%	13.5	225 ± 10%	16.5	170 ± 10%
10.6	326 ± 10%	13.6	223 ± 10%	16.6	169 ± 10%
10.7	322 ± 10%	13.7	221 ± 10%	16.7	168 ± 10%
10.8	318 ± 10%	13.8	219 ± 10%	16.8	167 ± 10%
10.9	314 ± 10%	13.9	217 ± 10%	16.9	166 ± 10%
11.0	310 ± 10%	14.0	215 ± 10%	17.0	165 ± 10%
11.1	306 ± 10%	14.1	213 ± 10%	17.1	163 ± 10%
11.2	302 ± 10%	14.2	211 ± 10%	17.2	161 ± 10%
11.3	298 ± 10%	14.3	209 ± 10%	17.3	159 ± 10%
11.4	294 ± 10%	14.4	207 ± 10%	17.4	157 ± 10%
11.5	290 ± 10%	14.5	205 ± 10%	17.5	155 ± 10%
11.6	286 ± 10%	14.6	203 ± 10%	17.6	154 ± 10%
11.7	282 ± 10%	14.7	201 ± 10%	17.7	153 ± 10%
11.8	278 ± 10%	14.8	199 ± 10%	17.8	152 ± 10%
11.9	274 ± 10%	14.9	197 ± 10%	17.9	151 ± 10%
12.0	270 ± 10%	15.0	195 ± 10%	18.0	150 ± 10%
12.1	267 ± 10%	15.1	193 ± 10%		

Fibrinogen (Continued):

INTERPRETATION:

Many conditions are associated with a decrease in fibrinogen, as noted in the list below. The dilution of 1:10 dilutes out most antithrombin. This measures thrombin clottable fibrinogen. The amount of plasma fibrinogen may be determined from a curve previously prepared from a plasma of known fibrinogen value. A variation of approximately 10 percent is present and should be reported as $\pm$ 10% of the value obtained. Low fibrinogen occurs as a result of a production defect which may be hereditary or due to severe liver disease. Intravascular conversion of plasma to serum is known as disseminated intravascular coagulation or consumptive coagulopathy. These conditions are:

1. Sanarelli-Schwartzman reaction
2. Purpura fulminans
3. Hemolytic-uremic syndrome (Gasser's syndrome)
4. Kasabach-Merritt syndrome
5. Septic shock
6. Incompatible hemolytic blood transfusion disease
7. Abruptio placentae
8. Dead fetus syndrome
9. Amniotic fluid embolism
10. Acute promyelocytic leukemia
11. Malaria
12. Septic abortion
13. Carcinoma
14. Meningococcemia
15. Waterhouse-friderichsen syndrome
16. Prostate gland surgery

Other conditions which will predominantly activate the fibrinolytic system are:

1. Preoperative anxiety
2. Pulmonary surgery
3. Neurosurgery
4. Open heart surgery

Conditions which simultaneous or cause coequal activation of clotting system and fibrinolytic system are:

1. Cirrhosis of liver
2. Hepatitis

Fibrinogen (Continued):

An increase in plasma fibrinogen occurs in the following conditions:

1. Acute infection
2. Collagen diseases. The plasma fibrinogen has been used to assess activity in both rheumatic carditis and rheumatoid arthritis.
3. Nephrosis. A very high concentration may be found.
4. Hepatitis (in the absence of severe liver damage)
5. Post-X-ray therapy (indicates tissue damage)
6. Burns (response to tissue injury)
7. Multiple Myeloma
8. Pregnancy
9. Various epithelial malignancies

FIBRINOGEN STABILIZING FACTOR XIII

PRINCIPLE: Fibrinogen in the presence of thrombin, calcium, and factor XIII forms a fibrin clot which is insoluble in urea. This will detect only a complete deficiency as only 1 to 2% factor XIII is necessary to form an insoluble clot.

SPECIMEN: 4.5 ml. whole blood added to 0.5 ml. 3.8% sodium citrate.

EQUIPMENT AND REAGENTS:

1. Sodium Citrate, 3.8%

2. $CaCl_2$, 0.025 M.
   Dilute 1.0% $CaCl_2$ 1:2.72.

3. Urea, 5.0 M.
   30.03 gm. are dissolved in distilled water in a 100 ml. volumetric flask and diluted to volume.

4. Thrombin
   Reconstitite 100 Units/ml. in Tris Buffer, pH 7.4.

PROCEDURE:

1. Draw blood and add 4.5 ml. to 0.5 ml. 3.8% citrate. Always draw a normal control.

2. Centrifuge samples immediately.

3. Place in 10 x 75 mm. tubes the following plasmas:
   a). 0.5 ml. Control citrated plasma
   b). 0.5 ml. Patient citrated plasma
   c). 0.5 ml. citrated plasma which is 95 parts patient and 5 parts control. (i.e. 0.95 ml. (0.475) patient citrated plasma; 0.05 ml. (0.025) control citrated plasma.) Mix well but gently.
   d). 0.5 ml. EDTA plasma - (optional). This will be a positive control.

4. Add 0.5 ml. 0.025 M. $CaCl_2$ to Tubes (a), (b), and (c). To (d) add 0.1 ml. reconstituted thrombin.

5. Let clot at 37°C. for 20 minutes.

Fibrinogen Stabilizing Factor XIII (Continued):

6. Pipette 5.0 ml. 5 M. Urea into four 16 x 100 mm. tubes.

7. Gently loosen clot with applicator stick and place in Urea.

8. Cap and leave at room temperature.

9. Observe clot at 1, 2, 3, and 24 hours.

RESULTS:

1. Control clot (Tube a) and mixed clot (Tube c) should not lyse before 24 hours.

2. Positive Control clot (Tube d) should lyse in 5 M. Urea as there is no calcium present in EDTA blood.

3. If mixed clot (Tube c) lyses before 24 hours, it suggests some other defect.

REFERENCE: Alami, S., Hampton, J., Race, G., Speer, R.: "Fibrin Stabilizing Factor, Factor XIII". Amer. J. Med. 44:1, 1968.

INTERPRETATION:

Clots which form in normal plasma are insoluble in 5 M urea due to the action of fibrin stabilizing factor. Disappearance of the clot is indicative of Factor XIII deficiency.

COUNTERELECTROPHORESIS TEST
FOR
FIBRINOGEN/FIBRIN DEGRADATION PRODUCTS

PRINCIPLE: Fibrin and fibrinogen split products are immunologically similar to fibrinogen. When subjected to electrophoresis in a negatively charged gel, antifibrinogen is moved toward the cathode. Negatively charged antigens migrate to the anode. At the point of antigen-antibody reaction, one or more precipitin lines will be formed.

SPECIMEN COLLECTION: Collect 8.0 ml. of blood by non-traumatic venipuncture after loosening the tourniquet. Dispense 5.0 ml. gently into collecting tube and mix by inverting gently. Blood will clot within a few seconds. Incubate at 37°C. for 10 minutes to ensure complete clotting. Ring clot and centrifuge. Remove serum. If test is not to be run within 8 hours, freeze serum at -20°C.

REAGENTS AND EQUIPMENT:

1. Collection Tubes
    Dilute bovine thrombin to 1000 U/ml. Aliquot 0.1 ml. in plastic tubes. Freeze at -20°C. Just prior to use, thaw briefly at 37°C. and add either 0.1 ml. 25% Epsilon amino caproic acid or 0.1 ml. Trasylol (5000 U/ml.). Trasylol is stored between 2° and 8°C. EACA is stored at room temperature.

2. Antiserum to Human Fibrinogen
    Store between 2° and 8°C.

3. Agar Gel Plates
    Store between 2° and 8°C. in plastic bag containing a sponge saturated with distilled water. Close bag tightly.

4. Capillary Tubes

5. Hyland Disposable Electrophoresis Base Units

6. Hyland Buffer
    Store between 2° and 8°C.

7. Hyland Electrophoresis Power Supply

8. Hyland Immuno-Illuminator

92

Counterelectrophoresis Test (Continued):

9. Controls
   Dilute fibrinogen to 50 ug./ml. Freeze at -20°C. in small aliquots. Thaw as needed for positive control. Negative control
   consists of serum collected from a normal person using same
   technique as the test subject. Aliquot and freeze.

PROCEDURE:

1. Remove the sponge wicks from the electrophoresis base units and
   add buffer to the indented line.

2. Replace sponges and depress two or three times to assure uniform
   saturation. They should expand to make firm contact with the
   electrodes and agar gel.

3. Number wells on back of agar plate beginning with the pair of
   wells nearest the Hyland name. Turn the plate to fill with the
   Hyland name backward on your right.

4. Allow excess moisture to evaporate, but do not allow plate to
   become dry. If wells contain moisture, remove it by carefully
   inserting a small piece of filter paper into the bottom of the
   well.

5. Of each pair of wells, fill the well on your right with patient
   serum or control. (This is the Cathode side.)

6. Fill the wells on the anode side with the antifibrinogen.

7. Wait about 2 minutes after filling wells. Then turn the plate
   over and place it on the base so that the agar gel makes firm
   contact with the sponges.

8. Insert the end of the electrophoresis cell closest to the sample
   wells (end with Hyland) into the permanent end cap (Cathode) of
   the power supply. Attach the removable end cap (Anode) on the
   power supply. Electrophorese at 40 milliamperes for 15 minutes.

9. Unplug the power supply and remove agar plate.

10. After 15 minutes read over the viewing box. Look for precipitin
    lines between the sample and antibody wells. They may be straight
    or curved and single or double. Very strong reactions will be
    visible in 15 minutes, but weaker reactions are not visible until
    later. Most will appear by 1½ hours. Do not report as negative
    for 3 hours.

Counterelectrophresis Test (Continued):

NORMAL VALUES: Less than 10 ug./ml.
                 No precipitin lines in 3 hours.

REFERENCES:

1. Lewis, J. H., Wilson, J. H. and Brandon, J. M.: "Counterelectrophoresis for Molecules Immunologically Similar to
   Fibrinogen". Am. J. Clin. Path. 58:400-403, 1972.

2. Rabaa, M. S., Bernier, G. M. and Ratnoff, O. D.: "Rapid
   Detection of Fibrinogen-related Antigens in Serum". J. Lab.
   Clin. Med. 81:476-483, 1973.

INTERPRETATION:

The clinical value for detecting fibrin degradation products in the
plasma is in the assessment of consumptive coagulopathy or disseminated intravascular coagulopathy.

A positive test with a decrease in platelets, intrinsic and extrinsic
factors, and fibrinogen is suggestive of disseminated intravascular
coagulopathy. A false positive test may occur in other conditions
associated with bleeding and clotting, such as postoperative state,
idiopathic thrombocytopenic purpura, bleeding gastrointestinal lesions, menstruation, phlebothrombosis, and pulmonary embolism.

LATEX TEST
FOR
FIBRINOGEN/FIBRIN DEGRADATION PRODUCTS

PRINCIPLE: Latex particles have been coated with antiserum to D and
E fragments. Fibrinogen or fibrin degradation products in the test
serum will cause macroscopic agglutination.

SPECIMEN COLLECTION: Collect 8.0 ml. of blood by non-traumatic tap
after loosening the tourniquet, and dispense 5.0 ml. gently to avoid
hemolysis. Mix by inverting gently. Blood will clot within a few
seconds. Ring the clot to allow retraction and place at 37°C. for
10 minutes to ensure complete clotting. Centrifuge and remove serum.

REAGENTS AND EQUIPMENT:

1. Glass Reaction Plate
    Clean by scrubbing with Bon Ami. Dry. Polish off. Rinse plate
    well with distilled water.

2. Viewing Box

3. Microhematocrit Capillary Tubes, plain

4. Applicator Sticks

5. Collection Tubes
    Containing Bovine Thrombin 0.1 ml. (1000 U./ml.) Prepare aliquots
    in 5.0 ml. plastic tubes and store at -20°C. Just prior to use,
    thaw briefly at 37°C. and add Trasylol 0.1 ml. (5000 U./ml.) or
    Epsilon amino caproic acid 0.1 ml. a 25% solution. The Trasylol
    is stored in the refrigerator while EACA is stored at room tem-
    perature.

6. Latex Suspension (Wellcome Reagents)
    Store in refrigerator. Bring to room temperature before using.

7. Glycine Buffer, pH 8.2.
    Refrigerate. Bring to room temperature before using.

8. Negative Control
    Normal serum diluted 1 to 5 with glycine buffer and frozen in
    0.2 ml. aliquots.

Latex Test (Continued):

9. Positive Control
Human fibrinogen diluted to 10 micrograms/ml. with glycine buffer.
Freeze in 0.2 ml. aliquots.

PROCEDURE:

1. Prepare a 1 to 5 dilution of patient's serum using 0.1 ml. of serum and 0.4 ml. of glycine buffer.

2. Using a microhematocrit capillary pipette, drop 1 drop of diluted test serum in a well of the reaction plate.

3. Put a drop of the positive control serum in another well.

4. Using a microhematocrit capillary, add a drop of well mixed latex suspension to each.

5. Mix and spread with applicator sticks.

6. Observe for 2 minutes only while tilting slide over viewing box.

7. If the 1 to 5 dilution is positive, make a 1 to 20 dilution with 0.1 ml. of the 1 to 5 dilution and 0.3 ml. of buffer.

8. Run the test again using a negative control and the 1 to 20 dilution.

NORMAL VALUES: About 5 micrograms/ml. in resting subjects.
Slightly higher with excercise and stress.

REFERENCES:

1. Garvey, M. B.: "The Detection of Fibrinogen/Fibrin Degradation Products by Means of a New Antibody-coated Latex Particle Am. J. Clin. Path. 25:680-682, 1972.

2. Pitcher, P. M.: "Preparation of a Rapid Slide Test for the Detection of F.D.P. in Serum". Proceedings of the Internation Society on Thrombosis and Haemostasis, (Oslo), pg. 282, 1971.

URINARY FIBRIN DEGRADATION PRODUCTS

PRINCIPLE: Latex particles have been coated with antiserum to D and

Latex Test (Continued):

and E fragments. Urinary fibrin/fibrinogen degradation products will cause macroscopic agglutination.

SPECIMEN: 5.0 ml. of urine.

REAGENTS AND EQUIPMENT:

In addition to Reagents and Equipment used in the Latex Test for Serum FDP, the following equipment will be needed:

1. Filter Paper, Whatman Glass Paper GF/B

2. Disposable Funnels

PROCEDURE:

1. Add 5.0 ml. of patient's urine to FDP Collection Tube. Mix and incubate at 37°C. for 30 minutes.

2. Filter through glass filter paper.

3. Using a capillary, drop 1 drop of undiluted urine in a well of the reaction plate.

4. Put a drop of the positive control in another well.

5. Using a microcapillary add a drop of well mixed latex suspesion to each.

6. Mix and spread with applicator sticks.

7. Observe for 2 minutes only while tilting gently over a view box.

8. If the undiluted specimen is positive, make a 1 to 5 dilution with 0.1 ml. of urine and 0.4 ml. of buffer.

9. Repeat the test using a negative control and the 1 to 5 dilution of urine.

REFERENCES:

1. Briggs, J. D., Prentice, C. R. M., Hutton, M. M., Kennedy, A. C., and McNicol, G. P.: "Serum and Urine Fibrinogen-Fibrin-related Antigen Levels in Renal Disease". Brit. Med. J. 4:82-85, 1972.

2. The other Journals cited for the Serum FDP.

Latex Test (Continued):

INTERPRETATION:

Macroscopic agglutination at 1 to 5 dilution indicates the presence
of fibrinogen degradation products/fibrin degradation products in
excess of 10 micrograms/ml. Agglutination in 1 to 20 dilution indicates agglutination in excess of 40 micrograms/ml. Positive undiluted
urine specimen indicates fibrinogen degradation products/fibrin degradation products in excess of 2 micrograms/ml. Positive 1 to 5 urine
specimen indicates degradation products in excess of 10 micrograms
per ml.

The clinical value for detecting fibrin degradation products is the
assessment of consumptive coagulopathy or disseminated intravascular
coagulopathy. The detection of split products in the urine is useful to identify renal transplant rejection.

A positive test with a decrease in platelets, intrinsic and extrinsic
factors, and fibrinogen is suggestive of disseminated intravascular
coagulopathy. A false positive test may occur in other conditions
associated with bleeding and clotting, such as postoperative state,
idiopathic thrombocytopenic purpura, bleeding gastrointestinal lesions
menstruation, phlebothrombosis, and pulmonary embolism.

SERUM FOLIC ACID ESTIMATION
USING LACTOBACILLUS CASEI

PRINCIPLE: Serum Folic Acid is determined utilizing the following microbiological procedure. The determination of serum folic acid is essential when a possible folic acid deficient macrocytic anemia is present.

SPECIMEN:

1. Serum samples arriving at the laboratory should be labelled and then placed in the deep freeze without delay, that is 30 minutes of receipt. They should not be unfrozen until time of assay.

2. If sample consists of clotted blood, the clot should be "rimmed" with a sterile, acid-washed rod. (A previously unused, sterile wooden applicator stick is also satisfactory.)

3. The tube is then centrifuged for 5 minutes at "3/4 speed", and the supernatant serum aspirated (using previously unused, capillary pipette, or an acid washed standard pipette).

4. This serum is placed in a sterile, acid-washed glass container (or disposable container), is labelled, and promptly placed in deep freeze.
   NOTE: Cap or plug for container must also be sterile, and should either be acid-washed, or washed twelve times in tap water, and rinsed three times in distilled water.

5. Record if serum sample is hemolyzed.

REAGENTS USED IN ASSAY:

1. Ascorbic Acid
   For each assay make up a fresh solution containing 180 mg. in 4.0 ml. distilled water or 270 mg. in 6.0 ml. of distilled water.

2. Pteroylglutamic Acid (Folic Acid)
   Make up fresh every 6 months and store in refrigerator.

   Stock Solution
   100 mg. (0.1 gm.) P.G.A.
   100 ml. sterile, distilled water
   Add 5.0 ml. of 0.1 N. NaOH.

   Be sure all crystals are thoroughly dissolved before proceeding to the Working Solution.

99

Serum Folic Acid Assay (Continued):

Working Solution
Take 10 ml. of Stock Solution and add to 90 ml. of distilled
water. Readjust pH to 7.0 with 0.06 N. H_2SO_4 (approximately
0.8 ml.).

0.06 N. H_2SO_4

a). 1.0 ml. concentrated H_2SO_4 (18 M. or 36 N.) + 35 ml.
     distilled water = 1.0 N. H_2SO_4
b). 1.0 ml. of 1.0 N. H_2SO_4 + 9.0 ml. distilled water
     = 0.1 N. H_2SO_4
c). 6.0 ml. of 0.1 N. H_2SO_4 + 4.0 ml. distilled water
     = 10 ml. of 0.06 N. H_2SO_4

This gives a Working Solution containing 10 mg./100 ml.
(0.1 mg./ml.) of P.G.A. or 100,000 ng./ml. This solution
should be made up in a 100 ml. flask that has been previously acid washed and sterilized. It should be stored
in the refrigerator at 4°C. for weekly use.

3. 0.1 M. Phosphate buffer for Folic Acid
    Make up as necessary and store in the refrigerator.

    Stock Solution
    0.2 M. NaH_2PO_4 · H_2O (Solution "A")
    Dissolve 13.8 gm. of the above in a 500 ml. volumetric flask
    and dilute to volume.
    0.2 M. Na_2HPO_4 (Solution "B")
    Dissolve 14.2 gm. of the above in a 500 ml. volumetric flask
    and dilute to volume.

    Working Solution
    Take 425 ml. of Solution A and 75 ml. of Solution B and mix
    well in a liter volumetric flask then dilute to volume with
    distilled water. This resulting solution is then adjusted
    with a pH meter to a pH of about 6.1. The final solution is
    1 liter of 0.1 M. Phosphate Buffer at pH 6.1.

4. 0.25 M. Phosphate Buffer containing 75 mg%. Ascorbic Acid
    Combine 150 ml. distilled water
            50 ml. Phosphate Buffer 0.1 M.
            150 mg. Ascorbic Acid

5. Folic Acid Medium (Difco #0822-15)
    Make up desired quantity each time.

Serum Folic Acid (Continued):

NOTE: All equipment (including stirrers) used in the preparation of these reagents must be acid-washed, or very thoroughly
washed (12 times in tap water, and then rinsed three times in
distilled water).

GENERAL COMMENTS: This is a microbiological assay and is dependent
upon meticulous attention to detail for results to be meaningful.

1. Trace contamination with folic acid will completely nullify the
   significance of the assay, and thus ALL equipment must be acid-
   washed or extremely thoroughly cleaned, washed 12 times in tap
   water and rinsed 3 times with distilled water.

2. Bacterial contamination is a problem that is dealt with by autoclaving. However, delays between the various steps of the assay
   will reduce the reliability of this technique. If any delay
   becomes necessary, it should always be timed to occur after an
   autoclaving and before the solutions are handled again.

3. Handling of the initial serum specimens should be minimal, and
   once deep frozen they should not be thawed out until time of
   assay.

4. Certain phases of the assay procedures are dependent upon very
   accurate pipette measurement. These are marked with an asterisk,
   "*".

PREPARATION OF BACTERIA FOR FOLIC ACID ASSAYS:

A. Initial Preparation and Subsequent Maintenance of Culture

   1. The initial basic cultures are prepared by rehydrating the
      lyophilized organisms, Lactobacillus casei.

      These organisms are placed in tubes containing the appropriate
      Difco Culture Broth and are then incubated at 37°C. for
      48 hours.

      These basic cultures are used for the first subcultures,
      and then are stored in the refrigerator for possible use if
      difficulties arise with subsequent cultures.

   2. Fresh agar stabs must be prepared every 2 weeks for Lacto-
      bacillus casei.

Serum Folic Acid (Continued):

>Using overnight broth culture, plunge flamed stab wire into culture and then down into 10 ml. of agar in one stab. Set up 2 agar cultures.
>
>Incubate at 37°C. for at least 48 hours, and then store in refrigerator.
>
>NOTE: Retain previously used stab for 2 further weeks.

B. Subcultures

1. Flame wire loop and place it down side of agar culture tube to cool it. Then place wire loop into the middle of the bacterial growth.

2. Put wire loop into 10 ml. of inoculum broth in a 40 ml. test tube and agitate. Set up 2 tubes.

3. Plug the broth tube with cottonwool and incubate at 37°C. overnight.

C. Harvesting Bacteria

1. Centrifuge the broth culture for 15 minutes at 2,000 rpm in the cold.

2. Pour off the broth leaving a pellet of bacteria.

3. Add sterile, distilled water to the 35 ml. mark and mix the bacterial pellet into this using a sterile, cottonwool plugged pipette.

4. Centrifuge for 15 minutes at 2,000 rpm in the cold and decant the water.

5. Add 5.0 ml. of sterile distilled water using a sterile pipette and resuspend the bacteria.

6. Take 0.6 ml. of this suspension and add it to 20 ml. of sterile distilled water. Thoroughly mix this dilute suspension by means of a sterile, cottonwool plugged pipette.

Serum Folic Acid (Continued):

7. Add *one drop of this dilute suspension into each assay tube (except the blank for each specimen) using a sterile cottonwool plugged Pasteur pipette.

D. Media and Equipment

1. Every 2 weeks prepare fresh "Difco" broth and agar for Lactobacillus casei (dark brown). These should be autoclaved in 40 ml. test tubes (150 x 20 mm.) in 10 ml. amounts using cottonwool plugs.

Special medium for the actual assay of folic acid is also provided by Difco, but these should be made up freshly for each assay.

Instructions on how to make up these preparations will be found on the label of the various media bottles. The particular Difco Code Numbers are as follows:

Lactobacillus casei

Broth   0901-15
Agar   0900-15
Medium   0822-15

2. All equipment used for bacterial preparation must be sterile, and when broth or agar stabs are inoculated, the mouths of the tubes should be flamed.

3. The wire loops and wire stabs used for the culture should be labelled and kept in a glass jar.

4. Always have spare vials of lyophilized Lactobacillus casei, subspecies rhamnous, stored in the refrigerator. (Can be obtained from: The American Type Culture Company, 12301 Parklawn Drive, Rockville, Maryland 20852)

5. Checking Bacteria
Every 4 weeks send spare broth culture tube (from sub-culture routine) to a Bacteriology Laboratory for a check on culture purity.

Serum Folic Acid (Continued):

AUTOCLAVE ROUTINE:

1. Check "Shut Out" Valve — open (counter-clockwise).

2. Check "By-Pass" Valve — closed (clockwise).

3. Liquid load selection (Drying time = 0).

4. Time selection adjusted.

5. Set temperature timing device.

6. Set pressure in "jacket" of autoclave (on left hand pressure dial) for the level required for particular run.

A. <u>First Autoclave</u> (15 lbs./square inch) - 118°C./3 Minutes

1. Set indicator at 240°F. (115°C.) - timing for 3 minutes.

2. Set pressure in jacket at <u>25 lbs. pressure</u> (Turn pressure reducing valve clockwise).

3. Close door - bringing up pressure inside chamber to 14 lbs. per square inch in 1 minute - then adjust pressure to 15 lbs. per square inch in both chambers (use pressure-reducing valve

4. When 3 minutes are completed and cooling starts, slowly reduce pressure in chamber by very gradually turning "By Pass" Valve <u>counterclockwise ¼ to ½ turn.</u>

Pressure down	1 minute 15 lbs.	- 11 lbs.
in 5 minutes	1 minute 11 lbs.	- 7 lbs.
by gradual	1 minute 7 lbs.	- 4 lbs.
reduction	1 minute 4 lbs.	- 2½ lbs.
	1 minute 2½ lbs.	- 1½ lbs.
Machine now turns off.		

B. <u>Second Autoclave</u> (10 lbs./square inch) - 115°C./6 minutes

1. Set indicator at 230°F. (110°C.) - timing for 6 minutes.

2. Set pressure in jacket at <u>15 lbs. pressure</u> (use Pressure-reducing Valve).

Serum Folic Acid (Continued):

3. Close door - bring pressure inside chamber to 9 lbs./square inch in 1 minute - then adjust to 10 lbs./square inch in both chambers (using Pressure-reducing Valve).

4. When 6 minutes are completed and cooling starts, slowly reduce pressure in chamber by very gradually turning "By Pass" Valve <u>counterclockwise ¼ to ½ turn</u>.

Pressure down	1 minute	10 lbs.	-	7 lbs.
in 5 minutes	1 minute	7 lbs.	-	5 lbs.
by gradual	1 minute	5 lbs.	-	3½ lbs.
reduction	1 minute	3½ lbs.	-	2½ lbs.
	1 minute	2½ lbs.	-	1½ lbs.

Machine now turns off.

PROCEDURE:

1. Prepare growth of <u>Lactobacillus casei</u> in broth the night before using (See "Bacterial Preparation").

2. Using 15 ml. graduated centrifuge tubes and take,

Total = 5.0 ml.
    0.2 ml. Ascorbic Acid Solution
    2.2 ml. 0.1 M. Phosphate Buffer
    2.1 ml. Distilled water
    0.5 ml. Serum* (add last)
Plug tubes with cotton.

3. Autoclave at 15 lbs. pressure for 3 minutes (See Autoclave Protocol).

4. Cool tubes in water bath.

5. While tubes are cooling, prepare Folic Acid Standard Curve.

Solution "1"   1.0 ml. Standard Solution (bulb pipette) in 99 ml. distilled water (1000 ng./ml.)

Solution "2"   1.0 ml. Solution "1" (bulb pipette) in 99 ml. distilled water (10 ng./ml.)

Solution "3"   2.5 ml. of Solution "2" in 97.5 ml. distilled water (0.25 ng./ml.)

Solution "4"   5.0 ml. of Solution "2" in 45 ml. distilled water (1.0 ng./ml.)

Serum Folic Acid (Continued):

6. Using only Solutions "3" and "4" (all measurements in ml.):

Row Number	1	2	3	4	5	6	7	8	9
*Solution "3"	0	0.1	0.2	0.4	0.8	0	0	0	0
*Solution "4"	0	0	0	0	0	0.4	0.6	0.8	1.0
Distilled water	1.0	0.9	0.8	0.6	0.2	0.6	0.4	0.2	0
Total P.G.A. (ng./ml.)	0	0.025	0.05	0.1	0.2	0.4	0.6	0.8	1.0

This gives a total volume of 1.0 ml. in each tube. The tubes must be set up in quadruplicate. Cover temporarily with parafilm

7. Now take autoclaved (and cooled) tubes from Step No. 4 and centrifuge at 3/4 speed for 10 minutes. Pour off the supernatant into clean tubes.

8. Using supernatant fluid, prepare unknowns for assay:

    1st Row: 0.25 ml.* supernatant + 0.75 ml. of distilled water.

    2nd Row: 0.50 ml.* supernatant + 0.50 ml. of distilled water.

    NOTE: Both rows should be done in quadruplicate, thus giving a total of 8 assays for each original serum specimen. (Careful marking of tubes with a felt tip marking pen is vital, e.g., Dixon's "Redimark".)

9. Add 1.0 ml. of 0.25 M. buffer, 75 mg%. ascorbic acid to each tube, both standards and unknowns.

10. Add 3.0 ml. of folic medium to each assay tube, both standards and unknowns. Plug and autoclave at 10 lbs. for 6 minutes.

11. After tubes have cooled, place one* drop of Lactobacillus casei in 3 of the 4 tubes of each serum dilution, the fourth tube being set aside as a blank. (This must be done with a sterile Pasteur pipette, taking care to avoid contamination and only inoculating with one drop).

12. Plug all tubes and incubate for 18 hours at 37°C. (including blanks).

Serum Folic Acid (Continued):

13. If growth is excessive it may be necessary to add 2.0 ml. of distilled water to each tube with an automatic syringe before reading.

14. Shake all tubes well before transferring fluid to cuvettes. Read at 600 nm. in a spectrophotometer. Read each dilution against its own blank which must be used to zero the instrument.

15. Plot Standard Curve on arithmetic graph paper (semilog) using spectrophotometric growth densities against the known amount of folic acid per tube.

16. CALCULATIONS:

Calculate the amount of Folic Acid in the unknown serum samples by reading directly from the Standard Curve (utilizing the mean value of the 3 Spectrophotometric readings on the 3 tubes of each dilution). Each serum sample will have 3 readings at dilutions of 1 in 40 (Row No.1) and 3 readings at dilutions of 1 in 20 (Row No. 2).

	Mean of 3 Photometer Readings	EXAMPLE Folic Acid (ng./ml.)	Dilution	Actual Folic Acid Value (ng./ml.)	Final Average
Row "1"	32	0.170	1:40	6.80	6.87
Row "2"	59	0.347	1:20	6.94	

NORMAL VALUES: 3 - 27 mgm./ml.

REFERENCES:

1. Waters, A. H. and Molin, D. L.: "Studies on the Folic Acid Activity of Human Serum", J. Clin. Path., 14:335, 1961.

2. Herbert, V., Fisher, R. and Koontz, B. J.: "The Assay and Nature of Folic Acid Activity in Human Serum", J. Clin. Invest., 40:81, 1961.

3. Baker, H., Herbert, V., Frank, O., Pasher, I., Hutner, S. H., Wasserman, L. R., and Sobotka, H.: "A Microbiological Method for Detecting Folic Acid Deficiency in Man", Clin. Chem., 5:275, 1959.

INTERPRETATION:

Refer to Interpretation section under Serum Vitamin B_{12} Assay Procedure on page 370.

DIAGNEX BLUE TEST FOR GASTRIC ACIDITY

PRINCIPLE: Diagnex Blue is a compound of Azure A dye with an Amber-
lite cation exchange resin which is ingested in granular form after
gastric stimulation by caffeine. If free acid is present (approximately gastric pH of 3), the dye is released from the complex and
absorbed and excreted in the urine. A characteristically blue or
blue-green colored urine results. If no free acid is present, no
ionic exchange occurs, the dye remains attached to the resin and
does not appear in the urine in the prescribed test period. Azure
A may be excreted in the urine in either its blue form or a conjugated colorless form, or both. To preclude a false negative test,
any colorless Azure A in the aliquot must be oxidized to the blue
form by acidification and boiling.

COLLECTION: The patient should be fasting. Obtain Diagnex Blue
drugs from Pharmacy. The patient urinates at the beginning of the
test and discards specimen. The two tablets supplied with test
material (caffeine sodium benzoate) are taken. Water need not be
restricted. One hour later the patient urinates again and discards
specimen. Stir the Diagnex Blue granules in one-quarter glass of
water and drink. The granules may not completely dissolve. Patient
should not chew undissolved granules. Two hours after taking granules, patient urinates again and all the urine is submitted to the
Clinical Laboratory.

EQUIPMENT AND REAGENTS:

1. Ascorbic Acid, 300 mg.

2. Diagnex Blue Comparator
   This comes with test kit of dye and can be obtained from Pharmacy.

3. HCl, 10%

4. Waterbath, boiling

PROCEDURE:

1. Dilute the urine sample with water to 300 ml.

2. Fill 3 test tubes with approximately 10 ml. of urine each. Use
   one tube as the test aliquots and prepare two control aliquots by
   adding about 300 mg. of ascorbic acid to the two tubes.

108

Diagnex Blue Test (Continued):

3. Place the test sample in the center slot of the comparator and the two control aliquots in the color standard slots. If at this step of the test, the color intensity of the test sample is equal to or is greater than that of the 0.6 mg. standard, the patient has secreted free gastric acid and the test is complete.

4. If the test sample is less intense in color than the 0.6 mg. standard, acidify with 2 drops of 10% HCl. This should adjust the pH of the urine to between 2 and 4. If a red pigment occurs, the test should be repeated with a fresh aliquot and a smaller amount of acid added as the red color indicates a pH of less than 2.

COMMENTS ON PROCEDURE:

1. When the color of the test urine falls between 0.6 gm. and 0.3 mg. standards, it is presumptive evidence of hypochlorhydria.

2. When the color is less intense than the 0.3 mg. standard, it is presumptive evidence of achlorhydria.

3. Caffeine is used as the stimulus and at times a stronger stimulant (histamine) may be required for gastric secretion.

4. Misleading results may occur in patients after gastric surgery, with malabsorption syndromes, liver disease, and renal insufficiency.

5. If the gastric secretion lacks free acid, the dye resin complex remains intact and no dye appears in the urine in the prescribed time. When the dye appears in the urine after this period, it is of no diagnostic significance.

6. The procedure for Diagnex Blue has been modified so that aliquots of urine containing Azure A can serve as controls by the addition of ascorbic acid which reduces the blue form of Azure A to the colorless form.

NORMAL VALUES: REPORT AS FOLLOWS
              Greater than 0.6 mg. Standard
              Between 0.3 and 0.6 mg. Standard
              Less than 0.3 mg. Standard

REFERENCE: Hoffman, W. S.: THE BIOCHEMISTRY OF CLINICAL MEDICINE, pg. 661, 1959.

Diagnex Blue Test (Continued):

INTERPRETATION:

The basal acid secretion for normal males is 1.3 to 4.0 mEq./L. per hour. Lower values occur in females and with aging. Low values occur in gastric cancer and benign gastric ulcer, higher values are present in duodenal ulcer. Extremely high acid output is present in patients with the Zollinger-Ellison Syndrome.

When the Histamine Test is utilized, the maximum rate of acid secretion is attained in 15 minutes and is maintained for 30 minutes. Basal levels are achieved in 60 minutes, the maximum acid output representing the sum of the acid outputs for the four 15 minute post histamine samples. This is the generally accepted expression of gastric acid secretion. The range for maximal acid output in normal males is 4.9 to 38.9 mEq. per hour.

A maximal acid output of greater than 210 mEq. per hour is found in about 40 percent of males with duodenal ulcer. Zollinger-Ellison syndrome patients have a high ratio of basal to maximal acid output. Ratios greater than 60 percent are indicative of this disorder.

Anacidity in the Histamine Test is found in adults with gastric cancer and pernicious anemia with atrophic gastritis. It is also found in conditions such as hypochromic anemia, rheumatoid arthritis, steatorrhea, aplastic anemia, and myxedema.

Surgeons utilize gastric acid analysis in determining the surgical procedure to be performed. Elevated maximal acid output indicates the need for gastric resection. Elevated basal secretion with slightly elevated maximal secretion is an indication for vagotomy.

GASTRIC ANALYSIS

PRINCIPLE: A measured amount of gastric sample is titrated with
0.1 N NaOH until the indicator Topfer's reagent (dimethylaminoazo-
benzene) is bright yellow (pH 4.0). This is the end point for "free
hydrochloric acid". To measure the amount of "combined acid" ...
weakly ionized protein salts, organic acids and free acidic groups
of protein ... phenolphthalein which changes from colorless to red
at pH 8.5 is used as the indicator and the titration continued to a
pink color.

REAGENTS:

1. Sodium Hydroxide, 0.1 N.

2. Topfer's Reagent, 0.5%
    0.5 gm. p-dimethylaminoazobenzene is placed in a 100 ml. volumet-
    ric flask and brought to volume with 95 percent ethyl alcohol.

3. Phenolphthalein, 1.0%
    In a 100 ml. volumetric flask dissolve 1.0 gm. of phenolphthalein
    in 95 percent alcohol.

PROCEDURE:

1. Macroscopic Examination

    A. Record volume of each specimen. Normal is 20 - 50 ml.

    B. Note color:

        1). Normally colorless
        2). Green from bile
        3). Faint red from blood
        4). Coffee-colored from altered blood remaining in stomach
             for some time

    C. Odor:

        1). Normally odorless or sour
        2). Fecal due to bowel obstruction or gastrocolic fistula.
        3). Pungent odor due to cancer or catarrhal gastritis

111

Gastric Analysis (Continued):

D. Appearance, normally three layers:

  1). Top - mucus
  2). Mid - opalescent fluid
  3). Lower - sediment residual food

2. Chemical Determination

  A. To 5.0 ml. gastric specimen in a porcelain evaporating dish,
      add 2 drops of Topfer's reagent.

    1). Lemon yellow color indicates <u>NO</u> free hydrochloric acid.
    2). If red or orange color, titrate with 0.1 N NaOH until
        lemon-yellow end point. Note volume of NaOH used. If
        less than 5.0 ml. of gastric sample is used, titrate
        with 0.01 N NaOH.

  B. To the above sample (after free HCl determination), add
      2 drops phenolphthalein. Continue titration with 0.1 N
      NaOH until pink color develops. Note volume of NaOH used.

3. CALCULATIONS:

Degrees acidity = ml. 0.1 N NaOH used x $\dfrac{100}{\text{Vol. gastric sample used in titration}}$

If 5.0 ml. gastric sample used:

Degrees (or units) = ml. NaOH used to yellow end point x 20
FREE HCL

Degrees (or units) = ml. NaOH used in both titrations x 20
TOTAL ACID

NORMAL VALUES: Since a broad range of normal values exist for free
hydrochloric acid in gastric juice, the primary
importance of quantitating free HCl is the demonstration of achlorhydria. The absence of free HCl after
histamine stimulation and the presence of stomach
lesions is strongly suggestive of stomach cancer.

Gastric Analysis (Continued):

REFERENCES:

1. Ham, T.: SYLLABUS OF LABORATORY EXAMINATION IN CLINICAL
   DIAGNOSIS, Harvard Univ. Press, pg. 310, 1958.

2. Hepler, O.: MANUAL OF CLINICAL LABORATORY METHODS, 4th Ed.,
   pgs. 97-105, 1966.

INTERPRETATION:

Refer to Gastric Analysis - The Histolog Test, page 116.

GASTRIC ANALYSIS
(The Histalog Test)

PRINCIPLE: A measured amount of gastric juice is titrated with
0.1 N. NaOH utilizing the pH Meter. The gastric juice is collected
after Histalog stimulation.

REAGENTS AND EQUIPMENT:

1. Sodium Hydroxide, 0.1 N.

2. Nasogastric tube

3. 20 ml. Glass Syringe

4. Centrifuge

5. pH Meter

6. Histalog, 1.7 mg./Kg. Body Weight

COMMENTS ON PROCEDURE:

1. Patient is fasted at least 12 hours before test.

2. A nasogastric tube is passed by the Technologist (pass tube to
   above 1 inch from the second to last black mark on the tube).

3. If any doubt as to position of tube, get it checked in X-ray.

PROCEDURE:

1. Ask patient to lie on left side, semi propped up.

2. Empty stomach and discard aspirate.

3. Make two 30 minute collections (samples 1 and 2) — viz:
   basal 1 hour collection. Aspirate by hand every 2 to 3 minutes,
   using a 20 ml. glass syringe. Do not aspirate too hard (an
   indication of this blood staining). If tube appears blocked,
   clear with 15 ml. of air, and then aspirate again.

4. Doctor gives I. M. histalog injection — using 1.7 mg./Kg.
   body weight.

Gastric Analysis, Histolog Test (Continued):

5. Make 5 x 15 minute collections (samples 3, 4, 5, 6, and 7) of gastric juice.

6. Remove nasogastric tube.

7. A careful check on the patient throughout the test should be maintained. If any serious change in patient's condition develops, doctor must be notified at once.

CALCULATIONS:

A. Measure and record volume and pH of aspiration samples (1) - (7). Also note bile, mucus and blood.

B. Take aliquots and centrifuge at "3/4 speed" for 15 minutes to get clear supernatant.

C. Take 5.0 ml. aliquots from each sample (less if necessary, but record volume used). Titrate with 0.1 N. NaOH to pH 7.4 (using pH meter).

D. Record volume of 0.1 N. NaOH used for each aliquot, and estimate mEq./L. of acid and total mEq. of acid in each sample.

Example:

1). 5.0 ml. aliquot from 38 ml. sample used 2.5 ml. 0.1 N. NaOH

2). Thus 5.0 ml. aliquot was equivalent to 0.25 mEq. NaOH

3). Thus 1000 ml. $= \dfrac{0.25}{5}$ x 1000 = 50 mEq. (viz: mEq./L.)

4). Total sample of 38 ml. $= \dfrac{50}{1000}$ x 38 = 1.9 mEq.

(Total acid in sample).

These figures represent acid in mEq.

NORMAL VALUES: See Clinical Interpretation.

REFERENCES:

1. Zaterka, S. and Neves, D. P.: "Maximal Gastric Secretion in Human Subjects after Histalog Stimulation", Gastroenterology, 47:251, 1964.

Gastric Analysis, Histolog Test (Continued):

2. Ward, S., Gillespie, I. E., Passaro, E. P., and Grossman, M. I.: "Comparison of Histalog and Histamine as Stimulants for Maximal Gastric Secretion in Human Subjects and in Dogs", Gastroenterology, 44:620, 1963.

3. "Effect of Large Doses of Histamine on Gastric Secretion of HCl: An Augmented Histamine Test", Brit. Med. Journal, 2:77, 1953.

INTERPRETATION:

The basal acid secretion for normal males is 1.3 to 4.0 mEq./L. per hour. Lower values occur in females and with aging. Low values occur in gastric cancer and benign gastric ulcer higher values are present in duodenal ulcer. Extremely high acid output is present in patients with the Zollinger-Ellison Syndrome.

When the Histamine Test is utilized, the maximum rate of acid secretion is attained in 15 minutes and is maintained for 30 minutes. Basal levels are achieved in 60 minutes, the maximum acid output representing the sum of the acid outputs for the four 15 minute post histamine samples. This is the generally accepted expression of gastric acid secretion. The range for maximal acid output in normal males is 4.9 to 38.9 mEq. per hour.

A maximal acid output of greater than 210 mEq. per hour is found in about 40 per cent of males with duodenal ulcer. Zollinger-Ellison Syndrome patients have a high ratio of basal to maximal acid output. Ratios greater than 60 per cent are indicative of this disorder.

Anacidity in the Histamine Test is found in adults with gastric cancer and pernicious anemia with atrophic gastritis. It is also found in conditions such as hypochromic anemia, rheumatoid arthritis, steatorrhea, aplastic anemia, and myxedema.

Surgeons utilize gastric acid analysis in determining the surgical procedure to be performed. Elevated maximal acid output indicates the need for gastric resection. Elevated basal secretion with slightly elevated maximal secretion is an indication for vagotomy.

GLUCOSE-6-PHOSPHATE DEHYDROGENASE
(U. V. Method on Red Cell Hemolysate)

PRINCIPLE: The enzyme G-6-PDH catalyzes the reaction which takes place when glucose-6-phosphate is converted to 6-phosphogluconic acid. In carbohydrate metabolism, this enzyme introduces the reaction which starts the pentose phosphate (hexose monophosphate) pathway. For this reason, an active and adequate concentration of G-6-PDH must be present in the red cell under certain conditions of stress. Low levels of G-6-PDH in the red cell have been associated for some time with hemolytic episodes in individuals following exposure to agents such as primaquine (and some other aromatic, heterocyclic structured medications) and fava beans.

G-6-PDH catalyzes the hydrogen transport reaction indicated beneath. The rate of formation of $NADPH_2$, which absorbs strongly at 340 nm. and 366 nm., is utilized as a measure of enzyme activity.

$$G-6-PDH$$
$$\text{Glucose-6-Phosphate} + NADP \rightleftharpoons \text{6-Phosphogluconate} + NADPH_2$$

SPECIMEN: Collect whole blood in sodium citrate or sodium heparin anticoagulant. This may be stored at refrigerator temperatures for up to 4 days. (See Specimen preparation under "Comments on Procedure.")

REAGENTS AND EQUIPMENT:

Available as Biochemica Test Combination TC-W 15993 (20 Determinations).

1. Triethanolamine Buffer, 0.05 M., pH 7.6
   Dissolve the contents of Bottle #1 in 100 ml. of redistilled water. Also contains 0.005 M. EDTA. Stable for one year at room temperature.

2. NADP, 0.01 M.
   Dissolve the contents of Bottle #2 in 2.0 ml. of redistilled water. Stable for four weeks at approximately 4°C.

3. Glucose-6-Phosphate, 0.031 M.
   Dissolve the contents of Bottle #3 in 1.5 ml. of redistilled water. Stable for four weeks at approximately 4°C.

4. Digitonin, approximately 0.02%
   Use the solution in Bottle #4 undiluted. Stable for one year at room temperature.

117

Glucose-6-Phosphate Dehydrogenase (Continued):

COMMENTS ON PROCEDURE:

1. Specimen Preparation
   a). Wash 0.2 ml. of whole blood three times with 2.0 ml. physio-
       logical saline. Centrifuge after each washing for ten min-
       utes at approximately 3000 rpm.
   b). Do a red count on 20 lambda of the packed cell button.
   c). Suspend the washed button in 0.5 ml. digitonin and allow to
       stand at 4°C. for 15 minutes. Recentrifuge for clear hemo-
       lysate.

2. Derivation of Factor (at 340 nm.):

$$\frac{0.001}{6.22} \times 10^6 \times \frac{1}{1} \times \frac{3.25}{0.10} \times \frac{6}{1} \times \frac{5}{1} = 15661$$

3. Refer to original methodology for G-6-PDH determination on serum.

PROCEDURE:

1. Into a 1.0 cm. square glass cuvette, pipette the following solutions: 3.0 ml. of triethanolamine buffer, 0.1 ml. of NADP, and
   0.1 ml. of hemolysate.

2. Mix the contents of the cuvette well by inversion and incubate in
   the waterbath at 25°C. for approximately five minutes.

3. Pipette 0.05 ml. of glucose-6-phosphate into the cuvette, mix,
   and determine the absorbance at 340 nm. or 366 nm. Immediately
   start stopwatch and record absorbance change in the temperature
   controlled cuvette at 1, 2, and 3 minutes. (Or scan for three
   minutes on a recorder.)

4. Determine the mean absorbance change per minute (ΔE/min.) against
   an air reference. Absorbance differences greater than 0.060/min.
   at 340 nm. or 0.030/min. at 366 nm. require a dilution of 1:10
   with physiological saline.

5. CALCULATION:

$\Delta E_{340 \text{ nm.}}$/min. x 15661 = milli-units (mU)/#RBC in 1.0 ml. blood.

$\Delta E_{366 \text{ nm.}}$/min. x 29600 = milli-units (mU)/#RBC in 1.0 ml. blood.

Glucose-6-Phosphate Dehydrogenase (Continued):

NORMAL VALUES: 120 - 240 mU./10^9 erythrocytes.

REFERENCES:

1. Kornberg, A., Colowick and Kaplan: METHODS IN ENZYMOLOGY, Vol. I, 322, Academic Press, 1955.

2. Bergemeyer: METHODS OF ENZYMATIC ANALYSIS, Academic Press, 1965.

3. Bishop: J. Lab. and Clin. Med., 68:149, 1966.

4. Batsakis and Brierre: INTERPRETIVE ENZYMOLOGY, C. Thomas, 1967.

INTERPRETATION:

During the last few years a number of hemolytic anemias have been investigated which are caused by inherited errors in the metabolism of glucose. The erythrocyte derives all its energy from the metabolism of glucose by the Embden-Meyerhof cycle along with the pentose monophosphate shunt. Red cells do not have all the tricarboxylic acid cycle components or the cytochrome oxidase system, but the mature red cell does possess a functioning Krebs cycle. Thus, over 90% of glucose consumption occurs through the Embden-Meyerhof anaerobic pathway. Glucose must be phosphorylated before it can be metabolized by the erythrocytes. A direct oxidative pathway of glucose metabolism is also present within the red cell, this is known as the pentose monophosphate shunt. Usually, less than 10% of glucose undergoes direct oxidation by this shunt. The primary function of the anaerobic cycle is to provide sufficient adenosine triphosphate for the necessary metabolism of the red cell. It has been demonstrated that many of the recognized abnormalities of red cells are associated with enzyme deficiencies which occur with increasing age of the red cells. Thus, it might be valuable to consider these conditions as metabolic abnormalities which are imposed on the normal aging process.

Young red cells usually possess higher levels of glycolytic enzymes. The older red cells usually have a lesser amount of these essential enzymes. Young red cells such as reticulocytes utilize more glucose and have more glycolytic enzymes. The aging red cells have a very rapid decrease in activity in G-6-PD activity. Along with this decrease in this important enzyme, there is a decrease in ATP as well as DPN or NAD. One group of investigators has demonstrated that

Glucose-6-Phosphate Dehydrogenase (Continued):

G-6-PD activity in reticulocytes is ten times greater than the activity in the older red cells.

Deficiency of glucose-6-phosphate dehydrogenase occurs on a worldwide basis. It may exist as a number of genetic variants related to different changes in enzyme structure. It is a common cause for neonatal jaundice and kernicterus in highly affected groups such as in the black race; it has been more commonly recognized as the cause of hemolytic anemia in patients who have taken various drugs.

The underlying mechanism and one laboratory test is as follows: Glucose-6-phosphate dehydrogenase is an essential enzyme in the pentose monophosphate shunt which produces TPNH. In the absence of sufficient TPNH, there is a marked reduction in available reduced glutathione. Although the role of reduced glutathione in preserving red cell integrity is not well understood, it appears to be an important one. The glutathione stability test was originally proposed by Beutler. Reduced glutathione sensitive cells are extremely sensitive to oxidation in the presence of drugs such as acetyl-phenylhydrazine. It has been demonstrated that this test is not as reliable in detecting heterozygous females since in one series, 30 to 50% false negative results occurred. The dye reduction test is based on the inability of sensitive red cells to reduce the dye, brilliant cresyl blue. It is also unsatisfactory for the detection of the female heterozygote with the disease. In this test, decolorization should be complete within one hundred minutes; partial decolorization at one hundred minutes indicates partial enzyme deficiency. Because of the qualitative nature of the test, intermediate results are sometimes obtained and are difficult to interpret; those samples showing no decolorization at 3 to 6 hours have virtually no enzyme activity. The direct estimation of glucose-6-phosphate dehydrogenase activity is the most informative method, in particular, with respect to the detection of the heterozygous patient. Normal values are 150 to 215 units per 100 ml. of red cells. Less than ten units per 100 ml. red cells is indicative of a glucose-6-phosphate dehydrogenase deficiency.

A deficiency of G-6-PD was recognized many years ago to be present throughout the world. (It was recognized in the black races and in the Sephardic Jews.) A hemolytic anemia may arise in patients with this enzyme deficiency; these patients usually become anemic when they are exposed to certain drugs or fava beans. Patients with G-6-PD deficiency may have a hemolytic crisis when drugs of the following types are taken:

1. Analgesics or antipyretics such as aspirin

Glucose-6-Phosphate Dehydrogenase (Continued):

2. Sulfa drugs such as Sulfapyridine or Sulfasoxazole (Gantrisin)
3. Antimalarias such as Primaquine, Pentaquine (Atabrine), or Quinine
4. Nitrofurantoin or Nitrofurazone
5. Other drugs such as Chloromycetin, PAS, and Quinidine

Recently, conditions such as viral hepatitis and diabetic acidosis have been shown to induce hemolytic anemia in patients with G-6-PD deficiency. It is thought that certain oxidants increase in the blood of patients with viral hepatitis or diabetic acidosis, and this leads to an acute hemolytic crisis.

The deficiency is more severe in the Middle East as in the Sephardic Jew than in the black races. It is unwise to use donor blood from patients who have severe G-6-PD deficiency for blood transfusion purposes from affected individuals from the Middle East. However, individuals in the United States who have G-6-PD deficiency of the minimal type may serve as blood donors.

Patients who have acute hemolytic anemia progress through various phases: the first phase in the acute hemolytic reaction may last two weeks, a 7 to 10 day recovery phase follows, and this is followed by an equilibrium phase in which the anemia disappears. The exact mechanism for the hemolysis is not clear; however, it has been suggested that because of the G-6-PD deficiency, there is a defect in the sodium pump of the red cell membrane and associated with this defect, there is a defective generation of ATP because of glutathione deficiency. The potassium loss of G-6-PD deficient red cells has been reported to be greater than that of normal red cells following incubation of these with drugs such as Primaquine. However, no significant differences in potassium content of G-6-PD deficient or normal red cells after incubation with acetyl-phenyl-hydrazine has been demonstrated. These experiments emphasize that there are differences in the type of injury induced by different drugs, and that no single explanation suffices to explain the mechanism of the hemolysis. More and more drugs are being implicated in the causation of hemolysis in patients who have G-6-PD deficiency.

Usually spontaneous hemolysis does not occur in the newborn with this enzyme deficiency. The administration of an offending drug to the mother with a G-6-PD deficient fetus prior to delivery is considered hazardous.

GLUTATHIONE REDUCTASE ASSAY

PRINCIPLE: GSSG reductase in the presence of TPNH converts the oxidized Glutathione to the reduced state. The disappearance of TPNH is followed spectrophotometrically.

SPECIMEN: 5.0 ml. whole blood that has been collected in EDTA, centrifuged, and the plasma and buffy coat removed.

EQUIPMENT AND REAGENTS:

1. 0.165 M. Tris, pH 7.5
   Also contains 1.0 Ml. KCl. Adjust pH using 10 N. and 1 N. HCl.

2. EDTA, 0.01 M., combination of Na$_2$ and Na$_3$ Stock
   Na$_2$ 0.1 M. - 3.7 gm./100 ml. pH approximately 4.0
   Na$_3$ 0.1 M. - 3.7 gm./100 ml. pH approximately 9.2
   Both of the above are combined to obtain a pH of 7.5. The final volume is diluted to 1:10 with distilled water to obtain 0.01 M.

3. TPNH, 0.001 M.
   Dissolve 30 mg. in 0.05 M. Tris pH 8.2 in a 25 ml. volumetric flask and dilute to volume. Make up 10 ml. (12 mg./10 ml.) in the Tris pH 8.2. This material is unstable and should be kept frozen.

4. GSSG, 0.025 M. (M.W. 612.6)
   Dissolve 0.0306 gm. per 2.0 ml. of distilled water.

5. Beckman 3.0 ml. Cuvettes

6. Beckman Spectrophotometer, 340 nm.

PRECAUTIONS:

1. Blood may be stored as whole blood refrigerated for a maximum of 48 hours.

2. pH or reagents must be within $\pm$ 0.05.

3. All enzyme reagents must be weighed quickly as they tend to be hydroscopic.

4. Working solutions of reagents (except buffers) should be kept frozen when not in use.

Glutathione Reductase Assay (Continued):

5. Keep reagents in an ice bucket when using - NOT AT ROOM TEMPERATURE!

6. TPNH must be made up each time the test is run as this is not reliably stable.

PROCEDURE:

A. Preparation of Hemolysate
   1. After collection of sample, wash ONCE using 5.0 ml. cold normal saline and after centrifuging remove supernatant.

   2. Remove 0.2 ml. packed red blood cells and place in a pyrex test tube. Freeze-thaw twice using dry ice-acetone mixture. Do Not allow the temperature of the hemolysate to exceed 10 - 15°C.

   3. Add 10 ml. distilled water to the hemolysate, swirl, and refrigerate for 15 minutes.

   4. Determine the hemoglobin concentration in Gm%. and then dilute the hemolysate with distilled water to give a final hemoglobin concentration of 0.20 gm%.

B. Test

	Blank	1) TPNH Control	2) Control	3) Patient
Tris 0.165 M., pH 7.5 containing 1 M. KCl	1.0	1.0	1.0	1.0
EDTA 0.01 M.	0.1	0.1	0.1	0.1
TPNH 0.001 M.	0.0	0.5	0.5	0.5
Hemolysate 0.2 Gm%. Control	0.5	0.5	0.5	0.0
Hemolysate 0.2 Gm%. Patient	0.0	0.0	0.0	0.5
Distilled Water	1.3	0.9	0.8	0.8

Mix contents well and take a base reading at 340 nm.

Add with shaking:
| GSSG 0.025 M. | 0.1 | 0.0 | 0.1 | 0.1 |

Take O.D. readings: 30 seconds, 1 minute, 5 minutes, 10 minutes and 30 minutes.

Glutathione Reductase Assay (Continued):

C. CALCULATIONS:

Measure the difference in O.D. between 30 seconds and 30 minutes. There will be a decrease in O.D. and it should be linear. Activity is calculated by multiply the ΔO.D. x 2900 and is expressed as micromoles of substrate per hour per 10 minutes RBC.

NORMAL VALUES: 600 - 1200 Units

REFERENCE: Waller, H.D.:   "Glutathione Reductase Deficiency".   In E. Beutler (Ed.) HEREDITARY DISORDERS OF ERYTHROCYTE METABOLISM, Grune & Stratton, pg. 185, 1968.

INTERPRETATION:

Several enzyme deficiencies affecting the nonglycolytic pathway occur in red cells.   Included in this group is glutathione reductase.   These deficient individuals cannot be corrected by in vitro glucose but may be corrected by ATP, and thus fall in the Dacie-Selwyn Type II catagory.   They may have a severe type of hemolytic anemia which frequently is drug induced.   The deficiency is diagnosed by tests similar to those for G-6-PD deficiency.

GUAIAC FILTER PAPER TEST FOR FECAL BLOOD
(Occult Blood Test)

PRINCIPLE: Hemoglobin catalytically decomposes hydrogen peroxide with the liberation of oxygen which in an acid solution oxidizes gum guaiac, a colorless phenol, to a blue-colored derivative. In feces, hematin, the iron-containing complex of protoporphyrin catalyzes the guaiac reaction but free iron and iron-free porphyrins do not.

REAGENTS:

1. Gum Guaiac, 20%
   20 gm. guaiac dissolved in 100 ml. 95% ethanol.

2. Glacial Acetic Acid

3. Hydrogen Peroxide, 3%
   Usable as long as it effervesces when placed in contact with blood.

4. Positive Control
   0.05 ml. venous blood to 50 ml. water. Approximately 1+ reaction will occur with guaiac.

COMMENTS ON PROCEDURE:

1. Test is merely qualitative.

2. Lots of gum guaiac vary in sensitivity.

3. Alcoholic solutions of gum guaiac and 3% hydrogen peroxide are unstable and need to be checked with known positive specimen or control.

PROCEDURE:

To a thin fecal smear and a positive control on filter paper, add 2 drops each of glacial acetic acid, gum guaiac and 3% hydrogen peroxide.

NORMAL VALUES: Report as Follows:

Trace - Faint blue or greenish-blue appearing in one minute.
1+   - Light blue appearing slowly.
2+   - Clear blue appearing fairly rapidly.

125

126

Guaiac Filter Paper Test (Continued):

3+   - Deep blue appearing almost immediately.
4+   - Deep blue appearing immediately.

REFERENCES:

1. Davidsohn, I. and Henry, J.: TODD-SANFORD CLINICAL DIAG-
   NOSIS BY LABORATORY METHODS. 14th Ed., W. B. Saunders Co.,
   Phil., pg. 784, 1979.

2. Ham, T.: A SYLLABUS OF LABORATORY EXAMINATIONS IN CLINICAL
   DIAGNOSIS, 1950.

INTERPRETATION:

Loss of 50 ml. of blood from the upper gastrointestinal tract
causes the stool to be dark black and tarry. Bleeding from lower
gastrointestinal tract will cause a red stool. Smaller amounts of
blood will not cause a color change in the stool, and bleeding in
the upper or lower gastrointestinal tract will remain undetected
unless an Occult Blood Test is performed. The test may be applied
to stool, urine or gastric juice. It is positive for hemoglobin
or myoglobin. For the stool test, the patient should not eat meat
for 3 days since meat contains myoglobin and hemoglobin. The
reagents differ chiefly in sensitivity. Orthotolidine is 1 to 10
times more sensitive than benzidine; benzidine 10 to 1000 times more
sensitive than Guaiac. False negative reactions may occur if excess
reducing substances such as Vitamin C are ingested.

SERUM HAPTOGLOBIN

PRINCIPLE: Haptoglobins are serum proteins which combine with hemoglobin or hemoglobin derivatives. The haptoglobin-hemoglobin complex enhances the peroxidase activity of the latter substance. Using hydrogen peroxide as the oxidizing substance and guaiacol as the hydrogen donor, the formation of tetraguaiacol is measured spectrophotometrically. The standardization is such that the haptoglobin content is measured as methemoglobin binding capacity.

SPECIMEN: 5.0 - 8.0 ml. clotted blood, separated, and refrigerated until run.

REAGENTS AND EQUIPMENT:

1. Guaiacol, liquid (Sigma Chemical)
   1.66 ml. guaiacol in a 500 ml. volumetric flask, add 50 ml. 1.0 M. acetic acid, swirl, add about 100 ml. deionized water. Mix well. When all the guaiacol is mixed, add about 250 ml. deionized water. pH to 4.0 using 1.0 M. NaOH (pH starts about 2.9 and requires about 7.0 to 8.0 ml. NaOH). Dilute to volume with deionized water. Refrigerate in a brown bottle. Good for 2 to 3 weeks.

2. 1.0 M. Acetic Acid
   54 ml. of 99 to 100% acetic acid diluted to 1000 ml. with deionized water.

3. Normal Serum for Standard Curve
   Lyophilized special chemistry control serum. Should be fairly fresh.

4. 0.15 M. NaCl, 0.85%
   8.5 gm. NaCl diluted to 1000 ml. with deionized water.

5. 0.1% $K_3Fe(CN)_6$
   0.1 gm. $K_3Fe(CN)_6$ diluted to 100 ml. with deionized water.

6. Methemoglobin Solution

   A. Assay the hemoglobin concentration of any hemolysate.

   B. Dilute hemolysate to 1.0 gm%. with deionized water.

Serum Haptoglobin   (Continued):

C.   In a 50 ml. volumetric flask place 2.5 ml. of the 1.0 gm%.
     hemolysate and 1.0 ml. of the 0.1% $K_3Fe(CN)_6$. Let sit for
     10 minutes. Dilute to volume with deionized water.

D.   Methemoglobin is not stable and must be made up each week.

7. <u>0.05 M. Hydrogen Peroxide</u>, 30%
    0.575 ml. H_2O_2 diluted to 100 ml. with deionized water. MUST
    BE USED WITHIN 30 MINUTES.

PROCEDURE:

1. <u>Standard Curve</u>. Run each week.

    A.   Pipette 5.0 ml. guaiacol into each of 9 tubes numbered
         Blank through 8.

    B.   Place in covered wath bath at room temperature.

Tube	Blank	1	2	3	4	5	6	7	8
Normal Serum	0	0	0.1	0.2	0.3	0.4	0.5	0.6	0.7
Saline	1.0	1.0	0.9	0.8	0.7	0.6	0.5	0.4	0.3
Met. Hgb.	0	1.0	1.0	1.0	1.0	1.0	1.0	1.0	1.0

    Mix well and let sit 10 - 20 minutes.

    C.   0.1 ml. of each of the above tubes is pipetted into the
         corresponding guaiacol tube.

    D.   1.0 ml. of the Working Solution of H_2O_2, which has been
         brought to room temperature, is immediately added, tubes
         mixed, and incubated <u>covered</u> for <u>8</u> minutes.

    E.   Read Standard Curve within <u>4</u> minutes at 470 nm. on the
         Beckman DU.

2. <u>Unknowns</u>. Always run a control sample.

    A.   Pipette 5.0 ml. guaiacol into each of two tubes for each
         serum. Place in water bath.

    B.   In a test tube combine 2.0 ml. 0.15 M. NaCl and 0.5 ml.
         serum. Mix well.

Serum Haptoglobin   (Continued):

C. Label two tubes for each serum: One Blank and One Test.

	Blank	Test
Dilute Serum	1.0	1.0
Met. Hgb.	0	1.0
Water	1.0	0

Mix well.

D. 0.1 ml. of each of the above samples is pipetted into the corresponding guaicol.

E. Immediately add:
1.0 ml. Working H_2O_2. Mix. Let sit covered for 8 minutes.
Read O.D. against water within 4 minutes.

3. CALCULATIONS:

A. Standard Curve

1). Substrate tube 1, Reagent Blank, from each of the following tubes.

2). Plot O.D. vs. tube number using linear graph paper.

3). Draw slope, usually using the first four points.

4). Draw straight line using points 6, 7, and 8.

5). The point at which these lines intersect is 50 mg%. haptoglobin binding capacity.

6). Calculate the value of each square by dividing 50 mg%. by the total number of squares. This is the factor for this curve and these reagents only.

B. Unknowns

1). Subtract the O.D. of the blank from the O.D. of the test.

2). From the graph, obtain the number of squares for each O.D.

3). Multiply the number of squares by the factor obtained in Step No. 6 above. This is the mg%. value of the dilute sample.

Serum Haptoglobin (Continued):

4). Multiply the mg%. value by 5 (dilution) to obtain the haptoglobin binding capacity in mg%.

NOTES AND PRECAUTIONS:

1. Methemoglobin solution is not stable and must be prepared each week. In case a stat haptoglobin is requested, assay it using the methemoglobin and its curve, then repeat the sample when a new curve is prepared.

2. Reconstitute lyophilized serum every 1 to 2 weeks.

3. Working H_2O_2 is not stable for more than 30 minutes. Stock as long as it is well covered, refrigerated and kept in a brown bottle. It appears to be stable until it is gone.

4. Guaiacol is light sensitive and tubes should be placed in a covered water bath as soon as they are pipetted. The stock solution is good for 2 to 3 weeks. Thereafter it becomes increasingly more sensitive.

5. The brownish tetraguaiacol color fades on standing. Samples must be read within 4 to 5 minutes.

6. The normal control can be any serum previously assayed and found to be within normal limits. This value should be within $\pm$ 10% in each successive run.

7. If curve reads lower than usual, make up new methemoglobin.

NORMAL VALUES: 53 - 150 mg%.

REFERENCE: Owen, J.A.: "A Simple Method for the Determination of Serum Haptoglobins", Am. J. Clin. Path., 13:163, 1960.

INTERPRETATION:

Males have higher levels of serum haptoglobin than females. Premature infants do not have haptoglobins and levels are low in the cord blood of most term infants. The amount of haptoglobin rises slowly throughout infancy and reaches adult levels by the age of 6 months.

Serum Haptoglobin   (Continued):

Haptoglobin levels are decreased in hemolytic anemia. The disappearance of haptoglobin is accentuated by its combination with free hemoglobin. Normally the amount of plasma haptoglobin is sufficient to combine with 3.0 gm. of hemoglobin. Serum haptoglobin thus combines with free hemoglobin to protect the renal tubule from damage. The measurement of haptoglobin is thus a valuable test to ascertain the presence of hemolytic anemia. Hemoglobinemia and hemoglobinuria are usually transient following hemolysis, but depressed haptoglobin levels persist for a longer period.

Other causes for low haptoglobin are loss into the urine due to nephrosis, decreased synthesis in liver disease, and hereditary deficiency frequently associated with Glucose-6-Phosphate Dehydrogenase deficiency.

An increase in haptoglobin occurs in inflammatory states, both acute and chronic. In acute infections, haptoglobin reaches a maximum in two weeks and returns to normal during the healing phase. Chronic infections such as tuberculosis may cause the haptoglobin level to be 300 mg%. Immunologic disease such as rheumatoid arthritis and glomerulonephritis, and metastatic carcinoma cause prominent elevations of plasma haptoglobins.

PCV (PACKED CELL VOLUME) OR HEMATOCRIT

PRINCIPLE: This is the percent of packed erythrocytes in a given volume of blood.

SPECIMEN: EDTA tube or capillary blood.

EQUIPMENT:

1. Heparinized and/or plain capillary tubes I.D. 1.1 - 1.2 mm.; length 75 mm.

2. Micro hematocrit centrifuge.

3. Sealer for capillary tubes.

COMMENTS ON PROCEDURE:

Microhematocrits are usually 1 to 1.5% lower than macro hematocrits.

PROCEDURE:

1. Mix specimen well, fill two capillary tubes approximately three-quarters full. (For EDTA blood use plain capillary tubes.) Seal

2. Spin for four minutes.

3. Read on micro-hematocrit reader, being sure to read below buffy coat layer.

NORMAL VALUES:
Birth - 2 weeks	50 $\pm$	10
14 - 60 days	42 $\pm$	7
3 months - 10 years	36 $\pm$	5
11 - 15 years	39 $\pm$	5
Adult Male	47 $\pm$	5
Adult Female	42 $\pm$	5

REFERENCE: Miale, John B.: LABORATORY MEDICINE HEMATOLOGY 4th. Ed. C. V. Mosby Co., St. Louis, pg. 1205, 1972.

PCV (Continued):

INTERPRETATION:

When anticoagulated whole blood is centrifuged, the packed red cell
mass is called the hematocrit and is identified as the percentage of
red cells per volume of whole blood. The normal values vary with
age and sex of the patient. There are two methods for determination
of the hematocrit, the micro and macro procedures. The micro procedure is the method of choice in a majority of laboratories.

ASCORBATE-PEROXIDATION OF HEMOGLOBIN

PRINCIPLE: The oxidative substance, sodium ascorbate, acts on the hemoglobin to produce methemoglobin and sulfhemoglobin. The sodium cyanide inhibits the catalase activity allowing sustained levels of H_2O_2. Normally the metabolism via the HMP pathway is sufficient to prevent methemoglobin and sulfhemoglobin accumulation; consequently, the sample remains red with only gradual darkening by four hours. Because of the lack of TPNH or the presence of unstable hemoglobin, an increase in the methemoglobin and sulfhemoglobin cause a mild to marked darkening (brown) color in $\frac{1}{2}$ to 3 or 4 hours, indicating a positive test.

SPECIMEN: 5.0 ml. whole blood collected in EDTA. Always include a normal control.

EQUIPMENT AND REAGENTS:

1. <u>Test Tubes</u>, 16 x 100 mm.
   Stoppered and stored at $-20^{\circ}C$. containing 10 mg. sodium ascorbate and 5.0 mg. glucose.

2. <u>Sodium Cyanide</u>, neutralized 0.1 M. (M.W. 49.01)
   0.49 gm./100 ml. pH to 7.4 before diluting to volume.

3. <u>Waterbath</u>, $37^{\circ}C$.

4. <u>Equipment to adjust Hematocrits</u>
   If below 20%. Should be adjusted to 30 to 40%.

5. <u>Glass Flask</u>, 25 ml.
   Containing glass beads to aerate the blood.

6. <u>Fresh EDTA anticoagulated blood</u>

PROCEDURE:

1. EDTA blood is aerated to bright red by gentle swirling in the flask containing the glass beads.

2. 2.0 ml. blood is added to the ascorbate-glucose mixture.

3. 2 Drops (0.1 ml.) neutralized 0.1 M. NaCN is added and gently mixed.

134

Ascorbate-Peroxidation of Hemoglobin (Continued):

4. Leave tubes unstoppered at 37°C. in waterbath. Occasionally agitate the mixture.

5. At 1, 2, 3 and 4 hours mix thoroughly and observe color.

RESULTS: Negative Test - Slow darkening of blood over 4 hours.
Positive Test - Suspension becomes brownish at ½ to 4 hours.

REFERENCES:

1. Jacob, H. S. and Jandl, J. H.: "Screening Test for G-6-PD Deficiency Employing Ascorbate and Cyanide". New Eng. J. Med. 274:1162, 1966.

2. Fairbanks, V. P.: "Unstable Hemoglobinopathies". Am. J. Med. 46:344, 1969.

3. Fairbanks, V. F.: "The Identification of Metabolic Errors Associated with Hemolytic Anemia". J. Amer. Med. Assoc. 208:316, 1969.

INTERPRETATION:

Positive results may be seen in:

1. G-6-PD deficiency (with or without reticulocytosis)
2. G-6-PD heterozygotes (with or without reticulocytosis)
3. Glutathione Reductase deficiency
4. Glutathione Peroxidase deficiency
5. Pyruvate Kinase deficiency
6. Unstable hemoglobins, Köln, Olmsted, Santa Ana
7. Premature or newborn infants (50%) due to transitory deficiency of glutathione peroxidase
8. False positive if there is increased in vitro hemolysis

FETAL HEMOGLOBIN

PRINCIPLE: Fetal hemoglobin is more resistant to denaturation by a strong alkali than other hemoglobins. Within one minute after adding alkali to a hemoglobin solution, most hemoglobins are denatured, but fetal hemoglobin is not. Potassium hydroxide is added to a solution containing a known amount of hemoglobin, and exactly one minute later denaturation is stopped by adding half-saturated ammonium sulfate. The ammonium sulfate lowers the pH and precipitates the denatured hemoglobin. After filtration, the amount of unaltered hemoglobin in the solution is measured and expressed as the percent of alkali resistant hemoglobin.

SPECIMEN: 1.0 ml. freshly drawn oxalated, versenated or citrated blood. Clotted blood may be used.

REAGENTS:

1. Alkaline Reagent
   To 10 ml. of exactly 1 N. KOH solution add exactly 110 ml. of distilled water. Store in refrigerator in a paraffin-lined bottle. The pH should be exactly 12.7. If a precipitate forms or if the solution becomes cloudy it must be discarded.

2. Precipitating Solution
   Anhydrous ammonium sulfate   37.7 gm.
   HCL, 10 N.   0.25 ml.
   Distilled water, q.s. to   100.0 ml.

3. Physiological Saline

4. Toluene (C. P.)

COMMENTS ON PROCEDURE:

1. The procedure must be followed exactly. The time interval, temperature, pH, and concentration of the reactants are critical. The test should be carried out between 19° to 21°C. The final supernatant solution must be filtered and examined immediately as fading will occur.

2. When blood from a markedly anemic person is used, or when the red cells are very hypochromic, prepare the initial hemoglobin solution by using a larger volume of packed cells and less distilled water.

136

Fetal Hemoglobin (Continued):

3. A positive fetal hemoglobin control of cord blood and a normal control should be run with each test.

PROCEDURE:

1. Preparation of Hemolysate
   A solution of hemoglobin containing 9 to 11 gm. of hemoglobin per 100 ml. is prepared from freshly drawn clotted, oxalated, or citrated blood. A convenient technic is as follows: place 10 ml. of freshly drawn blood in a 15 ml. graduated centrifuge tube containing two drops of a 20% solution of potassium oxalate. Centrifuge at 3000 rpm for 20 minutes. Draw off and discard the plasma. Add approximately 10 ml. of physiological saline to the packed cells. Mix and then centrifuge at 3000 rpm for 30 minutes. Draw off and discard the saline. Draw off the packed red cells until 2.0 ml. of packed cells remain in the tube. Add distilled water to the 4.0 ml. mark, followed by 0.8 ml. of toluene. Shake for 5 minutes. The tube is then centrifuged at 3000 rpm for 5 minutes. However, a better recovery of hemoglobin solution is obtained if the mixture is allowed to stand overnight in the refrigerator prior to centrifugation. Discard the upper two layers. Filter the clear red solution. The final solution should contain approximately 13 gm. of hemoglobin/100 ml. The exact concentration of hemoglobin can be determined and the solution adjusted if necessary.

2. Prepare a series of six test tubes with the following labels: "Fetal Hemoglobin Positive Control", "Total Positive Control", "Fetal Hemoglobin Negative Control", "Total Negative Control", "Patient Fetal Hemoglobin", "Total Patient Hemoglobin".

3. Pipette 1.6 ml. of the alkaline reagent into the serologic test tube labelled "Fetal Hemoglobin Positive Control".

4. Pipette 3.2 ml. of the alkaline reagent into the serologic test tubes labelled "Fetal Hemoglobin Normal Control" and "Patient Fetal Hemoglobin".

5. Pipette 5.0 ml. distilled water into the test tubes labelled "Total Positive Control", "Total Normal Control" and "Total Patient Hemoglobin".

6. Into the tubes prepared for "Total Hemoglobin's in Step 5 above, pipette 0.02 ml. of appropriate hemoglobin hemolysate. Mix contents well.

Fetal Hemoglobin (Continued):

7. Place the test tubes prepared in Steps 3 and 4 into a 20°C. water bath for 5 minutes.

8. Into the test tube labelled "Fetal Hemoglobin Positive Control" (Step 3) pipette 0.1 ml. of cord blood hemolysate. Rinse the pipette 6 times with the contents of the tube and shake gently for 10 seconds. Exactly one minute after introducing the hemo-globin into the alkaline reagent add 3.4 ml. of the "precipita-ting" solution. Mix by inversion 6 times. Filter through a double layer of filter paper immediately, retaining the filtrate. Quantitatively prepare a 1:2 dilution of this filtrate with dis-tilled water.

9. Pipette 0.2 ml. of appropriate hemolysate into the tubes label-led "Fetal Hemoglobin Normal Control" and "Patient Fetal Hemo-globin" (Step 4); rinse the pipette 6 times with the contents of the tube and shake gently for 10 seconds. Exactly one minute after introducing the hemoglobin into the alkaline reagent, add 6.8 ml. of the "precipitating" solution. Mix by inversion 6 times. Filter through a double layer of filter paper immediate-ly, retaining the filtrate.

10. Determine the optical density of all filtrates and total hemo-globin solutions (Step 6) at 540 nm. in a 19 x 105 mm. cuvette against distilled water. Multiply the optical density of the "Fetal Hemoglobin Positive Control" times 2.

11. CALCULATIONS:

$$\frac{\frac{\text{O.D. Fetal Hemoglobin}}{5}}{\text{O.D. of "Total" Hemoglobin Solution}} \times 100 = \% \text{ Fetal Hemoglobin present}$$

NORMAL VALUES:

1. Under the conditions of this test, normal adult hemoglobin (hemo-globin A) is completely denatured (precipitated) within one min-ute. Therefore, when only normal adult hemoglobin is present, the filtrate will be colorless. If more than 2.0% of the hemo-globin is alkali resistant (fetal hemoglobin), the final filtrate will be faintly brown to deeply red in color.

2. The amount of alkali-resistant hemoglobin may be quantitated by determining the amount of hemoglobin in the initial solution and

Fetal Hemoglobin (Continued):

in the final filtrate. The alkali-resistant hemoglobin is then expressed as a percent of the initial amount of hemoglobin. In normal adult subjects, 0.5 to 1.7% of the hemoglobin is alkali resistant.

REFERENCES:

1. Singer, K., Chernoff, A. I., and Singer, L.: "Studies on Abnormal Hemoglobins. I. The Demonstration in Sickle Cell Anemia and Other Hemorrhagic (Hematologic) Disorders by Means of Alkaline Denaturation". Blood 6:413, 1951.

2. Cartwright, G. E.: DIAGNOSTIC LABORATORY HEMATOLOGY, 3rd. Ed., Williams & Wilkins Co., Baltimore, Md., 1965.

3. Cooper, H. A. and Hoagland, H. C.: "Fetal Hemoglobin". Mayo Clin. Proc. 47:402-414, 1972.

INTERPRETATION:

A list of the conditions that, at one time or another, have been associated with elevations in the level of HbF is shown below.

1. Anemias
   Aplastic anemia (congenital and acquired)
   Pernicious anemia
   Hereditary spherocytosis
   Hereditary elliptocytosis
   Congenital nonspherocytic hemolytic anemia
   Erythropoietic porphyria
   Paroxysmal nocturnal hemoglobinuria
2. Myelofibrosis
3. Postirradiation fibrosis of marrow
4. Malignancies involving marrow
   Tumor metastasis
   Leukemia (especially those with an erythroleukemia
      component)
   Histiocytosis
   Plasmacytic myeloma
5. Hemoglobinopathies
   Quantitative (thalassemias, major and minor)
   Qualitative
      HbS
      HbC
      HbD
      HbE

Fetal Hemoglobin (Continued):

6. Hereditary persistence of fetal hemoglobin

Major series in which HbF levels have been measured in these condition are lacking in all except the hemoglobinopathies, particularly the thalassemias. Nevertheless, some interesting data - much of which await interpretation - have accumulated. In Fanconi's anemia, for instance, elevated levels of HbF have been documented, and these precede the onset of pancytopenia. However, pancytopenia has preceded the elevation of HbF values by several months in aplastic anemia

Thalassemias, characterized by a defect in the genetic control of the rate of globin synthesis, may have associated high levels of HbF. Of 130 patients with thalassemia minor, 54 percent had elevated levels of HbF, whereas 100 percent of 32 patients with thalassemia major had even higher elevations.

Because HbF is present as the major hemoglobin of the newborn and only small amounts of HbS are present, newborns even with the homozygous state have relatively few problems before the age of 3 months. As HbF values decrease and HbS synthesis increases, clinical manifestations of severe anemia, hepatomegaly, splenomegaly, and painful crises may be found.

HEMOGLOBIN
(Coulter Hemoglobinometer Method)

PRINCIPLE: Hemoglobin is a conjugated protein which contains 4 heme groups and globin. The heme is a metal complex consisting of an iron atom in the center of a porphyrin structure. The heme imparts to hemoglobin its red color.

Zap-oglobin contains potassium cyanide and converts hemoglobin to cyanmethemoglobin.

SPECIMEN: Capillary blood or EDTA tube.

REAGENTS:

1. Coulter autodilutor

2. Coulter hemoglobinometer

3. Sahli pipettes (0.02 ml.)

4. Isoton

5. Zap-oglobin

6. Cyanmethemoglobin S Standard (Coulter)

PROCEDURE:

1. Make a 1:501 dilution of blood to Isoton, as for a WBC count. For capillary blood, use 0.02 ml. blood to 10 ml. of Isoton.

2. Add three drops of Zap-oglobin.

3. Read WBC within 2 minutes.

4. Read hemoglobin within 5 minutes.

5. Read hemoglobin in grams directly from the machine.

6. Samples should be run in duplicate.

141

Hemoglobin (Continued):

STANDARDIZATION:

1. Follow procedure using 4C Control.

2. Use Cyanmethemoglobin Standard (Coulter) undiluted.   Reading should check with assay value on bottle.

NORMAL VALUES: Adult Male: 14.8 gm. $\pm$ 1.3
                Adult Female: 13.0 gm. $\pm$ 1.0
                Children: 12.0 gm. $\pm$ 2.0

REFERENCE: COULTER DIAGNOSTICS LITERATURE AND REAGENT ENCLOSURES.

INTERPRETATION:

See Interpretation Section of Hemoglobin under Cyanmethemoglobin Method on page 144.

HEMOGLOBIN
(Cyanmethemoglobin Method)

PRINCIPLE: Hemoglobin is a conjugated protein which contains 4 heme groups and globin. The heme is a metal complex consisting of an iron atom in the center of a porphyrin structure. The heme imparts to hemoglobin its red color.

The ferricyanide converts hemoglobin iron from ferrous to ferric state to form methemoglobin, which then combines with potassium cyanide to produce the stable pigment, cyanmethemoglobin.

SPECIMEN: Capillary blood or EDTA tube.

REAGENTS AND EQUIPMENT:

1. Coulter Autodilutor

2. Sahli Pipettes (0.02 ml.)

3. Drabkin's Reagent
   NaHCO$_3$ 1.0 gm.
   K Cyanide (KCN)   50.0 mg.
   K Ferricyanide (K$_3$Fe(CN)$_6$)   200.0 mg.
   Distilled water q.s. to   1000.0 ml.

4. Spectrophotometer, 540 nm.

PROCEDURE:

1. Make a 1:301 dilution of blood to Drabkin's reagent:
   a). For capillary blood use 0.02 ml. blood to 6.0 ml. of Drabkin's.
   b). For autodilutor use 0.33 ml. blood to 10 ml. of Drabkin's.

2. Mix thoroughly and allow to stand for at least 20 minutes before reading.

3. Read O.D. in Spectrophotometer at 540 nm. wavelength against a reagent blank.

4. Read equivalent hemoglobin from conversion table.

Hemoglobin (Continued):

CURVE PROCEDURE:

1. Using Ortho Acuglobin Hemoglobin Standard (warmed to room temperature), make 1:3 (25%), 1:1 (50%), 3.1 (75%), dilution with Drabkin's reagent. Read O.D. of these along with an undiluted standard at 540 nm.

2. The concentration of hemoglobin in undiluted Standard is equal to Assay Value on vial x dilution (301).

3. These values should form a straight line curve when plotted on ordinary graph paper.

A Factor for hemoglobin can be calculated by the following Procedure:

1. Read undiluted Ortho Acuglobin (warmed to room temperature) at 540 nm. against Drabkin's blank.

2. Assay Value of Standard x Dilution (301) = Factor O.D. of Standard

3. Factor x hemoglobin O.D. = Gm. Hemoglobin/100 ml.

NORMAL VALUES: Adult Male   16.0 gm. $\pm$ 2.0
                Adult Female   14.0 gm. $\pm$ 2.0
                Children   12.0 gm. $\pm$ 2.0
                Newborns   19.5 gm. $\pm$ 5.0

REFERENCES:

1. Wintrobe, Maxwell M.: CLINICAL HEMATOLOGY 6th. Ed., Lea & Febiger, Phil., pgs. 86, 429, 1967.

2. Miale, John B.: LABORATORY MEDICINE HEMATOLOGY 4th. Ed., C. V. Mosby Co., St. Louis, pgs. 593, 1214, 1216, 1972.

INTERPRETATION:

The assessment of anemia requires the determination of hemoglobin, hematocrit, and the red blood cell count to determine the indices of MCV, MCH, and MCHC. The hemoglobin varies with age. It is high at birth and decreases to adult levels during the first few weeks of life. A slight decrease in hemoglobin occurs in the elderly. Men have higher values than women. A diurnal variation is present with hemoglobin values approximately 1.0 gm./100 ml. lower late in the afternoon.

Hemoglobin (Continued):

The Cyanmethemoglobin procedure measures all forms of hemoglobin except sulfhemoglobin. Turbidity due to leukocytosis, macroglobulinemia and lipemia will cause spurious elevations of hemoglobin levels.

PLASMA HEMOGLOBIN

PRINCIPLE: This procedure is performed as a test for hemolytic anemia. In hemolysis, the plasma hemoglobin is elevated.

SPECIMEN: 5.0 ml. blood drawn in a siliconized syringe. See "Preparation of Specimen".

EQUIPMENT AND REAGENTS:

1. Benzidine Reagent, 1%
   1 gm. pure benzidine base placed in a 100 ml. volumetric flask, to which 90 ml. of glacial acetic acid is added and then diluted to volume with deionized water. This reagent should be kept in the refrigerator. The small amount of water keeps the reagent from solidifying at refrigerator temperatures.

2. Hydrogen Peroxide, 1.0%
   1 Part 3% hydrogen peroxide to 2 parts deionized water. Prepare fresh when test is run.

3. Standard Hemoglobin Solution
   a). Concentrated Standard
      2.0 ml. washed red blood cells. Lyse by freeze-thawing 2 times and add 6.0 ml. of 0.9% NaCl. Concentration should be 9 - 11 gm%. hemoglobin. Check concentration with cyanmethemoglobin procedure.

   b). Working Standard
      0.02 ml. concentrated standard diluted to 10 ml. with 0.9% NaCl. Concentration is 20 mg%. if concentrated standard is 10 gm%.

PREPARATION OF SPECIMEN:

1. A clean venipuncture with an 18 gauge siliconized needle is made and a few ml. of blood withdrawn. The tourniquet is removed and syringes switched. Using a 5.0 ml. siliconized syringe allow the blood to freely enter the syringe.

2. 4.5 ml. of blood is placed in a centrifuge tube containing 0.5 ml. 3.8% sodium citrate. Allow the blood to gently run down the side of the tube.

Plasma Hemoglobin (Continued):

3. Cap with parafilm and invert 2 times GENTLY.

4. Spin the sample 2000 to 2500 rpm for 10 minutes.

5. Remove the plasma into a clean tube and recentrifuge.

6. Recentrifuge and again remove the top portion of plasma.

7. Store the plasma at 4°C. until the test is run.

COMMENTS ON PROCEDURE:

1. Use only acid cleaned glassware.

2. All equipment must be sulfate-free.

3. Carbonates, acetates, lactates and cyanide cause non-specific darkening.

4. Lead and other heavy metals cause peculiar shades of color.

5. If the concentration of hemoglobin is very low:
   a). Increase concentration of benzidine (3 or 4%)
   b). Increase volume of unknown. It may be increased to 0.05 ml. without causing turbidity.
   c). Decrease the volume of the 10% acetic acid diluent

6. If the concentration of the unknown is too high:
   a). Read as cyanmethemoglobin
   b). Dilute unknown plasma with distilled water

PROCEDURE:

1. Run a standard and blank with each unknown.

2. 1.0 ml. of 1% Benzidine reagent is placed in a 15 ml. tube.

3. 0.02 ml. Standard or unknown is added to the appropriate tube.

4. 1.0 ml. of 1% hydrogen peroxide is added to each tube and contents mixed immediately.

5. When color change is completed (a pink-violet color) about 20 minutes, add 10 ml. 10% Acetic Acid diluent and mix by inversion.

Plasma Hemoglobin (Continued):

6. Allow to sit 10 minutes and read in a Beckman Spectrophotometer at a wavelength of 515 nm. or use a Beckman DU with a wavelength of 515 nm. with a slit width of 0.04.

7. CALCULATIONS:

$$\frac{O.D. \text{ Unknown}}{O.D. \text{ Standard}} \times \text{Concentration of Std.} \times \frac{10}{9} = \text{mg\%. Plasma Hemoglobin}$$

NORMAL VALUES: 0 - 2.0% Plasma Hemoglobin

REFERENCE: Brodine, C. E., Vertrees, K. M.: DIFFERENTIATION OF MYOGLOBINURIA AND HEMOGLOBINURIA IN HEMOGLOBIN, Edited by F. W. Sunderman & F. W. Sunderman, Jr., J. B. Lippincott Co., Phil., pg. 90, 1964.

INTERPRETATION:

It is important to identify an increase in serum, plasma or urine hemoglobin to aid in the diagnosis of hemolytic anemia. Elevated hemoglobin occurs in various hemolytic states. One must exclude the presence of erythrocytes by microscopy. Myoglobin may also cause a darker serum, plasma or urine and is soluble in 80 percent saturated ammonium sulfate solution while hemoglobin is insoluble. One may differentiate hemoglobin from myoglobin by an electrophoretic separation.

HEMOGLOBIN ELECTROPHORESIS

PRINCIPLE: This procedure may be used as a screening test for the presence of abnormal hemoglobins or may be adapted for quantitation of A_2 hemoglobin. The use of the Beckman Microzone system allows for speed of analysis and adequate clarity of fractions is achieved using the Gelman Sepraphore III supporting medium.

SPECIMEN: Anticoagulated whole blood specimen; generally collection is made in an EDTA Vacutainer tube but may be made in any anticoagulant. A minimum of 2.0 ml. is desirable, but collection may be made in large, heparinized capillary tubes when working with pediatric patients.

The specimen may be stored at refrigerator temperatures until the hemolysate is prepared.

A smear of the whole blood should be made at the time of specimen collection; clip the smear onto the laboratory requisition.

REAGENTS:

1. Hemoglobin Control Specimens
   In the absence of patient specimens of known abnormal hemoglobin types, commercial control specimens purchased from Hyland Laboratories may be used. These lyophilized specimens are not recommended for quantitation but are excellent for location of abnormal hemoglobins in the screening procedure. The following controls have been found adequate for most routine screening: A (normal), AC, AS, and E (A_2). Reconstitute vials and store according to the directions enclosed with the specimens. These specimens must be centrifuged in Toluene until completely clear, before use.

   A control specimen for fetal hemoglobin may be obtained by preparing a hemolysate of cord blood.

2. Cellulose Acetate
   Sepraphore III cellulose acetate strips may be obtained from the Gelman Co. in a "microzone" size; this size, 2.25 x 5.687 inches with perforations, must be specified when ordering.

Hemoglobin Electrophoresis (Continued):

3. Electrophoresis Buffer, TEB, pH 8.6
   Into a 1000 ml. volumetric flask place 12.1 gm. Tris, 0.92 gm.
   Boric Acid and 1.56 gm. EDTA. Bring to volume with deionized
   water and mix thoroughly. Store at refrigerator temperatures in
   a tightly capped polyethylene bottle. Stable indefinitely.

4. Ponceau S Stain, 0.2%
   Beckman Company "Fixative Dye Solution" may be used; reconstitute
   according to the directions on the bottle.

   The stain may also be prepared by the following procedure:
   Place 1.0 gm. of Ponceau Red S into a 500 ml. volumetric
   flask. Place 37.5 gm. of Trichloroacetic Acid in a beaker
   and dissolve it in approximately 150 ml. of deionized water.
   Quantitatively transfer the contents to the flask containing
   the dye. Place 37.5 gm. of Sulfosalicylic Acid in a beaker
   and dissolve it in approximately 150 ml. of deionized water.
   Quantitatively transfer the contents to the flask containing
   the dye. Bring this flask to volume with deionized water.
   Allow the contents to mix on a magnetic stirrer until the dye
   has completely gone into solution. Store in a polyethylene
   bottle; stable indefinitely at room temperature.

5. Destaining Solution, 5% Acetic Acid
   Place 950 ml. deionized water into a 1000 ml. graduated mixing
   cylinder. Add 50 ml. of Glacial Acetic Acid and mix thoroughly.
   Stable when stored capped.

6. Clearing Solution
   Prepare a 10 to 15% solution of Glacial Acetic Acid in Methanol.
   Too great a concentration of acid will soften the acetate strips
   until they are not easily manageable; too dilute an acid solution
   will not completely clear the membrane. This must be prepared
   just before use and should be fresh for each membrane to be cleare

7. Saline, 0.9%
   Place 9.0 gm. of NaCl into a 1000 ml. volumetric flask and bring
   to volume with deionized water. Mix thoroughly. Stable.

8. Methanol, 99.9%
   Reagent grade.

9. Toluene

Hemoglobin Electrophoresis (Continued):

EQUIPMENT:

1. Beckman Microzone Electrophoresis Cell

2. Beckman Duostat Power Supply

3. Beckman Sample Applicator

4. Glass Plate for membrane clearing

5. Coleman Jr. Spectrophotometer with 10 x 75 mm. cuvette adaptor

6. Coleman Cuvettes, 10 x 75 mm.
   Great care should be taken that the cuvettes be optically matched.

7. Chaney Syringe Pipettes
   a). One 2.0 ml. syringe gravimetrically calibrated to deliver
       exactly 1.5 ml. of fluid.
   b). One syringe pipette gravimetrically calibrated to deliver
       exactly 12 ml. of fluid.

8. Blotter Paper (Beckman Co.)

9. Coverslip Forceps

COMMENTS ON PROCEDURE:

1. Cleanliness of the specimen is very important to the accuracy of
   the screening and the quantitation procedures.

2. Speed of handling of the membrane both after application and after
   completion of the electrophoretic run will inhibit diffusion of
   the pattern.

3. Thorough drying of the membrane before attempting elution for
   quantitation is critical to ensure complete elution of the dye
   from the "A" fraction.

4. Use of a high intensity lamp for viewing the electrophoretic pattern while cutting yields much more reproducible results.

PROCEDURE:

A. Sample Preparation
   1. Centrifuge whole blood specimens for 10 minutes at 3500 rpm.

Hemoglobin Electrophoresis (Continued):

Aspirate off the plasma and white cell layers. Wash cells at least 3 times with normal saline, or until supernate is completely clear. Aspirate any remaining buffy coat off with each saline rinse.

2. To washed cells add an equal volume of distilled water and mix well to lyse cells. Add a small volume if hemoglobin is low.

3. Add 10 to 20% Toluene by volume and shake contents vigorously for several minutes. Caution: Too much Toluene may result in a colloidal suspension which is difficult to break. The sample may be centrifuged and electrophoresed, but, for best yield, allow tube to remain at refrigerator temperature overnight.

4. Centrifuge specimen at 3500 rpm for 10 minutes. Remove the hemolysate by inserting a capillary pipette beneath the Toluene-cell debris layer and withdrawing the clear hemolyzed layer.

5. If the hemolysate is not sparkling clear, shake with more Toluene and centrifuge again. Hemoglobin S and Thalassemia cells may be more resistant to hemolysis but generally will hemolyze by overnight exposure to distilled water at refrigerator temperatures.

6. Before electrophoresis, draw up some clean Toluene into a micro PCV capillary tube to about one-half the volume. Fill two-thirds of the remaining volume with the hemolysate to be analyzed. Seal the Toluene end of the tube with "critoseal" and centrifuge in the microcentrifuge for 5 minutes. If the hemolysate has been stored for more than a week, repeat the process by transferring the hemolysate into a tube of fresh Toluene.

7. The hemolysate may be stored in either one lot, or aliquoted into microcapillary tubes at refrigerator temperatures or frozen for several months. It has been found that a more scrupulous cleaning with Toluene is required as the specimen ages. A_2 values, particularly those that are elevated, appear to change (lower) as the period of storage lengthens.

8. Just prior to electrophoresis, break the critoseal on a cleared hemolysate and place a drop of the specimen on a clean

Hemoglobin Electrophoresis (Continued):

    square of parafilm. Cover with a small plastic cup to prevent evaporation.

B. Hemoglobin Electrophoresis
1. Handling the electrophoretic membrane with forceps, gently float it on the surface of the TEB buffer in a staining dish; allow the buffer to penetrate and wet the strip from the underside to avoid the trapping of air pockets. Submerge the membrane for maximum exposure to buffer; allow at least 15 minutes.

    For A$_2$ Quantitation
    Before carrying out the above procedure for pre-buffering, cut the electrophoretic membrane in half longitudinally.

2. Fill the Microzone Cell to the indicated mark with TEB buffer (see Reagent #3) and allow the fluid to equillibrate by filling the siphon.

3. Remove the saturated membrane or membrane halves from the pre-buffer solution with forceps, place between two blotters and press firmly with one stroke of the hand to remove excess surface moisture. Too much moisture will diffuse the hemoglobin pattern; too dry a membrane will cause an uneven electrophoretic pattern.

4. Still handling the blotted membrane with forceps, position it on the bridge which has been removed from the Microzone Cell. Position the membrane halves so that they are not touching on the cut sides. Place the bridge on anything which will allow the membrane ends to hang free and will be stable (i.e., a stack of staining dish lids).

5. Position the template on the bridge.

6. Sample application. Steps #3 to #6 should be completed rapidly. Dip the sample applicator tip through the drop of hemolysate, with the tip in the lowered position, breaking the surface tension. Blot off this first sample on some filter paper and repeat the sampling process. Press the red button to retract the applicator tip and position the applicator on the template in the groove most centrally located (the applicator tip should be at the extreme left of the membrane). Press the white button to lower the applicator tip onto the membrane and, after five seconds, depress the red button to

Hemoglobin Electrophoresis (Continued):

retract the tip. Complete this process smoothly without jig-
gling the applicator. Rinse tip with deionized water between
patients.

For A$_2$ Quantitation

Using a split membrane, reserve one membrane half for the
patient's specimen and one membrane half for the known normal
control. Apply the patient's specimen, in duplicate, at the
four template positions of the appropriate membrane half.
Apply the known normal control, in duplicate, at the four
template positions on the other membrane half.

For Hemoglobin Screening

Using a whole membrane, employ the basic application procedure
to place known hemoglobin controls and the patient's specimen
in individual template positions on the membrane. Rinse and
blot the applicator tip after each specimen.

7. Place the bridge on the Microzone Cell and cover with template
   and lid. Check the fluid level of the buffer and the ends
   of the membrane to ensure good contact.

8. Connect the Duostat to the cell and adjust the meter to constant voltage at 480 volts by placing the voltmeter at 0 -
   500 and constant voltage switch at 300 - 500 V.

   The starting current should be between 3 - 5 ma. (This may
   be checked by switching the ammeter to 0 - 15 ma. and the
   constant current switch to 2 - 30 ma.)

   Allow electrophoretic migration for 30 minutes.

9. After 30 minutes, turn off Duostat, immediately unplug the
   cell and remove the membrane from the bridge. Care must be
   taken to keep the membrane flat and free from touching any
   moisture which may have accumulated on the bridge; moisture
   running down the strip will smear the electrophoretic pattern.

10. With forceps, remove the membrane from the bridge and place
    it in the fixative dye solution for a minimum of 10 minutes.

11. Place the stained membrane in 5% Acetic Acid destaining sol-
    ution and wash with fresh aliquots of this solution until the
    membrane background and wash fluid are completely colorless.

Hemoglobin Electrophoresis (Continued):

12. For A_2 Quantitation

a). Remove the electrophoretic membrane from the Acetic Acid solution and transfer into deionized water. Rinse briefly to remove excess acid. Drain off fluid and place carefully on a clean blotter. After 1 to 2 minutes cover gently with another blotter to keep the membrane flat during drying. Allow the membrane to dry overnight, or, after approximately 15 minutes, place the membrane in a 90°C. oven for 15 to 30 minutes. The membrane will shrink some in size.

b). Using four clean test tubes which can contain at least 12 ml. of fluid, label them respectively "A control", "A_2 control", "A patient", and "A_2 patient".

c). Hold the dried membrane half against the high intensity lamp and, with a pair of small, sharp scissors, cut out the hemoglobin fractions.

d). Place the fractions into the appropriately labelled tubes, cutting them into small pieces to achieve maximum surface exposure.

e). Using the calibrated Chaney pipettes, deliver 1.5 ml. TEB Buffer into the tubes containing the A_2 fractions. Deliver 12 ml. TEB Buffer into the tubes containing the A fractions.

f). Mix all tubes gently (gently invert the "A" tubes 2 times) to avoid flocculating the membrane; allow the fractions to elute for approximately 30 minutes.

g). Again mix all tubes gently and transfer the contents into one of two matched Coleman cuvettes (10 x 75 mm.). Determine the optical density of the "A" and "A_2" fractions against a buffer blank at 520 nm.

h). CALCULATION
1). Multiply the optical density of the "A" tube by 8.
2). Add this value to the "A_2" optical density to obtain total hemoglobin optical density and multiply the result by 100 to obtain the percent A_2 hemoglobin in the specimen.

Hemoglobin Electrophoresis (Continued):

3). Example:

$$A = 0.249 \times 8 = 1.992$$
$$A_2 = 0.048$$
$$\% \ A_2 = \frac{0.048}{1.992 + 0.048} = 0.024 \times 100 = 2.4\%$$

NORMAL VALUE: Normal range for A_2 Hemoglobin is 2.03 to 3.07% with this method.

Two Standard Deviations of Precision = $\pm$ 0.12%

13. For Hemoglobin Screening
The destaining membrane is transferred to methanol for about one minute.
a). Prepare membrane for clearing by removing it from methanol (see Step #13) and transferring it to a staining dish containing a clean glass plate and the freshly prepared clearing solution (see Reagent #6).

b). Do not allow membrane to remain in clearing solution more than 45 to 60 seconds. Remove membrane and glass plate; squeegee excess moisture off of membrane with a gentle and complete stroke across the surface of the plate. Do not distort membrane pattern during this process.

c). Place plate and membrane in 100°C. oven for 15 minutes; remove cleared membrane and allow plate to cool.

d). Peel membrane off of glass plate and place in a plastic envelope for storage.

e). Examine membrane for abnormal hemoglobins. See example beneath.

f). Fetal hemoglobin may be identified if in sufficient quantity but may not be quantitated by this method. Refer to method for Fetal Hemoglobin Alkali Denaturation for quantitative measurement of this fraction.

g). Hemoglobin S and Hemoglobin D are indistinguishable in this method. In the absence of a positive sickle cell preparation one may refer to the method for Acid Solubility Test.

Hemoglobin Electrophoresis (Continued):

REFERENCE: Lehmann, H. and Huntsman, R.: MAN'S HEMOGLOBINS
Lippincott, Phil., 1966.

INTERPRETATION:

Certain hemoglobins migrate together and another test must be performed to specifically identify the hemoglobin. Many hemoglobins
migrate like hemoglobin S. See Table below. The commonest hemoglobin which migrates like hemoglobin S is hemoglobin D. These hemoglobins may be differentiated by the Dithionite Solubility Test.
See page 323. Hemoglobin S is insoluble in contrast to hemoglobin
D which is soluble.

HEMOGLOBINOPATHIES
ELECTROPHORETICALLY SIMILAR TO HEMOGLOBIN S

At pH 8.0 to 8.9	Under Other Specified Conditions
D	Russ
Flatbush	Shimonoseki
Zurich	Koln
Stanleyville, II	G (Philadelphia)
Sealy (Sinai, Hasharon)	G (Port Arthur)
P	G (Galveston)
Etobicoke	G (Texas)
Sabine	Alexandra
Gunhill	Zurich
Shimonoseki	E
Kokura	
Umi	
Leiden	
L Ferrara	
Lepore	
G (Coushatta)	
Memphis/S	

The hemoglobins which are readily separated are hemoglobins A, S, C,
H, F, and A_2. Hemoglobin A_2 is elevated in heterozygous Beta Thalassemia.

Homozygous Beta Thalassemia may have elevated or normal levels of
hemoglobin A_2. Hemoglobin A_2 is decreased in hemoglobin H disease.

Hemoglobin Electrophoresis (Continued):

The relative mobilities of hemoglobins are depicted in the following diagram.

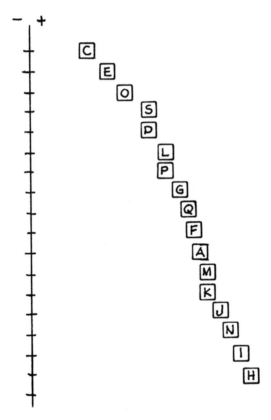

MIGRATIONS of HEMOGLOBINS IN AN ELECTROPHORETIC FIELD AT PH 8.6.

HEMOGLOBIN "H" INCLUSION BODIES

PRINCIPLE: Hemoglobin "H" is unstable and undergoes denaturation in the presence of brilliant cresyl blue dye.

SPECIMEN: 5.0 ml. of whole blood anticoagulated in EDTA.

REAGENTS:

1. Citrate - Saline Solution
   3% Sodium Citrate - 3.0 gm./100 ml. distilled water.
   0.85% NaCl - 0.85 gm./100 ml. distilled water.
   Mix 1 volume of sodium citrate with 4 volumes of NaCl.

2. Brilliant Cresyl Blue Dye, 1.0%
   1.0 gm. of brilliant cresyl blue dye dissolved in 100 ml. of sodium citrate - saline solution. Filter before using.

PROCEDURE:

1. Mix 1.0 ml. of anticoagulated whole blood with 1.0 ml. of the brilliant cresyl blue dye stain.

2. Allow the mixture to stand 3 hours at room temperature.

3. Smears should be made of the stained blood and allowed to dry.

4. Do not counterstain.

NORMAL VALUES: No inclusions present since there should be no unstable hemoglobin. If inclusions occur in 10 minutes, these are reticulocytes.

REFERENCE: Gabuzda, T. G.: "Hemoglobin H and The Red Cell". Blood 27:568, 1966.

INTERPRETATION:

Hemoglobin H inclusion bodies are blue-green spherical inclusions in almost every erythrocyte. The inclusions vary minimally in size and are diffuse throughout the erythrocyte. The pattern of a reticulocyte is different and the precipitate is blue-black.

159

Hemoglobin "H" Inclusion Bodies (Continued):

Hemoglobin H is an unstable hemoglobin and a positive slide occurs in one hour. Other unstable hemoglobins require a longer period of time to develop the precipitate. Alpha-thalassemia trait will cause inclusions in an occasional erythrocyte.

FERROHEMOGLOBIN SOLUBILITY TEST
(Goldberg Modification)

PRINCIPLE: The low solubility of reduced hemoglobin S in concentrated phosphate buffer is a valuable aid in differentiating this hemoglobin from hemoglobin D. Hemoglobin S is indistinguishable from hemoglobin D by electrophoresis, and the latter hemoglobin is usually suspected when the patient's erythrocytes do not sickle in the presence of a reducing agent.

SPECIMEN: 0.3 ml. of hemolysate which is prepared according to procedure under the "Hemoglobin Electrophoresis" Method.

REAGENTS:

1. Phosphate Buffer, 2.8 M.
   Place 21.7 gm. dibasic potassium phosphate (K_2HPO_4) and 16.9 gm. monobasic potassium phosphate (KH_2PO_4) in a 100 ml. volumetric flask. Dissolve and bring to volume in deionized water which is CO_2 free.

2. Sodium hydrosulfite ($Na_2S_2O_4$), 20 mg.
   Weigh out two 20 mg. aliquots of dry powder for each patient to be assayed.

PROCEDURE:

1. Prepare three small test tubes or flasks according to the following directions.

   A. Into a small test tube, pipette 1.8 ml. of phosphate buffer and add 20 mg. sodium hydrosulfite.

   B. Into a second small test tube, pipette 3.8 ml. of phosphate buffer and add 20 mg. sodium hydrosulfite.

   C. Into a small flask, pipette 20 ml. of deionized water.

2. Solubility Test Sample
   Add 0.2 ml. of patient hemolysate to the test tube (No. 1A.) containing 1.8 ml. of phosphate buffer. Mix well, and allow to stand for a minimum of 15 minutes. Filter the mixture through Watman Filter Paper No. 5.

161

Ferrohemoglobin Solubility Test (Continued):

3. Place 0.2 ml. of the filtrate from the proceding step into the test tube (1B.) containing 3.8 ml. of phosphate buffer and mix well.

4. Total Hemoglobin Sample
Add 0.1 ml. of patient hemolysate to the small beaker of deionized water prepared in step 1C. Mix well.

5. Determine the absorbance of both the solubility test sample (Step No. 3) and the total hemoglobin sample (Step No. 4) against a water reference in a spectrophotometer set at 415 nm.

6. CALCULATIONS:
Solubility, expressed as percent of the total hemoglobin, is calculated by dividing the absorbance of the solubility test sample by the absorbance of the total hemoglobin sample and multiplying by 100.

NORMAL VALUES:

1. Hemoglobin S-S (with varying amounts of fetal hemoglobin) will have low percent solubilities which are characteristic in the range of 6 - 23 percent.

2. Hemoglobin A-S or C-S will typically have solubilities in the range of 40 - 50 percent.

3. Hemoglobin A-A, A-D, A-C, C-C will gradually have solubilities above 90 percent.

REFERENCES:

1. Goldberg, C. A.: Clinical Chemistry, 4:146, 1958 (Primary Reference).

2. Itano, Harvey: Science, 117:89, 1953.

3. Itano, Harvey: Proceedings of the National Academy of Sciences, 37:775, 1951.

Ferrohemoglobin Solubility Test (Continued):

INTERPRETATION:

The Ferrohemoglobin Solubility Test is especially valuable to differentiate Hemoglobin D from S. Both S and D are indistinguishable electrophoretically since they travel similarly. However, Hemoglobin D is soluble and Hemoglobin S is insoluble in 2.8 M Phosphate Buffer. Hemoglobin A and C are also soluble.

SERUM OR URINE HEMOGLOBIN

PRINCIPLE: The reaction between benzidine, hydrogen peroxide and heme-containing pigments produces first a green, then a blue, and finally a permanent red color, the intensity of which is dependent upon the concentration of hemoglobin present.

SPECIMEN: Serum or urine only. EDTA tubes have too much hemolysis from the mixing for accurate results.

REAGENTS:

1. Benzidine Reagent, 1.0%
   Dissolve 1.0 gm. benzidine base in 90 ml. of glacial acetic acid and q.s. to 100 ml. with distilled water (demineralized). Keep reagent in refrigerator. COVER WITH PARAFILM BEFORE MIXING.

2. Hydrogen Peroxide, 1.0%
   Dilute 3% reagent to 1% using deionized water. Make up fresh before use.

3. Glacial Acetic Acid, 10%

4. Hemoglobin Standard, 20 mg%.
   Use low frozen hemoglobin control. Run another hemoglobin determination and use gm%. from hemoglobin chart. Add 20 cu. mm. (one Sahli pipette) frozen control to volume saline equal to the gm%.

   EXAMPLE:
   If frozen control is 7.6 gm%., add 20 cu. mm. to 7.6 ml. saline. This is a 20 mg%. standard.

5. Control, 30 mg%.
   Add 20 cu. mm. low frozen hemoglobin control (used above) to volume of saline equal to two-thirds of gm%. frozen control.

   EXAMPLE:
   If frozen control equals 7.6 gm%., two-thirds of 7.6 equals 5.1 ml Add 20 cu. mm. frozen control to 5.1 ml. saline. This solution will contain 30 mg%. hemoglobin.

Serum or Urine Hemoglobin (Continued):

PROCEDURE:

1. Spin or filter specimen to be tested.

2. Add 1.0 ml. benzidine reagent to tubes labelled Blank, Standard, Unknown, and Control.

3. With Sahli pipette, add 20 cu. mm. of hemoglobin standard to respective tube. If the urine is pink, add 20 cu. mm. to unknown tube. However, if the urine is yellow, add 0.1 ml. to unknown and divide the O.D. reading of the unknown by 5. Add 20 cu. mm. control to respective tube, add nothing to the blank. If a serum hemoglobin is being done, add 20 cu. mm. to respective tube.

4. Add 1.0 ml. of 1.0% H_2O_2 and mix immediately.

5. Let stand 20 minutes until color change is complete.

6. Add 10 ml. of 10% acetic acid and mix by inversion. Let stand 10 minutes.

7. If the urine hemoglobin is cloudy, make a separate blank using benzidine, urine, distilled water in place of H_2O_2, and 10% acetic acid. This need not set for 30 minutes.

8. Read at wavelength 515 nm. in clean cuvette. Use cuvettes which have been washed with deionized water and dried. Use these cuvettes for this hemoglobin method ONLY! Rinse with distilled water when through. Do not use cuvettes which have been used for cyanmethemoglobin determinations.

9. CALCULATIONS:

$$\frac{O.D. \text{ of Unknown}}{O.D. \text{ of Standard}} \times \text{Concentration of Standard} = \text{mg\%. Hemoglobin}$$

Plot calculated mg% for 30 mg% Control on chart with procedure in a notebook. If not within 27 - 33 mg%. range, repeat test using new benzidine reagent.

NORMAL VALUES: Serum: 0 - 2.0 mg%.
Urine: 0 - 2.0 mg%.

REFERENCE: Crosby, W. and Furth, F.: Blood, 11:380, 1956.

Serum or Urine Hemoglobin (Continued):

INTERPRETATION:

It is important to identify an increase in serum, plasma or urine hemoglobin to aid in the diagnosis of hemolytic anemia. Elevated hemoglobin occurs in various hemolytic states. One must exclude the presence of erythrocytes by microscopy. Myoglobin may also cause a darker serum, plasma or urine and is soluble in 80 percent saturated ammonium sulfate solution while hemoglobin is insoluble. One may differentiate hemoglobin from myoglobin by an electrophoretic separation.

THERMOLABILE HEMOGLOBIN

PRINCIPLE: The hemoglobin present in the cells of a Heinz Body hemolytic anemia is unstable and precipitates out of the hemolysate when exposed to heat.

SPECIMEN: 5.0 ml. whole blood from patient and control, heparinized, but may use any anticoagulant.

EQUIPMENT AND REAGENTS:

1. Normal Saline

2. Phosphate Buffer, pH 7.4, 0.1 M.
   Use Stock A 0.5 M KH_2PO_4 and Stock B 0.5 M Na_2HPO_4. Dilute each 1:5 with distilled water. Use 3.8 ml. of Stock A and 16.2 ml. of Stock B, combine together mixing well. Check the pH as it should be 7.4 and then dilute to 40 ml. with distilled water.

3. 50°C. Waterbath

PROCEDURE:

1. Place 1.0 ml. of blood in a 12 ml. centrifuge tube.

2. Centrifuge and discard serum.

3. Wash cells 2 times in 10 ml. normal saline.

4. Add distilled water to 5.0 ml. line.

5. Lyse cells by gentle mixing.

6. Add 5.0 ml. working buffer and mix.

7. Centrifuge tubes for 10 minutes at 3000 rpm.

8. Carfully remove upper 2.0 ml. of hemolysate and place in another tube.

9. Incubate the 2.0 ml. portions at 50°C. for 1 to 3 hours.

Thermolabile Hemoglobin (Continued):

10. Observe for a flocculent precipitate.

NORMAL VALUES: No Precipitate.
Positive Thermolabile Hemoglobin shows a flocculent precipitate within 10 minutes which increases over the next two hours.

REFERENCE: Dacie, J. V. et al: "Hereditary Heinz-Body Anemia", Brit. J. Hemat. 10:388, 1964.

INTERPRETATION:

Less than 1 percent of normal hemoglobin will precipitate when exposed to a temperature of 50°C. for one to three hours. The hemoglobin of a Heinz-Body type hemolytic anemia will precipitate during this exposure to 50°C. for one to three hours.

HEMOLYTIC SCREEN
FOR HEMOLYTIC ANEMIA

PRINCIPLE: To screen for possible causes of a hemolytic anemia.
Those that are 1) not primarily of intrinsic defects of a congenital
or acquired; 2) spherocytic or non-spherocytic nature.

SPECIMEN: 25 ml. clotted blood

EQUIPMENT AND REAGENTS:

1. Sterile 20 or 30 cc. syringes, plastic or siliconized

2. Thin-walled Needle, 19 gauge

3. 16 x 100 mm. Tubes at 37°C.

4. Sterile 25 ml. Erlenmeyer Flasks
    Containing 5 glass beads about 5mm. in diameter.

5. 37°C. Waterbath

6. 0.5% Methyl Violet in normal saline
    Filter prior to use.

7. Saline, 37°C. and 20°C.

8. 0.2 N. HCl

9. Coombs Sera

10. Anti-nongamma Sera

11. Glass slides and Coverslips

12. Micro Hematocrit blue-tipped Tubes and Centrifuge

13. Drabkin's Cyanmethemoglobin Solution

14. Sterile 5 cc. Screw-topped Vials

15. About 12 10 x 75 mm. Tubes

Hemolytic Screen (Continued):

SAMPLE COLLECTION:

1. Draw 25 ml. (15 ml. minimum) of blood.

2. Place 20 ml. into the two 16 x 100 mm. tubes and keep at 37°C. until clotted. Centrifuge and remove serum.

3. Defibrinate 5.0 ml. using sterile technique.

4. Place about 2.0 ml. of the sterile defibrinated blood in the sterile screw-topped vial and incubate for 48 hours at 37°C.

PROCEDURE:

I. HEINZ BODIES
    1. Place 2 drops of whole blood from the remaining defibrinated sample in a 10 x 75 mm. tube.

    2. Add 4 drops filtered 0.5% methyl violet stain and mix.

    3. Let sit 5 to 10 minutes and place a small drop on a glass slide and coverslip.

    4. Examine under oil immersion for Heinz Bodies.

II. COOMBS AND NON-GAMMA COOMBS
    1. The remaining defibrinated blood is placed in a 10 x 75 mm. tube, centrifuged, and the cells washed 3 times with 20°C. normal saline.

    2. Make a 2% suspension of some of the RBC.

    3. Put 2 drops of 2% RBC in each of two small tubes and fill with saline. Centrifuge and decant all the saline.

    4. Add 2 drops of Coombs sera to one tube and 2 drops anti-non-gamma Coombs sera to the other tube. Mix.

    5. Centrifuge lightly (1000 rpm for 15 seconds).

    6. Read for agglutination using a microscope. If positive, run a titer.

III. COMPLETE ANTIBODIES

Hemolytic Screen (Continued):

To perform test, use patient's serum from the clot. Use a 50 percent suspension of the 37°C. saline-washed cells.

Tube	1	2	3	4	5	6
Serum	0.5	0.5	0.5	0.5	0.5	0.5
1 Drop 0.2 N. HCl	0	0	+	+	0	0
1 Drop RBC	+	+	+	+	+	+

Incubation Time	Centrifuge Immediately	37°C. 90 Min.	37°C. 90 Min.	20°C. 90 Min.	4°C.* 90 Min.	4°C. 30 Min. 37°C. 60 Min.

1. Centrifuge all tubes lightly (1000 rpm for 15 seconds).

2. Compare serum to serum of Tube No. 1 for hemolysis.

3. Tap cells gently and observe for agglutination

4.* If positive for cold agglutinin titer.

IV. REPEAT HEINZ BODY PREP. ON 48 HOUR INCUBATED BLOOD

V. AUTOHEMOLYSIS - AFTER 48 HOURS INCUBATION

1. Determine the whole blood hemoglobin using 0.02 ml. blood in 5.0 ml. of Drabkins

2. Determine the microhemocrit.

3. Centrifuge remaining blood.

4. Place 0.2 ml. serum in 5.0 ml. of Drabkins.

5. Read whole blood and serum hemoglobins using the Coleman Jr. Spectrophotometer at a wavelength of 540 nm. Read O.D.

6. CALCULATIONS:

$$\% \text{ Autohemolysis} = \frac{100 - PCV \times O.D. \text{ Serum}}{O.D. \text{ Whole Blood} \times 10}$$

NOTES AND PRECAUTIONS:

1. Serum should be clotted at 37°C. and cells washed with 37°C. saline to avoid any influence from a cold agglutinin.

Hemolytic Screen (Continued):

2. Parts I., II., and III may be done on blood drawn at night or on weekends if it is absolutely necessary; however, studying stored red cells is not the best set of conditions.

3. When studying RBC's using the methyl violet stain for Heinz Bodies, the serum must be present to prevent massive crenation and agglutination of the RBC.

REFERENCE: Cartwright, G.: DIAGNOSTIC LABORATORY HEMATOLOGY 4th. Ed., Williams & Wilkins, Baltimore, pg. 275, 1968.

RESULTS AND INTERPRETATIONS:

I. Heinz Bodies
Heinz Bodies may be present in patients who have been splenectomized, are on certain drugs, are G-6-PD deficient or have a Heinz Body hemolytic anemia. If Heinz Bodies are not present initially but are apparent after 48 hour incubation, an abnormal hemoglobin may be present.

Care must be taken not to confuse Heinz Bodies with Howell-Jolly Bodies or inclusion bodies from Hemoglobin H. Both of these are visible on a Wright's stained smear.

II. Complete Antibodies

1. Control may have some agglutination present if a cold agglutinin with a wide thermal range is present.

2. 37°C. hemolysis here and not in No. 3 is indicative of a rare warm hemolysin. Agglutination here and not in No. 5 is indicative of a rare warm agglutinin.

3. 37°C. + Acid. Hemolysis here greater than in No. 2 is indicative of PNH. Confirming test should be done. Agglutination is same as for No. 2. Optimal conditions for PNH are 37°C., pH about 6.5 to 6.8, complement, calcium and magnesium.

4. 20°C. + Acid. Hemolysis here greater than that present in No. 3 (or No. 2), is indicative of a cold hemolysin. Optimal conditions are 20 to 26°C., acid and complement. Confirming test should be done. Agglutination may be due to a cold agglutinin with a wide thermal range.

5. 4°C. Hemolysis is probably a cold hemolysin, but this is not

Hemolytic Screen (Continued):

an optimal temperature. Agglutination is due to a cold agglutinin and must be titered using doubling dilutions of patient's sera in saline. See Method. Normals may have a titer of 1:64. Titers in the range of 512 to 2000 are probably due to infection, cold agglutinin disease rarely titers 8000 to 1×10^6. Often the higher the titer, the wider the thermal amplitude.

6. 4^0 and 37^0C. Hemolysis here is due to the rare cold-fixing warm hemolysin Donath-Landsteiner antibody. A confirming test must be done. Agglutination is probably a cold agglutinin which did not dissipate at 37^0C.

III. Autohemolysis
If increased, the complete test must be done to distinguish hereditary spherocytosis, hemolytic anemia, Dacie Types I, II, and III. See Methods.

COLD HEMOLYSIN SCREEN FOR HEMOLYTIC ANEMIA

PRINCIPLE: Serum with high titer cold agglutin antibody may also cause a cold hemolysin. Optimum pH for lysis is 6.5 to 6.8 at 20°C. in the presence of complement.

SPECIMEN: 5.0 ml. defibrinated blood and 10 ml. whole blood clotted at 37°C.

REAGENTS AND EQUIPMENT:

1. Normal Saline

2. 0.2 N. HCl

3. Centrifuge

4. Serofuge

5. 37°C. Waterbath

PROCEDURE:

1. Separate defibrinated RBC and serum.

2. Wash RBC 3 times with normal saline.

3. Make a 50% suspension of RBC in normal saline.

4. Separate clot and serum.

5. Label six test tubes (1 - 6) and follow procedure as directed below:

Tube	1	2	3	4	5	6
Patient Serum	0.5 ml.	0.5 ml.	0.5 ml.	0.5 ml.	0.5 ml.	0.5 ml
0.2 N. HCl	-	-	1 Drop	1 Drop	-	-
50% Patient's RBC	1 Drop	1 Drop	1 Drop	1 Drop	1 Drop	1 Drop
Incubation	Cent.	37°C.	37°C.	20°C.	4°C.	20°C.
	Immed.	90 Min.	90 Min.	90 Min.	90 Min.	90 Min

Centrifuge at 1000 rpm for 2 minutes.
Examine for lysis.

Results	0	0	0	+	∓	0
	Cont.					Cont.

174

Cold Hemolysin Screen for Hemolytic Anemia (Continued):

REFERENCE: Cartwright, G.:   DIAGNOSTIC LABORATORY HEMATOLOGY   4th.
             Ed., Williams & Wilkins, Baltimore, pgs. 274-275, 1965.

INTERPRETATION:

See Interpretation Section of the Cold Agglutinin Test on page 59.

HEINZ-EHRLICH BODIES

PRINCIPLE: Heinz-Ehrlich bodies are prominent in those hemolytic anemias produced by agents toxic to erythrocytes and in hemolytic disease of the newborn. They are the result of hereditary G-6-PD deficiency which is an intrinsic biochemical defect of the erythrocyte.

The Heinz-Ehrlich bodies are seen by phase microscopy or after staining with methyl violet or other basic dyes.

EQUIPMENT AND REAGENTS:

1. WBC pipette

2. Glass slides

3. Methyl Violet Solution
   Methyl violet   0.5 gm.
   Saline   100.0 ml.
   Filter before using.

COMMENTS ON PROCEDURE:

Heinz-Ehrlich bodies disappear if slide is fixed with either methyl or ethyl alcohol. Heinz-Ehrlich bodies are never found in reticulocytes.

PROCEDURE:

1. Mix equal volumes of blood and the dye solution in a WBC pipette.

2. Let stand for 15 minutes.

3. Mix and make smears.

4. Examine under oil for Heinz-Ehrlich bodies.

REFERENCES:

1. Miale, John B.: LABORATORY MEDICINE HEMATOLOGY 4th. Ed. C. V. Mosby Co., St. Louis, pg. 1227, 1972.

2. Fertman, M. H. and Fertman, M. B.: "Toxic Anemia and Heinz Bodies". Medicine 34:131, 1955.

Heinz-Ehrlich Bodies (Continued):

INTERPRETATION:

Heinz Bodies represent denatured precipitated hemoglobin and may be seen in certain hemoglobinopathies as well as in G-6-PD in the presence of oxidant drugs. A few are seen in splenectomized patients.

DRUGS AND INTERCURRENT ILLNESSES
KNOWN TO INDUCE HEMOLYTIC ANEMIA
IN G-6-PD DEFICIENT INDIVIDUALS

I. SPECIFIC DRUGS
Analgesics
Acetanilid
Acetophenetidin
Acetylsalicylic Acid

Antimalarials
Chloroquine
Pamaquine
Primaquine
Quinine

Nitrofurans
Nitrofurantoin
Nitrofurazone

Sulfonamides
N2 acetylsulfanilamide
Salicylazosulfapyridine
Sulfacetamide
Sulfamethoxypyridazine
Sulfanilamide
Sulfapyridine
Sulfisoxazole

II. MISCELLANEOUS DRUGS
Chloramphenicol
Dilantin
Dimercaprol (BAL)
Fava Beans
Isoniazid
Methylene Blue
Naphthalene
Para-aminosalicylic acid
Phenylhydrazine
Probenecid
Quinidine
Streptomycin
Vitamin K (water soluble analogues)

III. INTERCURRENT ILLNESSES
Cholecystitis
Chronic renal failure
Diabetic acidosis
Hepatitis
Infectious mononucleosis
Pneumococcal pneumonia
Septicemias

If drug-induced hemolysis is suspected, tests for Heinz bodies should be carried out as soon as possible since the cells in which hemoglobin has been precipitated disappear from the circulation within hours to days after the toxic drug exposure.

This is a more accurate means of documenting drug-induced hemolysis than G-6-PD assay. The latter merely demonstrates the potential susceptibility of the patient whereas Heinz Body preparation demonstrates the hemolytic event.

HEMOSIDERIN
(Prussian Blue Reaction)

PRINCIPLE: Colloidal iron oxide, hemosiderin, can be readily detected in urine sediment by the blue colored granules formed in reaction with potassium ferrocyanide (Prussian Blue Reaction).

REAGENTS:

1. HCl, 1%

2. Potassium Ferrocyanide, 2%, aqueous
   Rinse tube with HCl before running test.

PROCEDURE:

1. Centrifuge 10 ml. of urine at three-quarters speed for 10 minutes. Decant supernatant. To sediment add 10 ml. HCl - potassium ferrocyanide solution. 5 ml. HCl and 5 ml. potassium ferrocyanide are prepared just before use.

2. Suspend sediment in solution and let stand for 10 minutes.

3. Centrifuge and decant supernatant.

4. Examine sediment on glass slide with coverslip.

5. Report:

   a). Positive if intracellular granules* are present.
       Positive if only extracellular granules* are present.
   b). Report as "No Intracellular Granules Present".
   c). Negative if no granules* present.

ABNORMAL VALUE: Hemosiderin granules will appear blue and may be found in casts and epithelial cells.

REFERENCE: Page and Culver: A SYLLABUS OF LABORATORY EXAMINATIONS IN CLINICAL DIAGNOSIS, Harvard Univ. Press, pp. 85, 312, 318 - 319, 1961.

---

* Don't confuse Prussian Blue Reacting artifacts with granules.

Hemosiderin (Continued):

INTERPRETATION:

Hemosiderin will be found in renal tubule cells and casts in patients who have hemolytic anemia with subsequent hemoglobinuria and deposition of hemoglobin in renal tubular cells. Patients with hemochromatosis will have prussian blue stainable iron in renal tubular cells and epithelial casts in their urine.

HETEROPHILE
(Rapid Slide Differential Test - Monospot)

PRINCIPLE: Anti-sheep red cell or anti-horse red cell agglutinins
may be of three types; the agglutinin of infectious mononucleosis,
the agglutinin of serum sickness, and the agglutinin of a non-specific
type. This test indicates whether agglutinins are of the heterophile
type or not. Agglutinins of the serum sickness type are adsorbed by
both guinea pig kidney antigen and by the beef cell antigens. Agglutinins of the infectious mononucleosis type are adsorbed by the beef
cell antigens but not by the guinea pig kidney antigen. Agglutinins
of the non-specific type are adsorbed by the guinea pig kidney antigen and may or may not be adsorbed by the beef cell antigen. The
essence of the following test is that all of the agglutinins except
those of the heterophile of infectious mononucleosis are adsorbed
out of serum by guinea pig kidney antigen.

REAGENTS:

1. Monospot Reagent Kit
   This kit contains reagents for 20 tests. The following reagents
   are provided.
   a). Guinea Pig Kidney Antigen Suspension
       Reagent No. 1 (White Label); store at 2 to 8°C. and mix well
       before using.

   b). Beef Erythrocyte Stroma Antigen Suspension
       Reagent No. 2 (Blue Label); store at 2 to 8°C. Mix well.

   c). Horse Red Cells
       "Indicator Cells" preserved in sodium citrate. Store at
       2 to 8°C. These are used rather than sheep cells due to
       their greater sensitivity to the presence of the agglutinins.

   d). Positive Heterophile Control Serum
       Store at 2 to 8°C. Specimen is a weak positive reaction.

   e). Glass Slides and Calibrated Capillary Pipettes
       These are also supplied in the kit.

SPECIMEN: Two drops (0.10 ml.) of serum or plasma. The serum does
not need to be inactivated.

180

Heterophile - Monospot Test

COMMENTS ON PROCEDURE:

1. All reagents should be stored at 2 to 8°C. and should not be frozen.

2. Do not pick up or move the slide during the reaction period.

3. When the results of the spot test are questionable, they should be checked with the sheep agglutinin differential test.

4. The slides should be washed under running water; do not use detergent.

PROCEDURE:

1. The positive control serum provided in the kit is a "weak positive" reaction. The control serum should be used to check the reagents upon arrival in the laboratory and periodically during the dated life of the test. Use the control just as you would a patient serum specimen.

2. The Monospot kit supplies slides which have two squares, labeled No. I and No. II. Place on level surface under direct light source.

3. Invert the Indicator Cells several times and deliver 10 lambda of the cells to a corner of each square on a slide.

4. Place one drop of thoroughly mixed guinea pig kidney antigen (Reagent No. 1 - White Label) in the center of the square marked I.

5. Place one drop of thoroughly mixed beef erythrocyte antigen (Reagent No. 2 - Blue Label) in the center of the square marked II.

6. Add one drop of serum to the center of each square. Avoiding the Indicator Cells, mix the contents of the center of each square at least ten times with an applicator stick.

7. Blend in the Indicator cells thoroughly and evenly over the entire surface of each square.

8. Leaving the slide perfectly still, observe for agglutination for no longer than one minute after the final mixing.

Heterophile - Monospot Test (Continued):

RESULTS: If the agglutination is <u>stronger on</u> the <u>left side</u> of the slide (Box I), the test is considered <u>positive</u>.

If the agglutination is <u>stronger on</u> the <u>right side</u> of the slide (Box II), the test is considered <u>negative</u>.

REFERENCE: Miale, John B.: LABORATORY MEDICINE HEMATOLOGY 4th. Ed. C. V. Mosby Co., St. Louis, pg. 917, 1972.

INTERPRETATION:

The mononucleosis spot test is an excellent screening test for infectious mononucleosis. When we see patients with lymphadenopathy, we should consider infectious mononucleosis or other causes for lymphadenopathy. We must not place too much emphasis on a positive mononucleosis spot screening test result if other evidence, such as the routine blood smear or a sheep cell heterophil agglutination absorption test, does not suggest the diagnosis of infectious mononucleosis.

The mononucleosis spot test is a very sensitive test for infectious mononucleosis. Horse agglutinins are generally in higher titer than sheep cell agglutinins in patients with infectious mononucleosis. The spot test has also been found to yield positive results in patient with Burkitt's lymphoma, Hodgkin's disease, lymphocytic lymphoma, viral hepatitis, pancreatic cancer metastatic to the liver, and in test kits containing old horse red blood cells. In patients with clinical lymphoreticular disease not typical of infectious mononucleosis, a positive spot test result should be viewed with caution, and further evaluation and follow-up carried out.

HETEROPHILE
(Presumptive Test)

PRINCIPLE: The presence in sera of heterophilic agglutinins for sheep cells at a titer of 1:56 or greater is considered a positive presumptive test for infectious mononucleosis. A differential test is then done to absorb out all agglutinins which are due to serum sickness or are non-specific in origin. (See Differential Test.)

SPECIMEN: 0.2 ml. unhemolyzed serum which has been inactivated at 56°C. for 30 minutes. Hemolyzed serum is unsatisfactory.

EQUIPMENT AND REAGENTS:

1. Normal Saline, 0.85% NaCl

2. Sheep Red Blood Cells, 2% cell suspension

3. Waterbath, 56°C.

4. Test Tubes, disposable, 12 x 75 mm.

5. Centrifuge Tube, graduated
   For making sheep cell suspension

COMMENTS ON PROCEDURE:

1. Preliminary reading may be done after 15 minutes, but, the final reading should not be recorded until after 2 hours incubation.

2. Inactivation of serum must be for 30 minutes at 56°C. $\pm$ $\frac{1}{2}$°.

PROCEDURE:

1. Set up a row of 11 test tubes in a rack.

2. Add 0.4 ml. of normal saline to the first tube, and 0.25 ml. to the other ten tubes.

3. Add 0.1 ml. of inactivated serum to the first tube, mix the contents thoroughly, and transfer 0.25 ml. to the second tube. Continue mixing and transferring 0.25 ml. through the tenth tube. Discard the excess 0.25 ml. from the tenth tube.

Heterophile - Presumptive Test (Continued):

4. Tube No. 11 is the negative control and should contain only 0.25 ml. normal saline.

5. Add 0.1 ml. of the sheep cell suspension to all tubes and shake the rack to mix the contents of the tubes thoroughly. (See dilution chart for final dilutions.)

6. Allow the tubes to stand at room temperature for 2 hours.

7. Shake the rack of tubes to resuspend the sedimented red cells. Record the results; if no clumping is visible to the naked eye, place the tube horizontally on the stage of the microscope and examine with the low power objective.

Tube	Ml. Saline	Ml. Serum	Serum Dilutions	2% Sheep Cells Ml.	Final Serum Dilution
1	0.4	0.1	1:5	0.1	1:7
2	0.25	0.25 of 1:5	1:10	0.1	1:14
3	0.25	0.25 of 1:10	1:20	0.1	1:28
4	0.25	0.25 of 1:20	1:40	0.1	1:56
5	0.25	0.25 of 1:40	1:80	0.1	1:112
6	0.25	0.25 of 1:80	1:160	0.1	1:224
7	0.25	0.25 of 1:160	1:320	0.1	1:448
8	0.25	0.25 of 1:320	1:640	0.1	1:896
9	0.25	0.25 of 1:640	1:1280	0.1	1:1792
10	0.25	0.25 of 1:1280	1:2560	0.1	1:3584
11	0.25			0.1	Neg. Control

NORMAL VALUES:

A titer of 1:56 or higher is usually suggestive of infectious mononucleosis and the differential test is indicated. Anti-sheep red cell agglutinins in titers up to 1:56 may be found in normal persons.

REFERENCES:

1. Difco: SUPPLEMENTARY LITERATURE, Difco Laboratories, Detroit, 1966.

2. Davidsohn and Henry: TODD-SANFORD CLINICAL DIAGNOSIS BY LABORATORY METHODS, 14th Ed., W. B. Saunders Co., Phil. pg. 285, 1969.

Heterophile - Presumptive Test (Continued):

INTERPRETATION:

Various other conditions may be associated with an elevated presumptive titer of anti-sheep red cell agglutinins. These conditions are Burkitt's lymphoma, infectious hepatitis, post-immunization with vaccines produced in horses, and conditions associated with the EB virus.

HETEROPHIL
(Differential Test)

PRINCIPLE: Patients with serum having a heterophile presumptive
test titer of 1:56 or greater may have one of three types of agglutinins present; antisheep agglutinin of infectious mononucleosis, anti-
sheep agglutinins of serum sickness, and the non-specific type of
antisheep agglutinins found in serum of normal people. The following
differential adsorption test is used to differentiate between these
three types of agglutinins. Agglutinins of the serum sickness type
are adsorbed by both guinea pig kidney antigen and by the beef cell
antigens. Agglutinins of the infectious mononucleosis type are
adsorbed by the beef cell antigens, but, not by the guinea pig kidney
antigen. Agglutinins of the non-specific type are adsorbed by the
guinea pig kidney antigen and may or may not be adsorbed by the beef
cell antigen.

SPECIMEN: 0.5 ml. of unhemolyzed serum which has been inactivated
at 56°C. for 30 minutes. Hemolyzed serum is not acceptable.

REAGENTS AND EQUIPMENT:

1. Guinea Pig Kidney Antigen, Bacto Reagent #0476, 5.0 ml., dessicate
   Reconstitute the vial by adding 5.0 ml. volumetrically of distilled water. Dessicated vials should be stored at 2 to 10°C.

2. Beef Cell Antigen, Bacto Reagent #0475, 5.0 ml., dessicated
   Reconstitute the vial by adding 5.0 ml. volumetrically of distilled water. Store the dessicated vials at 2 to 10°C.

3. Normal Saline, 0.85% NaCl

4. Sheep Red Cells, 2% cell suspension

5. Waterbath, 56°C. $\pm$ ½°
   Temperature is critical.

6. Test Tubes, 12 x 75 mm., disposable

COMMENTS ON PROCEDURE:

1. It is essential that vials of antigen be well shaken so that the
   suspension is even.

Heterophile - Differential Test (Continued):

2. The antigen suspension should be pipetted with a large bore, 5.0 ml. pipette so that the particles do not aggregate at the tip and clog the pipette.

3. The antigen suspension should be pipetted promptly; the larger aggregates tend to settle out rapidly in a 5.0 ml. pipette.

4. The differential test should only be done in the presence of a positive presumptive test (i.e. titer of 1:56 or greater).

PROCEDURE:

1. Place two 12 x 75 mm. test tubes into a rack; one labeled "Guinea Pig Kidney", and one labeled "Beef Cell". A set should be prepared for each patient serum to be tested.

2. Shake each vial of antigen suspension thoroughly and place one ml. into the appropriately prepared tube from Step No. 1.

3. To each tube containing antigen, add 0.2 ml. of the patient's inactivated serum. Shake well.

4. Allow the serum to be exposed to the antigen suspension for three minutes at room temperature.

5. Centrifuge all tubes at 1500 rpm for 10 minutes.

6. Carefully transfer the supernatant fluid to clean test tubes with a capillary pipette.

7. Prepare two sets of eleven test tubes each, for every patient being analyzed. Label one set "Guinea Pig"; label the other set "Beef Cell".

8. Add 0.25 ml. of normal saline to all except the first tube in each set of 11 test tubes (prepared in Step No. 7).

9. Add 0.25 ml. of the supernatant fluid from Step No. 6 to the first tube in each set of appropriately labeled tubes.

10. Add 0.25 ml. of the supernatant fluid from Step No. 6 to the second tube in each set and mix well.

11. Transfer 0.25 ml. of the fluid from tube No. 2 to tube No. 3 in each set and continue mixing and transferring serially through

Heterophile - Differential Test (Continued):

the tenth tube. Discard 0.25 ml. from the tenth tube. The elevei th tube is a negative control. See the final serum dilutions on chart.

12. Add 0.1 ml. of a 2% sheep cell suspension to all tubes and shake well. Incubate test at room temperature for two hours.

13. After fifteen minutes shake all tubes to resuspend the sediment, and observe for clumping. Final reading should be made after two hours. If no clumping is visible to the naked eye, observe under the low power objective of the microscope. The titer is the reciprocal of the highest dilution showing clumping. See dilution chart.

DILUTION CHART:

Tube	Ml. Saline	Adsorbed Serum Supernatant Ml.	Serum Dilutions	Ml. Sheep Cells	Final Adsorbe Serum Diluti(
1		0.25	1:5	0.1	1:7
2	0.25	0.25	1:10	0.1	1:14
3	0.25	0.25 of 1:10	1:20	0.1	1:28
4	0.25	0.25 of 1:20	1:40	0.1	1:56
5	0.25	0.25 of 1:40	1:80	0.1	1:112
6	0.25	0.25 of 1:80	1:160	0.1	1:224
7	0.25	0.25 of 1:160	1:320	0.1	1:448
8	0.25	0.25 of 1:320	1:640	0.1	1:896
9	0.25	0.25 of 1:640	1:1280	0.1	1:1792
10	0.25	0.25 of 1:1280	1:2560	0.1	1:3584
11	0.25			0.1	Neg. Control

NORMAL VALUES:

	Titer of Unadsorbed Serum	Titer After Adsorption With:	
		Guinea Pig Antigen	Beef Cell Antigen
Neither Inf. Mono. nor Serum Sickness	0 to 1:112	0	±
Serum Sickness	1:56 to 1:224	0	0
Infectious Mono- nucleosis	1:28 to 1:3584 or higher	+	0

REFERENCES:

1. Difco, SUPPLEMENTARY LITERATURE, Difco Laboratories, Detroit, 1966.

Heterophile - Differential Test (Continued):

2. Davidsohn and Henry: TODD-SANFORD CLINICAL DIAGNOSIS BY
   LABORATORY METHODS, 14th Ed. W. B. Saunders Co., Phil.,
   pg. 286, 1969.

INTERPRETATION:

This test should be performed when the monospot test or heterophile
differential test is positive to differentiate infectious mononucleosis from other conditions which may cause a false positive monospot
test or presumptive test. See Interpretation of both of these procedures.

The patient has infectious mononucleosis if there is no absorption
of the serum anti-EB antibody by the extract of guinea pig kidney
and thus, no decrease in the antibody titer by two tubes. In contrast, conditions which are not infectious mononucleosis will have
a fall in titer by more than two tubes after absorption by guinea
pig antigen. The antibody titer in infectious mononucleosis falls
to 0 after absorption by the antigen of beef erythrocytes.

INTRAERYTHROCYTIC INCLUSIONS
(Reaction with Various Staining Techniques)

	Wright-Giemsa	Prussian Blue (Iron)	Crystal Violet	Brilliant Crystal Violet
Pappenheimer (Iron)	POSITIVE	POSITIVE	NEGATIVE	NEGATIVE
Howell-Jolly	POSITIVE	NEGATIVE	POSITIVE	POSITIVE
RNA Reticulocytes	NEGATIVE	NEGATIVE	POSITIVE	POSITIVE
Heinz-Ehrlich Precipitated Hemoglobin	NEGATIVE	NEGATIVE	POSITIVE	POSITIVE
Hemoglobin H	NEGATIVE	NEGATIVE	NEGATIVE	POSITIVE
Basophilic Stippling	POSITIVE	NEGATIVE	NEGATIVE	NEGATIVE
Cabot Rings	POSITIVE	NEGATIVE	POSITIVE	POSITIVE

REFERENCE: Miale, John B.: LABORATORY MEDICINE HEMATOLOGY 4th. Ed. C. V. Mosby Co., St. Louis, pg. 655-656, 1972.

INTERPRETATION:

Pappenheimer Bodies are iron granules in siderocytes while Howell-Jolly Bodies represent portions of the nucleus of a normoblast. Their presence in the peripheral blood results after splenectomy. The absence of a functional spleen results in the lack of the normal pitting function of the spleen. Reticulocytes contain stranded or punctate ribonucleic acid. Heinz-Ehrlich Bodies represent precipitated hemoglobin induced by oxidation of hemoglobin in the G-6-PD deficient or absent red blood cells. The oxidation of the hemoglobin is induced by drugs or intercurrent diseases, such as viral hepatitis, diabetic ketoacidosis, or bacterial infections, in which oxidants are present in the blood. Hemoglobin H is unstable and precipitates. Cabot Rings represent the rim of the nucleus of the normoblast and are especially found in pernicious anemia.

^{59}IRON PLASMA CLEARANCE,
ERYTHROCYTE INCORPORATION
AND PLASMA IRON TURNOVER

PRINCIPLE: This procedure is designed to measure the metabolism of iron by the red blood cell and the plasma clearance of iron. Radioactive iron is injected intravenously. Radioactive iron is injected intravenously. The rate of disappearance of radioactivity from the plasma and the subsequent increase in activity in the red blood cells are determined. The heart, liver, spleen, and sacral bones are scanned for iron incorporation and utilization.

SPECIMEN: 30 ml. of heparanized blood is collected under sterile conditions. A serum sample should also be obtained to determine serum iron and iron binding capacity.

REAGENTS AND EQUIPMENT:

1. ^{59}Iron, 10 Microcuries

2. Evans Blue Dye

3. Scintillation Counter

4. Microhematocrit Centrifuge and Reader

PROCEDURE:

1. Obtain 30 ml. of heparinized blood under sterile conditions and serum for a serum iron and TIBC determination.

2. Incubate 10 microcuries of ^{59}iron with 11 ml. of plasma for 30 minutes.

3. Reinject 10 ml. of the plasma intravenously into the patient.

4. Save 1.0 ml. of the incubated plasma for a zero time calculation.

5. Perform a blood volume determination with the Evans Blue Dye.

6. Obtain 2.0 ml. heparinized plasma from the patient at 15, 30, 45 minutes, 1 hour, 3 hours, 6 hours and 2 to 14 days after injection.

^{59}Iron Plasma Clearance (Continued):

7. CALCULATIONS:

1.0 ml. of saved plasma ^{59}Fe is diluted to 250 ml. and counted. With the calculated blood volume, the amount of radioactivity at zero time can be calculated. The subsequent values of radioactivity obtained are plotted either as absolute values on regular graph paper, or as a percent of the zero value on logarithm paper.

Zero time CPM/ml. plasma =

$$\frac{\text{CPM of diluted specimen/ml. x dilution x ml. injected}}{\text{Plasma Volume (ml.)}}$$

RESULTS:

1. Time at which the curve reaches one-half the value at time zero is the "Plasma Disappearance ½ (PT½)".

2. Plasma iron turnover (PIT) is determined as follows:

$$PIT = \frac{(0.693) \text{ (plasma volume in ml.) (serum Fe ug/ml.) 24 x 60}}{PT½ \text{ (minutes)}}$$

$$0.693 = \log_e$$

$$PIT \text{ (mg./100 ml. blood/day)} = \frac{\text{Serum Iron x Plasma Crit.}}{PT½ \text{ x 100}}$$

REFERENCE: Pollycove, M. and Mortimer, R.: "Quantitative Determinati of Iron Kinetics and Hemoglobin Synthesis in Human Subject J. Clin. Invest. 40:753, 1961.

INTERPRETATION:

The amount of ^{59}Fe that is metabolized in the red cells may be calculated by obtaining daily samples of whole blood from the patient. The iron utilization usually shows a rise at a relatively rapid rate for 2 to 7 days. Following that period, the radioactivity in erythrocytes remains at a relatively stable level. Normally there is 70 to 95 percent utilization in about 8 to 10 days.

	PIT	PT½	INCORPORATION
Iron Deficiency	Increased	Shortened	Increased
Chronic Disease	Increased	Shortened	Increased
Polycythemia	Increased	Shortened	Variable
Hemolytic Anemia	Increased	Shortened	Variable
Aplastic Anemia	Decreased	Prolonged	Decreased
Ineffective Erythro-poiesis	Increased	Shortened	Decreased

[59]Iron Plasma Clearance (Continued):

	PIT	PT½	INCORPORATION
Normal Value:	0.65±	60-120'	70-95%

Incorporation is variable in hemolytic anemia. The increased rate of destruction of red cells may never allow the maximal incorporation to be measured.

IRON STAIN FOR BONE MARROW

PRINCIPLE: The storage of iron can be estimated by the amount of hemosiderin present in the bone marrow. The hemosiderin gives a positive Prussian Blue reaction.

EQUIPMENT AND REAGENTS:

1. 10% Potassium Ferrocyanide (W/V)
   Weigh out 10 gm. of potassium ferrocyanide and dilute to volume in a 100 ml. volumetric flask with deionized water.

2. 20% HCL (V/V)
   Add 20 ml. concentrated HCl to a 100 ml. volumetric flask and dilute to volume with distilled water.

3. Approximate 0.2% Aqueous Safranin Solution
   Stock Safranin is 2.5% in 95% alcohol. (This is diluted to about 0.2% in water for the Working Solution.)

4. Coplin Staining Jars

COMMENTS ON PROCEDURE:

1. It is unnecessary to fix smears in methanol for iron stain.

2. It is necessary to have a spicule on smear used for iron stain.

3. Run a positive control with each fresh mixture of iron stain.

4. Date control and check by microscope for iron.

PROCEDURE:

1. Stain smears for 30 minutes in freshly mixed solution of 30 ml. of 10% potassium ferrocyanide and 30 ml. of 20% HCl.

2. Wash with water.

3. Counterstain with 0.2% Safranin Solution 5 - 10 minutes.

4. Wash with water and air dry.

Iron Stain for Bone Marrow (Continued):

REFERENCE: Miale, John B.:   LABORATORY MEDICINE HEMATOLOGY   4th. Ed.,
C. V. Mosby Co., St. Louis, pg. 1214, 1972.

NORMAL VALUES AND INTERPRETATION:

The assessment of iron in the marrow is useful in the diagnosis of
iron deficiency. The reticuloendothelial cell in the marrow obtains
iron from transferrin and transfers iron to the developing normoblast.
In iron deficiency, a marked decrease or absence of iron is present
in the reticuloendothelial cells. In addition, stainable iron in
sideroblasts is decreased in iron deficiency anemia.

Increased iron is present in reticuloendothelial cells and sideroblasts in various disorders, such as hemachromatosis, hemolytic anemia,
sideroblastic anemia and aplastic anemia. A heavy accumulation of
iron in reticuloendothelial cells is found in the anemia of chronic
disease. Sideroblasts are normoblasts which contain one or more
iron granules while ring sideroblasts are normoblasts with a ring of
iron surrounding the nucleus and are usually associated with sideroblastic or ineffective erythropoiesis. The iron is present in mitochondria surrounding the nucleus.

Exogenous iron may contaminate the bone marrow iron stain and is
recognized by the iron not being in the plane of the smear.

SERUM IRON AND TOTAL IRON-BINDING CAPACITY

PRINCIPLE: Serum iron is bound to the protein transferrin in the
ferric form. It can be directly measured without protein precipitation, by complexing the reduced form (Fe^{+2}) with magnesium bathophenantroline sulfonate. The three important steps for the reaction
are: 1). Dissociation of ferric iron from transferrin, 2). Reduction of ferric iron to ferrous iron, and 3). Complexing with
iron complexing agent. The simplicity and sensitivity of the method
is worth mentioning, since the reaction occurs in one tube, without
the problem of incomplete recovery due to coprecipitation or lack
of filtrate clarity. The entire reaction is also irreversible,
insuring complete recovery.

(TRANSFERRIN) $(Fe^{+3})_2 \rightleftharpoons$ TRANSFERRIN + $2Fe^{+3} \longrightarrow Fe^{+2}$

(red) $Fe \overset{\beta}{\underset{\beta}{\overset{\beta}{\longleftarrow}}}$ $\longleftarrow$ 3β (BATHOPHENANTROLINE)

The total iron-binding capacity (TIBC) of serum is the sum of the
serum iron plus the ferric iron that combines with transferrin
following the addition of ferric iron to the serum. The excess
ferric iron is removed by adsorption with magnesium carbonate.

SPECIMEN: UNHEMOLYZED, pipettable 2.0 ml. of serum is needed to
run both serum iron and total iron-binding capacity. A diurnal
variation has been found, which in general is higher in the morning and lower in the afternoon. It is therefore recommended that
fasting blood specimens be drawn for the determination. The serum
is stable in the refrigerator for one week, and for several weeks
in the freezer.

EQUIPMENT AND REAGENTS:

1. Iron Blank Reagent
   0.1 M. Hydroxylamine (reducing agent) in acetate buffer at
   pH 4.0 Available from American Monitor, Kit # R5350 (for 60
   determinations). Stable indefinitely at room temperature.

2. Iron Color Reagent
   Magnesium bathophenantroline sulfonate. Available from American Monitor, Kit # 5350 (for 60 determinations). Stable indefinitely at room temperature.

Serum Iron (Continued):

3. Iron Binding Reagent
   For use in the determination or iron-binding capacity of serum.
   500 micrograms of Ferric Chloride per 100 ml. in 1/200th M.
   HCl with Redox Preservative. American Monitor Kit # 5350.

4. Iron Adsorbent
   $MgCO_3$ powder, supplied in capsules, one capsule for each TIBC
   Test. American Monitor Kit # 5350.

5. Iron Working Standard
   200 micrograms per 100 ml. Dissolved in HCl with preservative.
   American Monitor Kit # 5350.

6. Calibration Curve
   Stock Iron Standard, 20 mg%. (20,000 ug%.). Transfer 1.404 gm.
   ferrous ammonium sulfate hexahydrate (MW. 392), Fe $(NH_4)_2$
   $(SO_4)_2$. $6H_2O$ to a one liter volumetric flask. Dissolve in
   about 800 ml. of deionized water. Add 0.5 ml. of concentrated
   sulfuric acid, and dilute to the mark. This solution is stable.
   Working standards of 100, 200, 300, 400, and 500 ug%. can be
   made by diluting 0.5, 1.0, 1.5, 2.0, and 2.5 ml. of the stock
   standard to 100 ml. with acidified (HCl) deionized water respectively. pH should be around 2.4.

7. Gilford Spectrophotometer 300 N.

NOTE: The lot number of color and of blank reagent should be the
same. Do not mix lots.

GLASSWARE: Glass pipettes should be rinsed with dilute HCl (10 ml.
concentrated HCl, q.s. to about 500 ml.) and rinsed several times
with deionized water.

PROCEDURE:

Serum Iron

1. Using disposable culture tubes, 75 x 12 mm., set up a
   "Standard Blank" and two tubes for "Standard".

2. For each serum, set up a "Test" and "Serum Blank".

3. Controls are Hyland Normal and Hyland Abnormal.

Serum Iron (Continued):

4. Pipette 0.5 ml. of water to "Standard Blank".
   Pipette 0.5 ml. of Std. or Stds. (Calibration Curve) to
   "Standard".
   Add 0.5 ml. serum to both "Test" and "Serum Blank".

5. Add 1.6 ml. of Blank Reagent to "Standard Blank" and "Serum
   Blank".
   Add 1.6 ml. of Color Reagent to "Standards" and "Test".
   Cover all tubes with parafilm, and mix well.

6. Incubate all tubes at 37°C. for 5 minutes.

7. Set the machine at 0.000 absorbance with water and read
   absorbance of "Blanks", "Standards", and "Tests" at 535 nm.
   Final product should be read as soon as possible.

CALCULATIONS: $\dfrac{\text{O.D. Test}}{\text{O.D. Standard}}$ x   200   =   ug Fe/100 ml.

TIBC

1. Pipette 1.0 ml. of serum into a 12 ml. glass stoppered
   centrifuge tube.
   Controls are Hyland Normal and Hyland Abnormal.

2. Add 2.0 ml. of Iron-Binding Reagent. Mix well, and let
   stand for 5 minutes.

3. Add $MgCO_3$ (one capsule). Stopper, and mix by inversion for
   2 minutes.

4. Centrifuge for at least 20 minutes.

5. Run 0.5 ml. of supernatant in place of serum for test and
   blank in the above procedure.

CALCULATIONS: $\dfrac{\text{O.D. Test}}{\text{O.D. Standard}}$ x   600   =   TIBC in ug./100 m

$\%$ Saturation = $\dfrac{\text{Fe}}{\text{TIBC}}$ x   100

Serum Iron (Continued):

NORMAL VALUES:

Serum Iron
Men   —   80 - 160 ug./100 ml.
Women —   60 - 135 ug./100 ml.

TIBC
250 - 350 ug./100 ml.

PROCEDURE FOR ULTRAMICRO SERUM IRON AND TOTAL IRON-BINDING CAPACITY

Serum Iron

1. Using disposable 3.0 ml. A.A. cups, set up a "Standard
    Blank" and 2 cups for "Standard".

2. For each serum, set up a "Test" and a "Serum Blank". Run
    the same controls.

3. Using a pre-calibrated Hamilton syringe, deliver 0.5 ml. of
    Blank Reagent to the "Standard Blank" and to all the Serum
    Blanks. Rinse well with deionized water, then with the color
    reagent, and dispense the same amount (0.5 ml.) of Color
    Reagent to the cups marked "Standards" and "Tests".

4. Pipette 100 ul. of water to the "Standard Blank".
    Pipette 100 ul. of Standard or Standards (Calibration
    Curve) to Standards. 100 ul. of serum is added to both
    Test and Blank.

5. Incubate the same way, and read in the Gilford Spectro-
    photometer 300 N with the micro cuvette.

TIBC

1. Pipette 0.5 ml. of serum into a 12 ml. glass stoppered
    centrifuge tube. Use the same controls.

2. Add 1.0 ml. of Iron-Binding reagent. Mix well, and let
    stand for 5 minutes.

3. Add $MgCO_3$ (one-half capsule). Stopper, and mix by inversion
    for 2 minutes.

Serum Iron (Continued):

4. Centrifuge for 20 minutes.

5. Run 0.1 ml. of supernatant in place of serum for test and blank in the above procedure.

CALCULATIONS: The same.

REFERENCES:

1. Goodwin, J. F., Murphy, B., and Guilemette, M.: Direct Measurement of Serum Iron and Binding Capacity. Clin. Chem. 12:2, 1966.

2. Levy, A. C., and Vitacca, P.: Direct Determination and Binding Capacity of Serum Iron. Clin. Chem. 7:241, 1961.

3. Ramsay, W. N. M.: Plasma Iron. Advances in Clin. Chem. 1:1, 1958.

INTERPRETATION:

The most common cause for a low serum iron is blood loss which may be gross or occult, especially from the urogenital or gastrointes-tinal tract. Malnutrition or malabsorption may contribute to low serum iron. Gastrointestinal lesions which may cause iron deficiency anemia are esophageal varices, peptic ulcer, gastric carcinoma or carcinoma of the colon. Other causes for decreased serum iron are chronic infection and azotemia.

Elevated serum iron is found in hemolytic anemia and acute hepatitis. Iron is released from the red blood cells and necrotic liver. Hemo-chromatosis and siderochrestic anemia may be associated with an elevated serum iron.

An increased iron binding capacity or unsaturated capacity is found in iron deficiency anemia, while a decreased iron binding or saturated capacity is found in loss due to nephrosis, hemochroma-tosis, azotemia, hereditary transferrin deficiency, hemolytic anemia and siderochrestic anemia.

ISOCITRATE DEHYDROGENASE
(U.V. Methodology)

PRINCIPLE: Mammalian tissue contains two isocitrate dehydrogenase enzymes; the one which is of clinical interest is that enzyme linked to NADP. The enzyme shows molecular heterogeneity, with four distinct isoenzymes being separated following electrophoresis. The activity of I.C.D. in man is found in greatest concentration in the liver, then heart, tumors and muscle. Abnormal I.C.D. activity is best considered as a relatively sensitive indicator of hepatocellular damage. Elevations of serum I.C.D. may also be found with myocardial infarction, but not consistently so, due to the rapid denaturation or "clearing" of the heart isoenzyme fraction in the body. Red cells and platelets also display significant I.C.D. activity.

The spectrophotometric determination is based upon the reaction indicated beneath. The reduction of NADP to $NADPH_2$ is followed spectrophotometrically at 340 nm. or 366 nm. $NADPH_2$ is strongly absorbant at the preceding wavelengths and its increase is proportional to I.C.D. concentration.

$$\text{Isocitrate + NADP} \underset{Mn^{++}}{\overset{I.C.D.}{\rightleftharpoons}} \text{Oxalosuccinate + } NADPH_2$$

Mn^{++} is an activator and is added to the reaction mixture along with the substrate.

SPECIMEN: 0.5 ml. of unhemolyzed serum. Do not use plasma specimens; anticoagulants interfere with enzyme activity.

REAGENTS AND EQUIPMENT:

Reagents for U.V. Method are available as Biochemica Test Combination TC-ID #15933 TIAA. One kit is sufficient for 25 determinations.

1. Triethanolamine Buffer, 0.1 M., pH 7.5 and DL-Isocitrate, 0.0046 M. Dissolve contents of bottle #1 in 75 ml. redistilled water. Stable for 3 months at approximately 4°C. Bottle also contains 0.052 M. NaCl.

2. NADP, 0.0001 M. and $MnSO_4$, 0.12 M. Dissolve contents of bottle #2 in 3.0 ml. of redistilled water. Stable for four weeks at approximately 4°C.

Isocitrate Dehydrogenase (Continued):

3. Waterbath, at 30°C.

4. Spectrophotometer, with temperature controlled cuvette well (30°C.)

PROCEDURE:

1. Into a glass cuvette of 1.0 cm. light path, pipette 2.5 ml. of buffer and isocitrate reagent.

2. Deliver 0.5 ml. of serum specimen into the cuvette containing reagent. Mix the contents and place the cuvette in a 30°C. waterbath for 5 minutes.

3. Deliver 0.1 ml. of NADP-MnSO$_4$ reagent into the cuvette and mix well by inversion.

4. Place cuvette in thermostated cuvette well and start recorder.

5. Monitor the change in absorbance for at least two consecutive minutes of linearity.

6. CALCULATIONS:

Calculations based on mean A change of 1 minute.

NADPH$_2$ at 340 nm. = 6.22 x 10^3 Liters/Mole x cm.

$$\frac{\Delta A}{\epsilon x d} \times 10^6 \times \frac{TV}{SV} \times \frac{1}{Time} = \text{I.U./L. or mU/ml.}$$

$$\frac{\Delta A}{1} \times \frac{1}{6.22 \times 10^3 \times 1} \times 10^6 \times \frac{3.1}{0.5} \times \frac{1}{1} = \text{mU/ml.}$$

$$\Delta A \times F = \text{mU/ml.}$$
$$F = 997$$

NOTE: Sera with absorbance changes per minute greater than 0.100 at 340 nm. should be diluted 1:10 with physiological saline and repeated on 0.5 ml. of this dilution. Multiply final answer x 10.

NORMAL RANGE: Up to 11 mU/ml.

Isocitrate Dehydrogenase (Continued):

REFERENCES:

1. Batsakis and Briere: INTERPRETIVE ENZYMOLOGY, C. Thomas, 1967.

2. Ochoa, in Colowick & Kaplan: METHODS IN ENZYMOLOGY, Vol. 1, Academic Press, pg. 699.

3. Wolfson: Proc. Soc. Exp. Biol. & Med., 92:231, 1957.

4. Wolfson, Ann: N. Y. Acad. Sci., 75:260, 1958.

5. Henry, J. B.: WORKSHOP ON CLINICAL ENZYMOLOGY; PRE-WORKSHOP MANUAL, ASCP, 1964.

6. Clin. Chem., 6:208, 1960 (Colorimetric Determination)

7. J. Lab. & Clin. Med., 62:148, 1963 (Colorimetric Determination).

8. Sterkel, R. & Wolfson: J. Lab. Clin. Med., 52:176, 1958.

9. Cohen: Ann. of Int. Med., 55:604, 1961.

INTERPRETATION:

Isocitric dehydrogenase is an ubiquitous enzyme which is present in the mitochondria of the cell. It occurs in two isoenzyme forms; a fast and a slow electrophoretic fraction. The liver contains the fast component, while the slow component is present in heart muscle. The slow portion is not as heat stable as the fast component. The enzyme is present in the liver, heart, skeletal muscle, and certain neoplasms. Activity has also been demonstrated in platelets and in erythrocytes; very little activity is demonstrable in normal plasma.

Heart isocitric dehydrogenase activity is heat labile; it is inactivated at 56°C. Isocitric dehydrogenase derived from a liver source, however, is heat stable at 56°C. After an acute myocardial infarct, the heat labile heart isoenzyme persists for a very short time in the blood; but with liver damage there is persistence of activity of isocitric dehydrogenase in the serum. An elevation of isocitric dehydrogenase is a sensitive indicator of parenchymal hepatic disease, but the enzyme activity cannot be used to differentiate various liver diseases. A normal isocitric dehydrogenase activity is usually found

Isocitrate Dehydrogenase (Continued):

after an acute myocardial infarct; however, if heart failure occurs as a complication, there may be an elevation due to the intense hepatic congestion with necrosis of centrilobular cells. Various lesions such as viral hepatitis, metastatic carcinoma, hepatoma, and severe congestive heart failure have caused an elevation of isocitric dehydrogenase. The enzyme activity is elevated early in the course of infectious hepatitis, it persists for approximately three weeks and then returns to normal with recovery from the illness. When isocitric dehydrogenase levels remain elevated, one may assume that there is persistence of the viral hepatitis.

It has been observed that isocitric dehydrogenase is elevated in patients with megaloblastic anemia, presumably the enzyme is produced in large amounts by the megaloblasts. This is the same situation that exists in pernicious anemia with serum elevations of LDH. Both isocitric dehydrogenase and LDH are mitochondrial enzymes, and staining the megaloblasts by the tetrazolium-formazan technique demonstrates a large amount of isocitric dehydrogenase and LDH activity in the megaloblasts. With proliferation of these cells, a large amount of enzyme activity will be contributed to the serum. In addition, intra-bone marrow destruction of megaloblasts results in elevated LDH. There are rare reports of elevations of isocitric dehydrogenase in patients who have carcinoma of the pancreas, carcinoma of the prostate, infarction of the placenta, and myeloid leukemia. Thus, this enzyme increase is from necrosis of the pancreas associated with carcinoma of this organ, from the placenta, from carcinoma of the prostate, and from myeloid leukemic cells which contribute it to the serum. Isocitric dehydrogenase activity is increased in the cerebrospinal fluid when there is a primary or metastatic carcinoma to the central nervous system, and in patients who have had cerebral infarction or an acute bacterial meningitis.

KLEIHAUER METHOD TO DETECT
FETAL RED BLOOD CELLS
IN MOTHERS BLOOD

PRINCIPLE: This method is utilized to detect fetal red blood cells in mothers blood. Adult hemoglobin is easily eluted from red blood cells by an acid phosphated buffer solution, while fetal hemoglobin is not eluted.

SPECIMEN: Thin smears of maternal venous blood collected in EDTA.

REAGENTS:

1. Dipotassium Hydrogen Phosphate-Citric Acid Solution
   Prepare a fresh solution of 0.16 M. dipotassium hydrogen phosphate in 0.18 M. citric acid. The pH of the solution should be 3.4 to 3.6.

2. Absolute Ethanol

3. Wright's-Giemsa Stain

PROCEDURE:

1. Prepare thin smears of maternal venous blood collected in EDTA.

2. The smears should be fixed with absolute ethanol for 2 minutes.

3. Immerse the fixed blood smears in acid phosphate buffer which should be at a temperature of 37°C.

4. Remove smears from the acid phosphate buffer after 5 minutes and wash in tap water for 30 seconds.

5. Dry rapidly.

6. Counterstain with Wright's-Giemsa Stain.

NORMAL VALUES: ABSENCE OF FETAL CELLS IN THE MATERNAL CIRCULATION

Reference: Kleihauer, E., and Betke, K.: "Elution Procedure for the Demonstration of Methemoglobin in Red Cells of Human Blood Smears". Nature 199:1196, 1963.

Kleihauer Method (Continued):

INTERPRETATION:

Maternal red blood cells appear as ghost forms with marked elution of hemoglobin in contrast to the fetal red blood cells which appear as well-stained dark forms.

LACTATE DEHYDROGENASE
(Wacker Method)

PRINCIPLE: LDH catalyzes the following reaction:

Lactate + NAD$^+$ $\rightleftharpoons$ Pyruvate + NADH + H$^+$

The reduction of NAD$^+$ proceeds at the same rate as the oxidation of
lactate and in equimolar amounts. The rate at which NADH is formed
can be determined by the increase in absorbance at 340 nm. This is
the forward reaction according to Wacker utilizing lactate as the
substrate at an alkaline pH.

SPECIMEN: 0.050 ml. (50 microliters) of hemolysis-free serum (or
body fluid) is required. Serum should be separated from cells soon
after clotting takes place. Specimens for LDH may be stored at room
temperature or 4°C. for several days.

REAGENTS AND EQUIPMENT:

1. Working Substrate
   Biochemica Test Combination LDH-L 10 Test Reagents are used.

   Contents of 10 Test System LDH-L vial:
   a). 150 mg. NAD/vial (7.10 mM after reconstitution)
   b). Stabilized 0.05 M. pyrophosphate buffer, pH 8.6;
        0.045 M. L-Lactate.

2. Spectrophotometer
   A. Gilford 222, 340 nm.
       This instrument is used when analyzing four samples at a
       time. Temperature control is by means of a 30°C. circulating
       waterbath. Rate of reaction is determined from the strip
       chart recorder set for 0.200 A. full scale and run at one
       inch per minute.

   B. Gilford 300N, 340 nm.
       This instrument is used when analyzing one sample at a time.
       The change in absorbance per minute is read from the Data
       Lister print-out. The instrument is used with the thermo-
       cuvette set at 30°C.

3. Bailey Microdilutor
   The sample syringe is set to pick up 0.050 ml. (50 microliters),
   and the reagent syringe is set to dispense 1.5 ml. of substrate.

LDH (Continued):

COMMENTS ON PROCEDURE:

1. Substrate exhaustion is rate limiting. The reaction will be linear for only a few minutes. DO NOT read after 5 minutes.

2. The reaction mixture and cuvette chamber must be at temperature before taking a reading.

3. During the run, the substrate and cuvettes are kept at 30°C. in the waterbath.

4. Dilute all specimens when ΔA is greater than 0.080/minute.

PROCEDURE:

1. With a microdilutor, take up 50 microliters of specimen, and flush with 1.5 ml. of pre-incubated substrate. Mix well and return to the waterbath.

2. Quickly dilute up 3 more specimens in the same manner.

3. When 4 specimens have been diluted, immediately dry cuvettes and place in Gilford 222 (normally takes about 45 seconds).

4. Quickly set the baseline of Specimen No. 1 with the slit, and No.'s 2, 3, and 4 with their OFF-SET knobs. Switch to "AUTO" and scan all 4 channels.

5. Record 2 to 3 minutes of linear reaction time at 340 nm. Determine ΔA/minute from recorder chart.

6. CALCULATIONS:

$$\text{I.U.} = \frac{\Delta A}{\varepsilon x d} \times 10^6 \times \frac{TV}{SV} \times \frac{1}{Time}$$

ε = Molar Extinction Coefficient

ε of NADH at 340 nm. = 6.22×10^3 Liter/Mole x cm.

d = Diameter of light path (1.0 cm.)

TV = Total Volume: 1.55 ml.

SV = Sample Volume: 0.05 ml.

LDH (Continued):

T = Time in minutes

10^6 converts Moles/Liter (or mMoles/ml.) into Micromoles/L. (or Millimicromoles/ml.)

1 I.U./Liter = 1 mU/ml.

THEREFORE:

$$\frac{\Delta A}{6.22 \times 10^3 \times 1} \times 10^6 \times \frac{1.55}{0.05} \times \frac{1}{1} = mU/ml.$$

When all conditions of the assay remain constant, a factor may be derived:

$$\frac{\Delta A}{1} \times \frac{1}{6.22 \times 10^3 \times 1} \times 10^6 \times \frac{1.55}{0.05} \times \frac{1}{1} = mU/ml.$$

$\Delta A \times F = mU/ml.$ at 30°C.

F = 4984

We report results as mU/ml. at 37°C.

I.U. at 37°C. = mU/ml. at 30°C. x Temperature Conversion Factor. Temperature Conversion Factor = 2 (For this Laboratory).

NORMAL VALUES: 85 - 200 mU/ml. (For this Laboratory)

REFERENCES:

1. Wacker, W. E. C., Ulmer, D. D., and Valu, B. L.: New Eng. J. Med., 255:449, 1956.

2. Amador, C. L., Dorfman, D., and Wacker, W. E. C.: Clin. Chem., 9:391, 1963.

3. Gay, R. J., McComb, R. B., and Bowers, C. N., Jr.: Clin. Chem., 14:740, 1968.

LDH (Continued):

INTERPRETATION:

Lactic dehydrogenase acts in the glycolytic cycle to catalyze the conversion of lactic and pyruvic acid. This enzyme also may catalyze the reduction of other keto acids, and it is widely distributed in the body. The isoenzymes of lactic dehydrogenase are composed of two basic units. Each of the isoenzymes contain four of the units in one of five different combinations. These five different forms of the enzyme differ in their mobility in an electrophoretic field, with the pattern of lactic dehydrogenase related to the metabolic activity of the tissue. The isoenzyme which exhibits optimal activity where there are high levels of lactic acid predominates in those cells where this intermediate tends to be present. The isoenzyme which acts on pyruvic acid is usually present in greater amounts in those tissues which have a richer supply of oxygen. Lactic dehydrogenase isoenzymes are tetramers formed from various combinations of two types of subunits.

The stabilities of LDH isoenzymes must be considered before electrophoresis. LDH_5 is heat labile in contrast to LDH_1. Thermal stability during storage is important because with storage LDH_5 disappears. LDH_1 concentration remains constant at $4^\circ C.$, $-20^\circ C.$, and $25^\circ C.$ for one month. At $-20^\circ C.$, there is a rapid loss of LDH_4 and LDH_5 (two days) and after 8 to 10 days LDH_2 and LDH_3 are severely decreased at $25^\circ C$. There is no decrease in LDH_2, LDH_3, LDH_4, and LDH_5 for ten days. After more storage LDH_2 and LDH_3 decrease with a marked decrease in LDH_4 and LDH_5.

The best way to store sera is at room temperature avoiding excessive heat and bacterial contamination.

Lactic dehydrogenase is an intracellular enzyme. Usually an increase in the serum level of the enzyme is present where there is cellular death and leakage of enzyme from the cell. In addition, when neoplastic cells proliferate, the serum lactic dehydrogenase will be elevated Strenuous exercise may increase the serum lactic dehydrogenase from skeletal muscle. Furthermore, the enzyme is elevated post-partum due to muscle exertion incurred during labor.

The level of serum lactic dehydrogenase is not influenced by meals. Lactic dehydrogenase is somewhat higher in infants and children. Hemolysis will increase the serum lactic dehydrogenase because a large amount of enzyme is present within red cells. It remains stable in stored serum.

LDH (Continued):

Oxalate inhibits lactic dehydrogenase. Thus, it is advisable to utilize serum rather than plasma in determining lactic dehydrogenase. Inhibitors of lactic dehydrogenase are present in urine, and these should be removed by dialysis if lactic dehydrogenase is determined in the urine.

The causes for an increase in serum lactic dehydrogenase are:

1. Acute myocardial infarction
2. Acute leukemia
3. Pernicious anemia
4. Acute pulmonary infarction
5. Malignant neoplasms
6. Acute renal infarction
7. Hepatic disease
8. Sprue
9. Skeletal muscle necrosis
10. Shock with necrosis of various major organs

The causes for a decrease in serum lactic dehydrogenase are:

1. Clofibrate
2. Oxalate anticoagulant

As previously mentioned, lactic dehydrogenase exists as five isoenzymes. A sixth isoenzyme has been identified in testicular tissue. When the isoenzymes are electrophoretically separated, it has been demonstrated that isoenzyme one travels between albumin and alpha-1 globulin; LDH_2 travels with alpha-1 globulin; LDH_3 travels with beta globulin; LDH_4 travels with the fast gamma globulin; and LDH_5 travels with the slow gamma globulin.

The total serum lactic dehydrogenase may be increased in many different conditions as listed above. In order to determine which tissue is diseased, it is recommended that the total lactic dehydrogenase be separated into its isoenzymes. Separation into isoenzymes is best accomplished by electrophoresis. However, various other methods are available to separate these isoenzymes. Lactic dehydrogenase-one is heat stable while lactic dehydrogenase-five is heat labile. The heat stability-lability test is performed by diluting the serum with buffer at pH 7.4 and incubating the serum for thirty minutes at 65°C. If lactic dehydrogenase persists, this indicates heat stable LDH_1. Lactic dehydrogenase-one reacts with the substrate for alpha-hydroxybutyrate dehydrogenase. However, the other LDH isoenzymes show

LDH (Continued):

progressive decreasing activity. Thus, alpha-hydroxybutyrate dehydrogenase is considered similar to LDH_1. Another less used procedure for the chemical fractionation of lactic dehydrogenase is based on the fact that lactic dehydrogenase-one reacts best at low substrate concentrations of either lactate or pyruvate and is not inhibited by urea. In contrast, LDH_5 reacts best at high substrate concentrations and is inhibited by urea.

A review of the localization of the various isoenzymes is as follows: Lactic dehydrogenase of heart is one and two, as is reticuloendothelial tissue lactic dehydrogenase and kidney cortex. Lactic dehydrogenase of the lung and placenta is two and three. Lactic dehydrogenase of the pancreas is four and five, as is lactic dehydrogenase of the liver and skeletal muscle. When lactic dehydrogenase four and five are frozen, there is loss of activity. Repeated freezing and thawing of LDH may cause dissociation and recombination of the H and M subunits, and thus, for practical purposes storage at 4°C. is recommended.

Patients who suffer an acute myocardial infarction have an elevation of lactic dehydrogenase within the first 12 hours after the onset of the infarct. A peak is reached within 72 hours, and there is persistence of elevation for seven days. Alpha-hydroxybutyrate dehydrogenase may persist for two weeks, thus if the elevation of GOT or lactic dehydrogenase or CPK is missed and a myocardial infarct is suspected, alpha-hydroxybutyrate dehydrogenase should be determined, and this serum elevation will persist for as long as two weeks. If there is an elevation of lactic dehydrogenase, there is an indication that a myocardial infarct has occurred. Generally coronary insufficiency without infarction does not cause elevation in enzyme activity. The increase in serum lactic dehydrogenase is proportional to the size of the myocardial infarction. It may also increase to a greater extent if the patient has sustained congestive heart failure associated with the myocardial infarct. In patients who suffer an acute pulmonary infarct, an elevation of lactic dehydrogenase-two and three occurs. Generally GOT and CPK are normal.

In patients with liver disease, total lactic dehydrogenase will increase with hepatocellular damage. The elevation is usually due to LDH_4 and LDH_5, especially 5. However, there are other causes for an elevation of LDH_5 such as skeletal muscle necrosis or proliferation of malignant neoplasms.

LDH (Continued):

Various hepatic lesions may result in an elevated LDH_5. These include congestive heart failure with necrosis of the centrilobular cells, acute and chronic active hepatitis, and carcinoma metastatic to the liver. Lactic dehydrogenase is increased with necrosis of skeletal muscle. The necrosis may result from trauma or due to inflammatory lesions. Usually LDH_5 is increased.

Patients with infarction of the renal cortex have an increase in serum lactic dehydrogenase. The LDH_1 and 2 fractions are usually elevated. Furthermore, there has been recent interest in the measurement of lactic dehydrogenase in the urine which may result from the presence of necrosis of the renal cortex or due to carcinoma of the kidney. Inhibitors of lactic dehydrogenase must be removed from the urine before determination. Other urinary tract conditions will cause an elevated lactic dehydrogenase in the urine. These include acute cystitis, acute pyelonephritis, and acute glomerulonephritis.

Malignant neoplasms produce lactic dehydrogenase 2, 3, 4, and 5. Various malignant neoplasms will present with an elevated lactic dehydrogenase in the serum. This is usually due to proliferation of neoplastic cells containing the enzymes. Furthermore, patients with leukemia such as acute or chronic granulocytic leukemia, and acute or chronic myelomonocytic leukemia may present with an elevated lactic dehydrogenase in the serum. Various lymphomas also may present with elevated serum lactic dehydrogenase. The use of LDH as a screening test for leukemia or cancer is not entirely reliable since various series differ in the incidence of elevated lactic dehydrogenase in the serum. The reported incidences vary from 40 to 90 percent. Various anemias, especially megaloblastic anemias such as pernicious anemia result in an elevated lactic dehydrogenase. The enzyme is produced and released from the megaloblasts. Destruction of the megaloblasts also accounts for the elevation of LDH. By utilizing the tetrazolium formazan technique and staining sections of bone marrow from patients with pernicious anemia, it has been shown that lactic dehydrogenase is present in abundant amounts in the cytoplasm of the megaloblasts. Treatment with vitamin B_{12} causes a rapid decrease in the serum lactic dehydrogenase. Patients with hemolytic anemia may also have an elevated lactic dehydrogenase since there is an abundant amount of lactic dehydrogenase in the red cell.

Only a minimal elevation of lactic dehydrogenase occurs during pregnancy. This is only found during labor and shortly after. The elevation occurs for approximately two days after delivery and then becomes normal. The elevation may be due to the increased muscular

LDH (Continued):

activity during labor or it may be due to necrosis of the placenta. Isoenzymes 3 and 4 may be elevated. The activity of lactic dehydrogenase may be elevated if there is an abruptio placenta. This elevation is on the basis of necrosis of the placenta. The rise in lactic dehydrogenase is also related to the presence of blood clot associated with the abruptio placenta. The highest lactic dehydrogenase levels have been found in patients who have hypofibrinogenemia induced by various abnormal pregnancy conditions. An elevation of lactic dehydrogenase has been found in patients with choriocarcinoma and hydatidform mole. Lactic dehydrogenase of the umbilical cord blood is greater than the activity in the blood of the normal adult. The activity rises during the first two days of life and returns to normal about the first week after birth. The activity in the umbilical cord blood is higher in jaundiced babies. An exchange transfusion which is utilized in erythroblastosis causes an decline in lactic dehydrogenase associated with a decrease in jaundice.

Lactic dehydrogenase isoenzymes 2 and 3 are elevated in the spinal fluid when there are destructive lesions of the central nervous system. In addition, there is an elevation of lactic dehydrogenase in the spinal fluid in Tay-Sachs disease with the level of lactic dehydrogenase in the spinal fluid reaching its highest level in the second year of the disease, then it declines to normal. In contrast, lactic dehydrogenase of the spinal fluid is normal in Niemann-Pick disease. In addition, there is elevation of lactic dehydrogenase in the spinal fluid in patients who have infarction of the cerebral cortex, tuberculous leptomeningitis, convulsive disorders, and hemorrhage into the cerebral cortex.

Lactic dehydrogenase is elevated in the gastric juice of patients with pernicious anemia. It is also elevated in patients with carcinoma of the stomach. It is not elevated in the gastric juice in patients with peptic ulceration.

Lactic dehydrogenase is present in increased amounts in synovial fluid in patients who have rheumatoid arthritis. The increased lactic dehydrogenase in this condition in the synovial fluid results from the increased number of cells in the synovial fluid producing lactic dehydrogenase.

Lactic dehydrogenase is present in effusions in elevated amounts which are exudates. Recent reports indicate that determination of lactic dehydrogenase in an effusion is one of the better methods of differentiating a transudate from an exudate. The increased level of lactic dehydrogenase in exudates reflects the greater cell count of

LDH (Continued):

an exudate over that of a transudate. Thus, effusions which are
exudates and are caused by a malignant neoplasm metastatic to the
mesothelial surface or the presence of an inflammatory or immunological disease will be characterized by increased numbers of cells in
the effusion with a resultant increased level of lactic dehydrogenase
in the fluid. Approximately 25 percent of all transudates may give a
slight rise in the lactic dehydrogenase which might be secondary to
an increase in the lactic dehydrogenase in the serum. The effusion
LDH/serum LDH ratio would be greater than one in a malignant effusion.

LDH ISOENZYMES BY ELECTROPHORESIS

PRINCIPLE: The isoenzymes of lactate dehydrogenase are separated by electrophoresis on agarose, thin-gel plates. Following electrophoresis, a reagent film consisting of sodium lactate and the coenzyme, nicotinamide adenine dinucleotide (NAD^+), is spread over the gel surface. According to the following reaction, NAD is reduced to NADH, which is fluorescent.

$$
\begin{array}{ccccccc}
COO^- & & & & COO^- & & \\
CHOH & + & NAD^+ \underset{\longleftarrow}{\overset{LDH}{\longrightarrow}} & & C=O & + \quad NADH \quad + \quad H^+ \\
CH_3 & & & & CH_3 & & \\
\end{array}
$$

$$\text{Lactate} \qquad\qquad\qquad\qquad \text{Pyruvate}$$

The intensity of fluorescence of each of the five fractions is directly proportional to the concentration. The relative fluorescence of the fractions is determined by scanning the gel strips in a specially adapted door for the Turner Fluorometer.

SPECIMEN: 1.0 microliter of unhemolyzed serum. Should be stored at room temperature if unable to perform analysis on day of specimen collection. Analysis should be made within three days of specimen collection. Do not freeze samples.

EQUIPMENT AND SUPPLIES:

Unless otherwise specified, the following equipment is obtained through Analytical Chemists, Inc., Palo Alto, California. The ACI part numbers are indicated in parentheses.

1. Cassette Electrophoresis Cell and Power Supply (#1-3300)
   1 set required.

2. Quantitative Microliter Sample Dispenser (Elevitch), (#1-4100)
   A modified 10 microliter Hamilton syringe. 1 each required.
   Disposable Sample Tips (#1-4110) (100 tips/vial)

3. Electrophoresis Buffer, Barbital, pH 8.6 (#1-5100)
   0.05 M. with 0.035% EDTA. 2 sets required.

4. Film Cutter (#1-4300)
   1 each required.

LDH Isoenzymes (Continued):

5. Incubator/Oven (#1-3500)

6. Agarose UNIVERSAL Electrophoresis Film[R] (#1-1000-96)
   12 Films (96 Determinations) per package.

7. Fluorometric Lactate Dehydrogenase Isoenzyme Substrate (#1-1500)
   One package is enough for 96 determinations.

8. Sta-Moist Paper (#1-3550)
   100 Sheets/package, for use in incubator.

9. Turner Fluorometer (#111 - G. K. Turner Associates, 2524 Pulgas
   Ave., Palo Alto, California)

   Prepare the fluorometer as follows:
   Filter Selection:
       Primary: 365 nm.
       Secondary: 410 nm.

10. Turner Strip Scanning Door, Automatic (#110-525)
    Designed to fit the above fluorometer.

11. Varian Chart Recorder, Model G-22, 10 mv. - Varian Associates
                                          Palo Alto, California

12. Chart Paper for above Recorder #5A (#00-940507-01)
    Varian Aerograph 2700 Mitchell Dr., Walnut Creek, California.

13. Tablet of Scratch Paper, 8½ x 11 inches, lined.

14. Labelling Tape (3 MM white pressure sensitive tape 1 inch width)

PROCEDURE:

1. Determine Total LDH value for all specimens. Samples with a
   Total LDH of 200 I.U. yield optimal tracings. Dilute samples
   with values greater than 200 I.U. with saline or isoenzyme buffer
   so that the dilution falls in the optimal range. The dilution
   need not be exact; drop-counting with a Pasteur pipette is satisfactory. If the value is much lower than 100 I.U., a double
   application can be made.

2. Each film has eight (8) numbered strip positions. In this laboratory, we conventionally run all samples in duplicate (reporting

LDH Isoenzymes (Continued):

averaged results) and reserve positions No. 1 and No. 8 for Control Serum. Assign strip positions to each specimen and record these together with pertinent sample identification information in a log or workbook.

3. The plastic bag enclosing each box of films contains a small amount of EDTA solution which acts as bacteriostatic and to maintain moisture. Save the tape on the plastic bag and use it to reseal the package. Remove the box of films carefully so as not to spill the EDTA. Handle the individual films carefully, avoiding pressure on the soft (film) side. If necessary, rinse the film with a small amount of distilled water and drain and wipe gently. Reseal the box of unused films into the plastic bag.

4. Arrange the work area for application: have on hand
   a). A clean pad of lined tablet paper
   b). Appropriately diluted samples
   c). Hamilton or Elevitch syringe with a clean disposable tip for each sample.

5. Peel the film from its rigid plastic backing, which may be discarded. Place the film, agarose side up, on the lined paper. The film may be secured in place by taping to the paper at the corners. The numbered edge of the film with the application troughs is the cathode (negative) edge. (See Diagram Below)

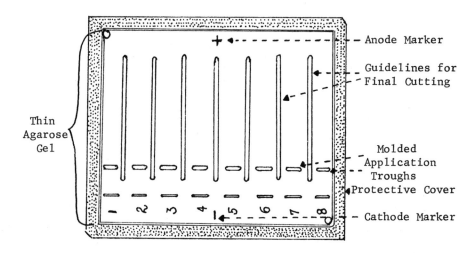

LDH Isoenzymes (Continued):

6. Apply 1.0 microliter of appropriately diluted specimen to each of
    the assigned troughs. Dispense the aliquot of sample in several
    consecutive portions, allowing each portion to soak into the gel.
    This will minimize the application artifact. Fill each position;
    if there are extra spaces, fill these with repeat samples or
    additional controls.

7. While waiting for the application to be completely absorbed into
    the gel, prepare the electrophoresis box. Connect the cassette
    to the power supply with the banana plugs. Measure 190 ml. of
    buffer with a graduated cylinder and add to the cassette, tilting
    the cassette to equilibrate the liquid level between the chambers.
    Cover with a pair of discarded film backings to protect from
    evaporation and contamination.

8. When the application troughs look "dry", pick up the film by the
    protective backing and flex into a "U" or trough shape with the
    protective cover on the outside and the agarose gel on the inside
    or concave aspect. Anode and Cathode markers will be opposite
    each other. Insert the flexed film into the trough holder in the
    electrophoresis box lid, being certain that the + and - markers
    on the film correspond to the + and - markings on the lid. (The
    lid markings are engraved on the outside of the lid. We have
    found it useful to clearly mark the inside of the lid with a
    bright wax marker crayon). Make sure that the film is snuggly
    inserted and that its edges are caught and held in place by the
    lip or "gutter" of the holder.

9. Invert the lid over the box and position gently to avoid splash-
    ing of the buffer. Placement of the lid trips the "ON" switch
    and the signal light turns a bright red. Electrophorese for
    35 minutes.

10. Ten (10) minutes before the end of the run, prepare the substrate.
    Add 2.0 ml. of refrigerated lactate to frozen dispenser bottle
    containing 10 mg. NAD. Make sure to replace the dispenser cap
    firmly so that it will not pop off or leak when using the dispen-
    ser as a drop-bottle. Store the light-sensitive substrate in
    the dark until ready to use. (Substrate saved frozen from prev-
    ious few days may be reused). Soak STA-MOIST paper to saturation
    with distilled water and pre-warm in the incubator at 38°C.

11. At the end of the 35 minute run, remove the lid vertically;
    again avoid splashing of the buffer. Place on a piece of

LDH Isoenzymes (Continued):

absorbant toweling to drain. At the end of the run, the anode
pH is about 8.2 and the cathode pH about 9.0 in contrast to the
initial uniform pH of 8.6. Before removing film from lid, blot
excess liquid from edges with a piece of clean tissue, but do
not scar the agarose gel. Remove from lid maintaining the "U"-
shape and release gradually to avoid spraying of condensation from
plastic protector. Blot away any excess liquid, but do not touch
the agarose gel.

12. Place the film, agarose side up, on a clean lined paper pad with
    the cathode side away from the operator. Tape the anode (near)
    edge to the paper, aligning the film edge with the lines on the
    paper which serve as a guide during application of the substrate.

13. Turn on the fluorometer and recorder to warm up at this time.

14. Using the dropper bottle in which it has been prepared, distribute
    16 - 20 drops of the NAD-Lactate Substrate (about 0.6 ml.) near to
    and parallel to the anode edge of the agarose. Lay a plastic
    5.0 ml. serological pipette along the drops, parallel to the edge
    and resting lightly on the agarose, so that the drops coalesce
    into a line along and ahead of the pipette. Check visually to
    see that the meniscus formed is continuous from side to side.
    Holding the pipette ends lightly between the fingertips, raise
    the pipette slightly off the agarose, but not enough to break the
    meniscus or separate the substrate from the agarose. Very slowly
    advance the pipette towards the cathode, pushing the substrate
    forward without touching the gel with the pipette. Watch the
    lateral edges to check that the meniscus is showing through the
    pipette. Keep the pipette parallel to the lines on the paper and
    advance right off the cathode end onto the paper. The process
    should be slow enough so that only a small amount of substrate
    is pushed off, and the bulk of it is absorbed by the end of the
    application.

15. As soon as the substrate is absorbed, place the film, agarose side
    up, on the wet filter paper on the incubator shelf, the shelf is
    removable for convenience. "Float" the film onto saturated filter
    paper laying down first at one edge to avoid trapping air bubbles
    (insulators). Uniform heating is essential. Plug in shelf for
    15 minutes. During this time turn on the oven to pre-heat.

16. When incubation is complete, remove film and dry the plastic side
    before transferring it to the removable oven shelf. Lay the film

LDH Isoenzymes (Continued):

on the shelf so that the anode-cathode axis is at right angles to a line extended from the banana plugs on the shelf. In this position the film can be held in place by elastic bands placed over the film edges and the shelf (the plastic tends to flex). Dry for 12 minutes. Remove to a dark, dust-free area until ready to scan.

17. View the film under an ultra-violet source to locate the extremes of the fluorescing patterns; mark the edges on the protective backing; trim along mark leaving a clearance of about 2.0 cm. from the pattern ends. (Careful trimming and taping will permit four pattern strips to be loaded onto the scanning drum simultaneously.) Take a strip of 1-inch white paper tape the same length as the protective backing (4½ inch) and place it so that ¼ inch of its width adheres to the film (the unused application troughs make a handy guide for positioning.) Place film and tape on the cutter and split the tape in half lengthwise. Position the trimmed-off strip of tape on the opposite side of the film, again allowing ¼ inch to overlap and press firmly into place. When the film is positioned gel-side up and with the application slots towards the operator, the left-most side of the film is position No. 1. It is advisable to number the positions on the labelling tape before cutting apart.

18. Line up the untaped edge of position No. 1 on the cutter plate and trim away just the protective backing without cutting into the agarose. Roll the cutter blade firmly and allow the tape to hold the film firmly in place. Release the film and tape carefully so that the agarose is not pulled away from the backing. Realign the film so that the interstrip division line is on the edge of the cutter plate and trim off the first pattern strip. Leaving the rest of the film in position on the cutter, take strip position No. 1 and apply it to the rotating drum of the fluorometer.

19. Hold the strip so that the application trough is on the right and position it on the drum so that the right-hand tape margin lines up with the marker "1A" on the vertical face of the drum. The drum width is exactly wide enough to seat the film, so it is important that the sides of the strips be cut parallel. Neither film nor tape must be allowed to project over the metal rim of the drum channel; the clearance as the drum rotates is extremely narrow and any projections will catch and tear or crumple the film.

LDH Isoenzymes (Continued):

20. Cut the next strip, No. 2 and again keeping the application-trough end to the right, position the strip on the drum to the left of strip No. 1, allowing the tape to overlap somewhat. In this manner four trimmed strips will fit onto the drum which normally will hold only three full-length strips.

21. The Turner Fluorometer should be allowed to warm-up for half an hour; after turning Power to "ON" and activating the "START" toggle switch, check visually for the blue light of the mercury vapor lamp. The Varian recorder is warmed up with the voltage switch (left hand toggle switch) at "STANDBY". The recorder pen is activated by the "RECORD" switch on the fluorometer. Chart speed is controlled by the right-hand toggle switch on the recorder and is left at "LOW". Chart motion is stopped and started by the left-hand toggle switch of the recorder and is used in the "HIGH" position. The scanning drum may be rotated manually in either direction by means of the knurled knob underneath the drum housing. When scanning automatically the drum moves counterclockwise until it hits the automatic stop. While scanning, the red indicator light in front of the drum is ON, when stopped, the light goes OUT. To reactivate scanning, the drum is rotated manually counterclockwise (approximately 3/4 turn of the knurled knob). In the starting position, the notation "OA" will be visible in the window on the top of the drum cover. Rotation is stopped or started by turning the "SAMPLE" toggle switch on the fluorometer to "ON".

22. After loading the strips onto the drum, replace the drum cover. Rotate the drum until the letters "OA" appear in the window. Set all switches on the fluorometer and recorder to "running" position. The light on the drum should be "ON". Rotate the drum manually, clockwise, until the light goes out and then back again, counterclockwise until the light just comes ON again. This places the drum in the starting position. One complete rotation takes approximately ten minutes.

23. Monitor the recorder during the scan for pattern and sensitivity. The pattern should stay between 0 - 10 on the recorder scale. Generally, if the specimens have been prediluted, no adjustment of the sensitivity will be needed. Label the tracings as they appear.

24. If the pattern goes off scale, the sensitivity must be readjusted and the tracing repeated. Sensitivity is controlled by the knurled knob on the top left of the drum housing. If the setting

LDH Isoenzymes (Continued):

of this knob is changed, the baseline adjustment (Blank-Adjust knob on top of fluorometer) must also be reset.

EVALUATION OF TRACINGS:

1. Draw the baseline. Application artefacts and various chemicals in medications can cause irregularities.

2. Draw a perpendicular line from each peak to the baseline; measure the height in mm. and record. The five peaks are equally based isosceles triangles, so that their comparative areas are proportional to their heights.

3. CALCULATIONS:

Calculate the percent of each fraction by the following formula:

$$\frac{\text{Height of fraction in mm.}}{\text{Total of all fractions in mm.}} \times 100 = \text{Fraction \%}$$

Average the duplicates and then multiply each percentage by the total LDH. This gives International Units per fraction. Report both the International Units and the percentage of Total.

4. INTERPRETATION:

Fractions are numbered from one-to-five, beginning at the anode. Fraction one is generally considered LDH of cardiac origin. Fractions four and five are primarily of liver origin.

NORMAL VALUES:

	Fraction 1	Fraction 2	Fraction 3	Fraction 4	Fraction 5
%:	17 - 27%	28 - 38%	19 - 27%	5 - 16%	5 - 16%
LDH:	Up to 54 I.U.	76 I.U.	54 I.U.	32 I.U.	32 I.U.

REFERENCES:

1. Methodology available through Analytical Chemist, Inc.

2. Elevitch, F.: PROGRESS IN CLINICAL PATHOLOGY, Ed. by Stefanini, Grune and Stratton, 1966.

LDH Isoenzymes (Continued):

INTERPRETATION:

Refer to Interpretation section under Lactate Dehydrogenase (Wacker Method) on page 210.

LEUKOCYTE ALKALINE PHOSPHATASE

PRINCIPLE: The enzyme, alkaline phosphatase, is found in neutrophilic granulocytes. The cytochemical demonstration of alkaline phosphatase depends on the formation of a colored precipitate at the site of hydrolysis of the substrate. Naphthol is liberated from the substrate Naphthol phosphate. This is coupled with a diazonium salt, Fast Blue, forming blue granules in the cells which contain alkaline phosphatase.

REAGENTS:

1. Formalin-Methanol Fixative
   Mix equal parts formaldehyde and absolute methyl alcohol. Store in the freezer and keep tightly covered.

2. Naphthol AS-MX Phosphate Concentrate, pH 8.6
   Purchased from Sigma Chemical Company, Stock #MX-L. Store in the refrigerator.

3. Fast Blue RR Salt (Sigma Chemical Company, Stock #FBSO25)
   Store in the refrigerator.

4. Ammonia Water, 0.2% aqueous

5. PVP
   20% aqueous polyvinyl pyrrolidine and polyvinyl acetate.

PROCEDURE:

1. Blood smears should be thin, dry, made without anticoagulant, and fixed within 2 hours.

2. Controls are fixed with each batch of slides. They are obtained from obstetrical patients or females using birth control pills.

3. Slides are immersed in fixative for 30 seconds. Rinse gently but well in cold running tap water. Air dry. If slides are not to be stained the same day, they should be refrigerated.

4. Pipette 2.0 ml. Naphthol AS-MX Phosphate Concentrate into a Coplin jar.

5. Add 48 ml. of distilled water.

Leukocyte Alkaline Phosphatase (Continued):

6. Empty contents of one Fast Blue RR Salt capsule (25 mg.) into the same Coplin jar. Stir to dissolve.

7. Immediately immerse slides into solution for thirty minutes.

8. Remove slides and wash in tap water. Allow to drain.

9. Counterstain 8 to 10 minutes in freshly filtered hematoxylin.

10. Pour off hematoxylin. Rinse slides with dilute ammonia water.

11. Rinse with running tap water until excess stain is washed off. Allow to drain and air dry.

12. Mount slides with PVP and coverslip to preserve stain. For routine use, smears may be examined unmounted. These must be discarded after scoring since immersion oil causes fading.

NORMAL VALUES: Scores of 50 to 150 as determined in our Laboratory. Each Laboratory should, however, determine its own normal range.

REFERENCES:

1. Kaplow, L. S.: "Cytochemistry of Leukocyte Alkaline Phosphatase". Amer. J. of Clin. Path. 39:439, 1963.

2. Blood, 10:1023, 1955.

3. Wintrobe, M. M.: CLINICAL HEMATOLOGY, 6th Ed., Lea & Febiger, Phil., pg. 449-450, 1967.

4. SIGMA TECHNICAL BULLETIN, #85, 1971.

INTERPRETATION:

Alkaline phosphatase activity is shown as blue granules in the cytoplasm of mature neutrophils. Other cells show no activity.

With the use of oil immersion, 100 consecutive segmented and band form neutrophils are rated 0 to 4^+ on the basis of the quantity and intensity of the precipitated dye within the cells. The score is the sum of these grades.

Leukocyte Alkaline Phosphatase (Continued):

Leukocyte alkaline phosphatase is increased in leukemoid states, pregnancy, acute lymphocytic leukemia and active Hodgkin's disease. It is increased in polycythemia vera and myeloproliferative syndrome.

It is decreased in acute and chronic myelogenous leukemia, acute monocytic leukemia, infectious mononucleosis, paroxysmal nocturnal hemoglobinuria, and congenital hypophosphatasia.

It is normal in secondary polycythemia, chronic lymphocytic leukemia, and multiple myeloma.

LEUKOCYTE BLOOD SMEAR

PRINCIPLE: The leukocyte differential expresses in percent the relative number of various types of leukocytes in the peripheral blood.

EQUIPMENT AND REAGENTS:

1. Wright's-Giemsa Stain

2. Blood Smears

PROCEDURE:

1. Stain smear according to Wright-Geimsa method.

2. On thin part of smear, count 100 white cells on counts ranging from 3,000 to 15,000. Above 15,000, count 200 cells and below 3,000 count 50 cells and multiply or divide results by 2 to give report in percent.

3. The abnormal cells should be identified if possible.

4. Two hundred cells should be counted on all abnormal differentials and the slide saved for the Pathologist.

5. Red cell morphology should be done on all patients. This should be reported in quantitative estimates as slight, moderate, or marked hypochromia. All other characteristics given in ranges as: 1 - 2, 2 - 4, etc. Use macrocyte and microcyte instead of anisocytosis. Use bizarre, elongated, tear drop, etc., instead of poikilocytosis.

6. Platelet estimations are done along with red cell morphology, using the terms decreased, normal, and increased.

7. All abnormalities should be noted.

REFERENCE: Miale, John B.: LABORATORY MEDICINE HEMATOLOGY 4th. Ed., C. V. Mosby Co., St. Louis, pgs. 905-907, 1209-1210, 1972.

Leukocyte Blood Smear (Continued):

NORMAL VALUES AND INTERPRETATION:

Adults		Children up to Age 8 Years
Neutrophils	56 ± 15	45
Bands	8 ± 2	8
Eosinophils	2 - 3	2 - 3
Basophils	0 - 1	0 - 1
Lymphocytes	34 ± 10	42
Monocytes	4 - 6	4 - 8

ABSOLUTE VALUES

Adults		Children up to Age 8 Years
Neutrophils	3800 cu. mm.	3700 cu. mm.
Bands	620 cu. mm.	660 cu. mm.
Eosinophils	200 cu. mm.	200 cu. mm.
Basophils	40 cu. mm.	50 cu. mm.
Lymphocytes	2500 cu. mm.	3500 cu. mm.
Monocytes	450 cu. mm.	750 cu. mm.

LEUKOCYTE COUNTS
(Coulter Counter)

PRINCIPLE: Blood is diluted 1:500 in 0.85% saline. Saponin is then added to lyse all non-nucleated cells. By means of a mercury syphon, a specific volume of this suspension is forced through an orifice (100 microns). Internal and external electrodes maintain a current in the orifice. A particle entering the orifice, changes the resistance, and a pulse is generated, which is proportional in magnitude to the size of the particle.

EQUIPMENT AND REAGENTS:

1. Coulter Counter

2. Plastic Vials

3. 0.85% Saline or Isoton

4. Saponin
   Diluted as directed on bottle, filter-freeze in small aliquots.

5. Coulter Autodilutor
   Sahli pipettes and 10 ml. pipettes may be used.

SOURCES OR ERROR:

1. Unclean equipment. The Coulter should be cleaned each day. The count should not be left standing in the Coulter but flushed through with saline. After about a dozen counts a saline rinse should be put through.

2. Clogged equipment. Debris may clog the orifice causing false counts or stopping the count entirely. This may be noted by an erratic pattern on the screen, slowing of the mercury, and a change in the cadence of the count.

3. Incomplete lysing. This may be prevented by counting at least two counts from the first vial or counting until a reproducible count is obtained.

4. Lysing of WBC. The dilution should not be saponized more than 15 minutes before counting.

230

Leukocyte Counts (Continued):

5. **Dilution error.** Always dilute two vials and the readings should check within 10%.

6. **Bubbles in the dilution.** Do not count foamy dilutions.

7. **Air leak in the stand.** This may be seen by watching the mercury, which will complete its circuit much faster than it should. Also air bubbles will appear in the stand, below the upper stopcock.

PROCEDURE:

1. Check the background count of the Coulter Counter as for RBC.

2. Make a 1:500 dilution using 20 lambda of blood and 10 ml. of saline.

3. Add three drops of saponin to this dilution and mix at once. Do not shake vigorously.

4. Aperture current setting should be 5. The threshhold setting is determined by calibration. Proper setting will be found taped on the face of the Coulter.

5. The solution is again mixed by swirling, and the cup is placed on the stand. The stopcock is opened and the mercury dropped below the start electrode. The stopcock is closed and the count is made.

6. The count which appears on the Coulter should be rounded off to the nearest hundred. Counts of over 20,000 must be corrected for coincidence. Use the same chart that is used for red counts.

7. Counts of more than 50,000 should be diluted until the count falls below 50,000.

8. Counts of less than 1,000 should be rediluted, using 0.1 ml. of blood in 10 ml. of saline and the resulting count divided by 5.

9. When more than 10 nucleated red cells per hundred leukocytes are counted on the differential, the leukocyte count must be corrected.

$$WBC = \frac{WBC \ (Observed \ Count) \ x \ 100}{(100 + nucleated \ RBC)}$$

NORMAL VALUES AND INTERPRETATION:

Adults	4.5 - 11.0	thousand/mm^3
Newborn	9.0 - 38.0	thousand/mm^3

Leukocyte Counts (Continued):

1 Year	6.0 - 17.0 thousand/mm^3
4 Years	5.0 - 15.5 thousand/mm^3
8 Years	4.5 - 13.5 thousand/mm^3
18 Years	4.5 - 12.5 thousand/mm^3
21 Years	4.5 - 11.0 thousand/mm^3

REFERENCE: Miale, John B.: LABORATORY MEDICINE HEMATOLOGY 4th. Ed.
C. V. Mosby Co., St. Louis, pgs. 904, 1201-1202, 1972.

LEUKOCYTE COUNTS
(Hemocytometer Method)

PRINCIPLE: Whole blood is diluted in an acid solution. The dilution fluid lyses all non-nucleated cells. When the blood smear shows nucleated erythrocytes, the leukocyte count must be corrected.

REAGENTS AND EQUIPMENT:

1. 1% HCl in water

2. WBC pipettes $\pm$ 1%

3. Aspirator

4. Hemocytometer and coverslip

PROCEDURE:

1. Fill the WBC pipettes to the 0.5 mark with blood and dilute to the 11 mark with 1% HCl. This makes a 1:20 dilution. Dilute 2 pipettes.

2. Shake the pipettes for 3 minutes. Discard the first 2 drops from each pipette.

3. Fill hemocytometer chambers and let settle for 1 minute.

4. For a leukocyte count the four large corner squares are counted. These are 1 square mm. each.

5. Calculate the leukocyte count as follows:

$$WBC/mm^3 = \frac{\text{Cells counted x 10 (depth) x 20 (dilution}}{4 \text{ (sq. mm. counted)}}$$

6. When more than 10 nucleated erythrocytes per 100 leukocytes are counted, the leukocyte count must be corrected.

$$\text{Corrected WBC} = \text{WBC (observed count) x } \frac{100}{100 + NRBC}$$

NORMAL VALUES AND INTERPRETATION:

Men	4.5 thousand - 11.0 thousand/mm^3
Women	4.5 thousand - 11.0 thousand/mm^3

233

Leukocyte Counts (Continued):

$$
\begin{array}{lll}
\text{Children - Newborn} & 9,000 & - 38,000/\text{mm}^3 \\
\text{1 Year} & 6,000 & - 17,000/\text{mm}^3 \\
\text{4 Years} & 5,000 & - 15,000/\text{mm}^3 \\
\text{8 Years} & 4,500 & - 13,500/\text{mm}^3 \\
\text{18 Years} & 4,500 & - 12,500/\text{mm}^3 \\
\text{21 Years} & 4,500 & - 11,000/\text{mm}^3 \\
\end{array}
$$

REFERENCE: Miale, John B.: LABORATORY MEDICINE HEMATOLOGY 4th. Ed.
C. V. Mosby Co., St. Louis, pgs. 904, 1200-1201, 1972.

DEMONSTRATION OF L. E. CELLS

PRINCIPLE: The formation of L. E. cells depends on the L. E. plasma factor found in the blood and other body fluids of patients with Lupus Erythematosus. When leukocytes and the L. E. plasma factor are mixed and incubated, the plasma factor produces a depolymerization of DNA in the nucleus of some cells. This is accompanied by the liberation of nuclear material which appears as free homogeneous globular masses. The typical L. E. cell is formed when these masses are ingested by the neutrophils.

SPECIMEN: 10 ml. of heparinized blood (Vacutainer #3200 Ka containing 0.5 ml. heparin.

REAGENTS AND EQUIPMENT:

1. B-D Vacutainer containing 0.5 ml. heparin

2. Wintrobe Hematocrit Tubes and Fillers

3. Tube Rotator

4. 37°C. Incubator

5. Glass Beads

6. Centrifuge, International

7. Wright's Stain and Buffer

PROCEDURE:

1. Place 2 to 3 glass beads in tube of blood and rotate in a 37°C. incubator for 1 hour.

2. Spin for 15 minutes in an International Clinical Centrifuge at full speed.

3. Remove buffy coat and place in Wintrobe Hematocrit Tubes.

4. Spin in International Clinical Centrifuge at full speed for 10 minutes.

5. Remove the buffy coat and make smears.

Demonstration of L. E. Cells (Continued):

6. Stain with Wright's stain and buffer only. Do not put through the Giemsa counterstain.

7. A total of 3 slides are scanned by at least two technologists.

NORMAL VALUES: Absence of the characteristic L. E. phenomena.

REFERENCES:

1. Miale, John B.: LABORATORY MEDICINE HEMATOLOGY 4th. Ed., C. V. Mosby Co., St. Louis, pg. 1265, 1972.

2. Magath, T. B. and Winkle, V.: "L. E. Cells Technique in Blood". A. Jour. Clin. Path. 22:586, 1952.

INTERPRETATION:

The L. E. cell has a typical appearance when the preparation is stained with Wright's stain. It is usually a neutrophil distended by an intracytoplasmic homogeneous red-purple body. The nucleus is compressed to one side, and the paler homogeneous body usually occupies most of the cell. Tart cells are mononuclear cells with ingested nuclei and do not indicate lupus. The inclusions are darker and retain some nuclear structure. Erythrocyte phagocytosis may also be seen on smears and is easily distinguished from lupus.

Extracellular homogeneous material may be found on smears either positive or negative for L. E. cells.

Rosettes are formed when neutrophils surround one of these extracellular homogeneous masses. Extracellular homogeneous masses and rosettes should be reported. Phagocytosis of both red and white cells should also be reported. L. E. cells may occasionally be found in conditions other than disseminated lupus erythematosus. These are rheumatoid arthritis, chronic active hepatitis (Lupoid Hepatitis), glomerulonephritis, rheumatic fever, hypersensitivity to drugs, such as Procaineamide, Apresoline, and anticonvulsant drugs. Usually the L. E. cells disappear with discontinuation of the drug. However, a latent L. E. condition may become overt with the utilization of these drugs and the condition may persist after discontinuation of the drug.

MALARIA SMEARS

PRINCIPLE: Malarial parasites in the blood stain with a Giemsa stain.

SPECIMEN: The specimen should be obtained during the febrile state.
Thin and thick blood films or saponin hemolysis smears are made.

REAGENTS: Wright-Giemsa Stain

COMMENTS ON PROCEDURE:

1. Thin and thick films or films prepared by saponin hemolysis are
   made. These are stained using the technique for staining differentials.

2. Two technologists should scan at least two different slides for
   malarial parasites.

PROCEDURE:

A. Thin Film
   1. Prepare a regular blood film and stain with Wright-Giemsa
      stain.

   2. Examine for 15 minutes under oil immersion.

B. Thick Film
   1. Place a drop of blood in the center of a slide.

   2. Allow it to spread out to three to four times the original
      area of drop.

   3. Dry the blood for 1 to 2 hours at room temperature. Do not
      fix the slide.

   4. Stain the slide with Wright-Giemsa stain.

   5. Examine by oil immersion.

C. Saponin Hemolysis
   1. Add 1.5 ml. of 1.0% Saponin in 0.9% Saline to 2.0 ml. anti-
      coagulated whole blood. Allow to stand 1 minute.

   2. Centrifuge for 1 minute.

Malaria Smears (Continued):

3. Remove and centrifuge supernate 10 minutes.

4. Dry and stain with Wright-Giemsa stain the sediments from each centrifugation.

5. This procedure gives a high concentration of parasites.

NORMAL VALUES: No Parasites Seen on the Blood Films or the Concentrates.

REFERENCE: Keffer, G.: "Malaria Parasites, Saponin Hemolysis Concentration". Am. J. Clin. Path. 46:155, 1966.

INTERPRETATION:

It is important to identify the type of malaria to institute appropriate therapy. Thus, rapid accurate identification of gametocytes, schizont forms and trophozoites is essential.

METHEMOGLOBIN

PRINCIPLE: The absorbance of methemoglobin in whole blood is measured at 640 nm. after which NaCN converts any methemoglobin present to cyanmethemoglobin which reduces the absorbance at this wavelength. The total hemoglobin is determined by converting all types of hemoglobin present to methemoglobin by the addition of potassium ferricyanide, and then all methemoglobin is converted to cyanmethemoglobin by the addition of NaCN and the absorbance of this is determined at 540 nm.

SPECIMEN: 1.0 ml. anticoagulated whole blood.

REAGENTS:

1. 0.02 M. KH_2PO_4 - NaOH Buffer, pH 6.6
   Place 3.4 gm. of KH_2PO_4 in a 500 ml. volumetric flask. Add about 125 ml. of distilled water. Add 44.2 ml. of 0.19 M. NaOH. Mix well. Dilute to volume. This solution is 0.05 M. Check pH.

2. Working 0.02 M. Phosphate Buffer
   Place 400 ml. of the Stock Solution in a 1 liter volumetric flask. Dilute to volume with distilled water.

3. KH_2PO_4 - NaOH Buffer, 0.05 M., pH 6.6
   Place 13.6 gm. KH_2PO_4 in a 2 liter volumetric flask. Add about 500 ml. distilled water. Add 177 ml. of 0.19 M. NaOH. Mix well. Dilute to volume with distilled water. Check pH.

4. Potassium Ferricyanide, 0.6 M.
   10 gm. K_3FeCN_6 is placed in a 50 ml. volumetric flask. Dilute to volume with distilled water. Keep refrigerated in a brown bottle. Stable for several months.

PRECAUTION: Blood must be fresh. Not more than 1 hour old. Also if hematocrit is less than 30% add 0.2 ml. of blood rather than 0.1 ml. as is called for in the procedure.

PROCEDURE:

1. 10 ml. of 0.02 M. phosphate buffer is mixed with 0.1 ml. blood. Read at 640 nm. on a Beckman Spectrophotometer between 2.5 and 5 minutes using buffer as the blank. This is called R_1.

2. Add 1 drop of 0.4 M. NaCN (16 - 20 drops/ml.) to each sample and blank. Read at 640 nm. on the Beckman Spectrophotometer. This is called R_2.

239

Methemoglobin (Continued):

3. Add 8.0 ml. of 0.05 M. Phosphate buffer to another cuvette.
   Add 2.0 ml. of sample from Step 2. Also to the Blank. Add
   1 drop of 0.6 M. potassium ferricyanide and 1 drop 0.4 M. sodium
   cyanide. Mix well and allow to stand for at least 10 minutes.
   Read at 540 nm. in the Beckman Spectrophotometer. This is called
   R_3.

4. CALCULATIONS:

   $R_1 - R_2$ in O.D. Units is directly proportional to the amount of
   methemoglobin present.

   $$\frac{R_1 - R_2}{R_3} \times 100 = \%\text{Methemoglobin}$$

   $$\frac{\text{Gms\%. Hemoglobin} \times \%\text{Methemoglobin}}{100} = \text{Gm\%. Methemoglobin}$$

STANDARDIZATION:

1. Place 1.0 ml. of any sample of whole blood in a 100 ml. volumetric
   flask and bring to volume with 0.02 M. Phosphate Buffer, pH 6.6.
   Place hemolysate in a 250 ml. Erlenmeyer flask and add 6.24 mg.
   potassium ferricyanide. This converts all hemoglobin to methemoglobin.

2. Make several dilutions from the hemolysate and use 10 ml. of the
   various dilutions to obtain R_1 and R_2.

3. Use 2.0 ml. of the Solution from R_2 to obtain R_3.

4. Translate R_3 into Gm%. hemoglobin using the factor derived from
   standardizing the hemoglobin method.

5. The Gm%. hemoglobin of each dilution is equal to the Gm%. Methemoglobin originally present since 100% of the pigment was in the
   form of Methemoglobin.

6. Construct a Standard Curve relating $R_1 - R_2$ in O.D. Units to
   Gm%. Methemoglobin.

NORMAL VALUES: 1 - 2%.

Methemoglobin (Continued):

REFERENCE: Davidsohn, I. and Henry, R.: CLINICAL DIAGNOSIS BY
LABORATORY METHODS, 14th. Ed., W. B. Saunders Co., Phil.,
pg. 135-136, 1969.

INTERPRETATION:

Methemoglobin is a derivative of hemoglobin. It is produced when Fe^{++} is oxidized to Fe^{+++}. Methemoglobin is inactive and unable to combine with oxygen. Thus, there is hinderance of transfer of oxygen and a functional anemia occurs. Cyanosis is present due to decreased oxygen-carrying capacity. The normal methemoglobin level is 0.24 gm. per 100 ml. Methemoglobin is reduced to hemoglobin by NADH reductase and hereditary NADH reductase deficiency results in methemoglobinemia. At levels of 10 to 25 percent no symptoms are demonstrated clinically while at 35 to 50 percent dyspnea and headache may be present. A 70 percent level is probably a lethal level. Methemoglobin occurs secondary to drugs and chemicals, such as benzene, nitrites, phenacetin, Gram-negative nitrite-producing bacteria and sulfa drugs. The treatment for methemoglobin consists of administration of reducing agents such as methylene blue or ascorbic acid.

SERUM MURAMIDASE

PRINCIPLE: Muramidase is released into the blood upon the destruction of granulocytes and monocytes. The lytic activity of this enzyme on a bacterial cell suspension is measured by following the optical density change over a given time. An index of granulocytic-monocytic turnover can then be calculated from the ug/ml. and the absolute granulocyte-monocyte white count.

SPECIMEN: 5.0 ml. serum, EDTA Lavender Top tube for white blood count and blood smears for differential counting.

EQUIPMENT AND REAGENTS:

1. Phosphate Buffer, 0.5 M., pH 6.2 (Difco #0464)
   Stable if refrigerated.

2. Stock Standard (Crystallized Egg White Enzyme) (Difco #0465)
   Stable for 2 years. Add 20 mg%. to the phosphate buffer. Mix immediately but DO NOT SHAKE! Freeze immediately in 1.0 ml. aliquots. Stable for about 10 months.

3. Substrate Micrococcus lysodeikticus Suspension (Difco #0461)
   70 mg. cells ADD (175 mg)
   90 ml. Phosphate buffer (225 ml.)
   10 ml. 1.0% NaCl (25 ml.)
   Should give an O.D. of about .300. This develops a distinctive odor in 7 to 10 days but appears to be stable if refrigerated, until gone. Mix well before using. It is a suspension.

4. Spectrophotometer, Coleman Jr., Wavelength 645 nm.

COMMENTS ON PROCEDURE:

1. The Standard is not stable once it is thawed so it must be run immediately.

2. All serums are run at a 1:2 dilution, if the ΔO.D. is greater than the 20 ug/ml. Standard, dilute serum further and rerun.

3. Duplicates should be run on all samples though not side/by side. This attempts to avoid partiality in reading O.D. Duplicate ΔO.D. should be within .008 or less.

242

Serum Muramidase (Continued):

4. The WBC and differential must be drawn at the same time the serum is drawn.

5. Serum samples diluted seem to be quite linear, and it is possible to estimate further dilutions of very high samples. The dilutions of serums are not linear to the undiluted samples.

6. Serums seem stable with repeated freezing and thawing, but not too stable if kept at room temperature for any length of time.

7. Serums may sit on the clots up to 24 hours before there is much change; however, it is best to separate them and freeze them as soon as possible.

8. On 5 Controls, there did not seem to be much difference between serum and versenated blood. Serum is preferable except under extreme conditions.

9. The ΔO.D. of a buffer-substrate blank at 8 minutes is about .003.

STANDARD CURVE:

1. Place eight 15 x 100 mm. tubes in a rack numbering 4, 8, 16, 20; 4, 8, 16, and 20.

2. 4.0 ml. of substrate is placed in each tube.

3. Prepare all tubes prior to thawing standard. Thaw standard with warmth from hand and run immediately as it deteriorates within a few minutes.

Buffer	Standard	Concentration
2.45	0.05	4 ug/ml.
2.40	0.10	8 ug/ml.
2.30	0.20	16 ug/ml.
2.25	0.25	20 ug/ml.

4. At Zero time, pipette 0.5 ml. of sample into substrate, mix by shaking.

5. At 30 seconds, take baseline reading using buffer as blank.

6. At 1 minute pipette next sample and mix.

Serum Muramidase (Continued):

7. At 1 minute 30 seconds, take baseline O.D. of sample No. 2.

8. Continue in this manner with remaining samples. The duplicate on No. 4 is pipetted at 7 minutes, baseline O.D. at 7 minutes 30 seconds.

9. At 8 minutes, read final O.D. of sample No. 1 after thorough shaking. At 9 minutes No. 2 and etc...

10. Using linear graph paper plot O.D. vs. Concentration of Standard.

11. Correct line through zero by drawing parallel line through zero.

PROCEDURE:

1. Always run normal control serum along with patient serum.

2. Always dilute all serum samples 1:2 with buffer prior to assaying.

3. Number tubes in rack 1, 2, 3, 4; 1, 2, 3, 4.

4. Proceed as with Standard Curve, Steps 4 through 9.

5. Calculate the O.D. for each sample averaging the duplicate values

6. CALCULATIONS:

   a). From the Standard Curve obtain the ug/ml. value.

   b). Multiply by the dilution of the serum.

   c). Record the WBC and the total number of granulocytes (PMN's, bands, myelocytes, promyelocytes) and monocytes.

   d). Calculate the absolute granulocyte-monocyte number.
Total WBC x Total G-M = Absolute #G-M.

   e). Muramidase Index = $\dfrac{\text{ug/ml.}}{\text{Absolute \#G-M}}$

      i.e.: WBC 5.0, Total No. Granulocytes and Monocytes 55%
ug/ml. = 20
5.0 x 55 = 2.75

$$\text{Index} = \frac{20.0}{2.75} = 7.3$$

Serum Muramidase (Continued):

f). Corrected Values:
    1). Subtract 5 ug/ml. from the Muramidase Value.
    2). Recalculate Index using corrected ug/ml. Value.

REPORT: ug/ml.
    Differential
    Index
    Corrected ug/ml.
    Corrected Index

NORMAL VALUES: Range - 15 to 48 ug/ml.
                Index - 3 to 12

                Corrected Range: 10 - 43 ug/ml.
                Corrected Index: 2.4 - 10.9

REFERENCES:

1. Hammonds, F., Quaglino, D., Hayhoe, F. J. J.: "Blastic
   Crisis of Chronic Granulocytic Leukemia. Cytochemical Cyto-
   genetic and Autoradiographic Studies in Four Cases". Brit.
   Med. J. 1:1275, 1964.

2. Finch, S. C., Lamphere, J. P., Jablon, S.: "The Relationship
   of Serum Lysozyme to Leukocytes and Other Constitutional Factors". Yale J. Biol. Med. 36:350, 1964.

3. Perillie, P. E., Kaplan, S. S., Lekowitz, E., Rogoway, W.,
   Finch, S. C.: "Studies of Muramidase (Lysozyme) in Leukemia".
   J. Amer. Med. Assoc. 203:317, 1968.

INTERPRETATION:

Muramidase is a lysosomal enzyme found normally in cells such as the
monocyte and the myeloid cell series. The major part of muramidase
in the serum is derived from granulocytes. Patients with acute monocytic leukemia and other diseases in which monocytosis occurs may
develop elevated muramidase activity in the serum and the urine. The
serum enzyme is markedly elevated in acute monocytic leukemia and
moderately elevated in acute and chronic myeloid leukemia. It is
usually normal or low in lymphocytic leukemia; thus, it is easy to
exclude acute lymphocytic leukemia if the muramidase level is elevated.
The muramidase activity in the serum varies with the total white blood
cell count. In monocytic or myeloid leukemia, the elevated enzyme

Serum Muramidase (Continued):

values return to normal when a remission occurs. With a relapse, the serum muramidase will increase again and this rise may precede development of overt symptoms; renal disease, tuberculosis, and sarcoidosis will cause an increased serum and urine muramidase level. Muramidase may cause damage to renal tubules with renal insufficiency.

According to Briggs in J. Histochem. and Cytochem. 14:167, 1966, progranulocytes, neutrophilic myelocytes, neutrophilic bands, neutrophilic segmented and monocytes contain from 2+ to 4+ activity. All other cells were negative or showed only trace amounts. Therefore, only the above cells should be included in calculating the absolute number of cells. DO NOT include blasts, eosinophils, basophils, or lymphocytes.

NITRO BLUE TETRAZOLIUM PROCEDURE

PRINCIPLE: This test is a rapid laboratory aid in confirming or ruling out bacterial infection in febrile illnesses of adults.

Tetrazolium salts have been used in histochemical studies of various enzymes. At the site of enzyme activity, colorless tetrazolium salts are reduced to water insoluble formazan which can be seen as blue-black deposits.

During the course of acute bacterial infection, normal neutrophils phagocytize bacteria and are bactericidal. This capacity is demonstrated in the cytoplasm of peripheral neutrophils by an increased spontaneous reduction of the colorless nitro blue tetrazolium (NBT) to the blue-black formazan crystals.

SPECIMEN: 3.0 ml. blood drawn very slowly in a plastic syringe and placed in a plastic tube containing 100 units sodium heparin. Rotate gently to prevent clotting, and process within one hour.

EQUIPMENT AND REAGENTS:

1. 1.0 ml. pipette, 1 in 1/10

2. 13 x 75 mm. covered plastic tubes

3. Coverslips, slides, and permount

4. Wright's stain

5. 37°C. waterbath

6. Stock Phosphate Buffered Saline (PBS), pH 7.3
   NaCl   8.5 gm.
   Na_2HPO_4 1.17 gm.
   $NaH_2PO_4 \cdot H_2O$ 0.22 gm.
   Distilled water q.s. to 1 liter
   Stable in refrigerator.

7. Working Phosphate Buffered Solution, pH 7.2 - 7.3
   Stock PBS   10 ml.
   Distilled water 90 ml.
   NaCl   8.5 gm.
   Stable in refrigerator.

Nitro Blue Tetrazolium Procedure (Continued):

8. 0.2% NBT (Nitro blue tetrazolium), TOXIC - HANDLE WITH CARE!
   NBT crystals   0.2 gm.
   Distilled water   q.s. to 100 ml.

   Place 0.2 gm. NBT crystals into a 100 ml. volumetric flask. Add
   80 ml. distilled water, dissolve, and q.s. to 100 ml. with distilled water. Store in brown bottle as is very LIGHT SENSITIVE.
   Stable indefinitely when refrigerated.

PROCEDURE:

1. Mix just before use: one part 0.2% NBT and one part working
   phosphate buffer in an amount necessary for the number of tests
   ordered. Using a 1.0 ml. pipette, deliver 0.1 ml. PBS-NBT mixture into a clean plastic tube with cover. To this tube, add
   0.1 ml. heparinized whole blood. Rotate gently.

2. Place covered tube in a 37°C. waterbath for 30 minutes, shaking
   gently several times during incubation.

3. Make coverslip preparations.

4. Counterstain with Wright's and Giemsa stains.

5. Mount coverslip to slide using permount.

6. Two technologists count 100 neutrophils; match within 10%.

NORMAL VALUES: Count Positive: Neutrophils with 1 large blue-black
                                crystal.
               Count Negative: Neutrophils which are lightly stipple
                                or void of blue-black crystals.

   NOTE: a). If WBC is below 3,000 cu. mm., spin down tube for 3
               minutes, and prepare as above using the buffy coat.

          b). Monocytes, eosinophils, and platelets also form
               crystals; do not count them as positive.

          c). Equivocal cells are neutrophils with positive plate-
               lets adjacent. Do not count this cell as positive or
               negative; i. e. ignore it!

          d). Write normal values on slip.

Nitro Blue Tetrazolium Procedure (Continued):

e). False negatives could be due to prior therapy.

f). Generally, positives go to negative within one to fifteen days after treatment.

REFERENCES:

1. Matula, G. & Paterson, P.: New Eng. J. Med. 285:311-317, 1971.

2. Park, B. H., et al: The Lancet 2:532-534, 1968.

INTERPRETATION:

The percentage of NBT positive neutrophils is low in normal individuals and is less than 10 percent. Patients with fever on drugs (such as cortisone and antibiotics), localized bacterial infections, viral infections, postsurgical condition, hemolytic anemia, and diabetes mellitus also have counts less than 10 percent. The following conditions cause the percentage of neutrophils to be greater than 10 percent: systemic bacterial infections, infants up to the age of two months, systemic fungal infections, and Hodgkin's disease with fever due to bacterial or fungal infection. Nonfebrile Hodgkin's patients have a score less than 10 percent.

The major clinical advantage of the NBT stain is to alert the physician to the possibility of systemic bacterial infection long before microbiologic data is available. A positive NBT score returning to normal after antibiotic therapy would indicate that treatment was successful. The lack of reduction of NBT in granulomatous disease is characteristic. The neutrophils in this disease are able to phagocytize bacteria but are unable to destroy them. A positive NBT test depends on increase in NADH oxidase activity of neutrophils induced by bacteria and neutrophils which can reduce NBT dye. The advantages of the NBT test are to make an early diagnosis of systemic bacterial or fungal disease and to exclude viral or other febrile disease. It may be useful to monitor and detect early bacterial infection in transplant patients. It also may be the only supportive evidence for bacterial infection when appropriate bacterial cultures are negative.

OSMOTIC FRAGILITY

PRINCIPLE: Erythrocytes are placed in varying solutions of saline. In hypotonic solutions the cells take up fluid until an equilibrium is reached or the cells rupture. In some hemolytic anemias the resistance of the red cells to hypotonic solutions is reduced, and in others it is increased.

SPECIMEN: Whole blood collected in EDTA or heparin.

REAGENTS:

1. Buffered Stock Saline, 10%
   NaCl   180.00 gm.
   Na$_2$HPO$_4$ 27.31 gm.
   NaH$_2$PO$_4$ 4.36 gm.
   Dissolve in distilled water and dilute to 2000 ml.

2. Working Saline Solutions
   Dilute from Stock Solution.
   0.85%
   0.70%
   0.60%
   0.52%
   0.50%
   0.48%
   0.44%
   0.42%
   0.40%
   0.38%
   0.36%
   0.32%
   0.28%
   0.16%
   0.10%

PROCEDURE:

1. Pipette 4.0 ml. volumes of each of the above working saline solutions into test tubes. (Pipette one set for each patient and each control).

2. Add 0.02 ml. of blood and mix gently. For the control, use normal blood with normal red cell morphology.

250

Osmotic Fragility (Continued):

3. Incubate tubes at room temperature for 45 minutes.

4. Centrifuge the tubes at 2,000 rpm for 10 minutes.

5. Remove the tubes from the centrifuge carefully to avoid disturbing the cells in the bottom of the tube.

6. Observe visually for initial and complete hemolysis.

7. Transfer the supernatant red cell free solution from each tube to cuvettes and read optical density at 540 nm. Use distilled water for the blank. (Read on the Coleman Jr. using 10 x 75 mm. cuvettes.)

CALCULATIONS:

Calculate the percent hemolysis in each saline concentration:

B = O.D. of the tube with the saline concentration of 0.85% (This will indicate hemolysis due to mechanical trauma.)
C = O.D. of the tube in which 100% hemolysis has occurred.
U = O.D. of each unknown tube.

$$\frac{U - B}{C - B} \times 100 = \% \text{ Hemolysis}$$

A Graph for each patient must be plotted with the saline concentrations along the (horizontal) ordinate, and the % hemolysis along the (vertical) abscissa. Plot the normal control on the same graph.

NORMAL VALUES: Initial Hemolysis 0.44 - 0.02 (Saline Concentration)
                  Complete Hemolysis 0.32 - 0.02 (Saline Concentration)

REFERENCES:

1. Miale, John B.: LABORATORY MEDICINE HEMATOLOGY, 4th. Ed. C. V. Mosby Co., St. Louis, pgs. 649-650; 786-787; 1225-1226, 1972.

2. Dacie, J. V.: HEMOLYTIC ANEMIAS, PART 1. THE CONGENITAL ANEMIAS, 2nd. Ed., Grune & Stratton, Inc. New York, pg. 35-42, 1960.

Osmotic Fragility (Continued):

INTERPRETATION:

The erythrocyte abnormality which is associated with increased osmotic fragility is hereditary spherocytosis. Autoincubation enhances the increased osmotic fragility. The erythrocytes of patients with autoimmune hemolytic anemia also exhibit increased osmotic fragility. The erythrocytes of thalassemia, sickle cell disease, liver disease, and iron deficiency are associated with increased resistance to hemolysis with saline.

ACTIVATED PARTIAL THROMBOPLASTIN TIME

PRINCIPLE: The Activated Partial Thromboplastin Time (PTT) is a
screening test for the entire coagulation mechanism except Factor VII,
Factor XIII, and platelets. Fresh citrated plasma provides all the
factors necessary for the intrinsic clotting mechanism, except ionic
calcium (removed by the citrate) and platelet factor (removed by centrifugation of the platelets). By adding brain lipids which replace
platelet phospholipid and calcium to the plasma, with Celite to enhance
reproducibility by providing maximal glass contact activation, we can
detect deficiencies of all the clotting factors except those mentioned
above. Fibrinogen (Factor I) deficiency is detected by the PTT, but
it picks up only pronounced deficiencies of 100 mg%. or less and will
miss moderate or borderline deficiencies.

SPECIMEN: Whole blood is collected in acid citrate (1 part acid
citrate to 9 parts blood). Centrifuge to obtain platelet-free plasma.
Remove plasma and freeze in 2 aliquots.

COMMENTS ON PROCEDURE:

1. All specimens must be frozen. This shortens the PTT slightly
    and normals are based on frozen specimens.

2. Fibrometer cups should be prewarmed at least ten minutes.

3. The fibrometer probe must be dipped in 0.1 N. HCl and wiped with
    a kimwipe before each test. This removes protein build-up on the
    probes that gives false low values.

EQUIPMENT AND REAGENTS:

1. Ice Water Bath

2. Fibrometer

3. Stopwatch

4. Verify Normal
    Reconstitute with 0.5 ml. distilled water. Do not shake. Let
    stand at room temperature 20 minutes before mixing. Then mix and
    put in ice water bath. (May be reconstituted and frozen in ad-
    vance to expedite procedure.)

253

Activated PTT (Continued):

5. Platelin
   Reconstitute with 2.5 ml. distilled water. Shake well. Incubate at 37°C. for 8 minutes before using. Do not use after 30 minutes.

6. $CaCl_2$, 0.025 M.
   Prewarm to 37°C.

7. HCl, 0.1 N.

8. Acid Citrate
   2 parts 0.1 M. citric acid to 3 parts 0.1 M. Na_3 citrate.

PROCEDURE:

1. Thaw one tube of each sample by putting into 37°C. bath. Remove as soon as it thaws, and put into ice water bath.

2. Mix platelin well with a 0.2 ml. pipette to resuspend the Celite. Blow 0.1 ml. into first cup. Add 0.1 ml. plasma (with gun off) and start stopwatch.

3. Mix thoroughly by shaking fibrometer cup. Return to fibrometer.

4. At about 4.5 minutes mix cup again by shaking and position for probe.

5. At exactly 5 minutes, with gun on, add 0.1 ml. of 0.025 M. $CaCl_2$.

6. Run in duplicate.

NORMAL VALUES: 26 - 39 seconds
                  (Report control value and normal range)

REFERENCES:

1. Langdell, R. D., Wagner, R. H., and Brinkhous, K. M.:   J. Lab. and Clin. Med., 41:637, 1953.

2. Proctor, R. R. and Rapaport, S. I.:   Amer. J. Clin. Path., 36:212, 1961.

3. Struver, G. P. and Bittner, D. L.:   Amer. J. Clin. Path., 38:473, 1962.

4. Lenahan, J. G. and Phillips, G. E.:   Clin. Chem., 12:269, 1966.

Activated PTT (Continued):

INTERPRETATION:

The primary value of determining the PTT is to detect abnormalities of the intrinsic system. However, as stated in the section of the principle of the test, other deficiencies in the coagulation system will be manifested by a prolonged PTT. Thus, congenital deficiency of Factors XII, XI, IX, and VIII, consumption in disseminated intravascular coagulation, or inhibition of these factors by acquired inhibitors will result in a prolonged PTT. A deficiency of V and X will also prolong the PTT.

Thus, deficiencies of clotting factors of 25-30% or less will prolong the activated PTT (except platelet phospholipid, Factor VII, and Factor XIII). PTT's are prolonged by heparin and circulating anticoagulants. Inhibitors are detected by the 1:1 (1:2) dilution of normal plasma with patient plasma. If the PTT is not corrected, an inhibitor is indicated. If the PTT is corrected with normal plasma, a factor deficiency is indicated. Adsorbed plasma and aged serum can be used to give a probable identification of the deficiency if the PTT Time is sufficiently prolonged. Slightly prolonged times are not easily identified in this way.

WHOLE BLOOD PARTIAL THROMBOPLASTIN TIME

PRINCIPLE: The Activated Partial Thromboplastin Time (PTT) is a screening test for the entire coagulation mechanism, excluding Factor VII and platelets. The whole blood PTT performed on the fibrometer is more accurate for monitoring heparin therapy than the Lee-White, because it eliminates variation in surface activation, phospholipid release from platelet, temperature, and end-point detection.

SPECIMEN: Whole blood is collected in acid citrate (1 part acid citrate to 9 parts blood). Perform test within 2 hours. Blood is maintained at room temperature.

COMMENTS ON PROCEDURE:

1. Fibrometer cups should be prewarmed at least 10 minutes.

2. The fibrometer probe must be dipped in 0.1 N. HCl and wiped with a kimwipe before each test. This removes protein build-up on the probes that give false low values.

EQUIPMENT AND REAGENTS:

1. Fibrometer

2. Stopwatch

3. Verify Normal
   Reconstitute with 0.5 ml. distilled water. Do not shake. Let stand at room temperature 20 minutes before mixing.
   a). Run test at once, OR
   b). Put in ice bath for use within 30 minutes, OR
   c). Freeze for use at a later time

4. Platelin plus Activator
   Reconstitute with 2.5 ml. distilled water. Shake well. Incubate at 37°C. for 8 minutes before using. Platelin is stable for about 30 minutes. Values then become shorter. Therefore, a new vial must be reconstituted for each series of tests.

5. CaCl$_2$, 0.015 M.
   Prewarm to 37°C.

6. HCl, 0.1 N.

256

Whole Blood PTT (Continued):

7. Acid Citrate
   2 parts 0.1 M. citric acid to 3 parts 0.1 M. Na$_3$ citrate.

PROCEDURE:

1. Mix platelin well with a 0.2 ml. pipette to resuspend the Celite.
   Blow 0.1 ml. into first cup. Add 0.1 ml. whole blood (with gun
   off), and start stopwatch.

2. Mix thoroughly by shaking fibrometer cup for 10 seconds. Return
   to heat block.

3. At about 4.5 minutes, mix cup again by shaking, and position for
   probe.

4. At exactly 5 minutes, with gun on, add 0.1 ml. of 0.015 CaCl$_2$.

5. Run in duplicate.

6. Run Verify Normal in same way. Control values for current lot
   number will be posted.

NORMAL VALUES: 28 - 39 seconds (mean 33.6 seconds)
                 Report control value and normal range.

REFERENCES:

1. Degnan, J. J., Karasik, S. A., and Lenahan, J.: "Laboratory
   Control of Heparin Therapy with the Activated Partial Throm-
   boplastin Test". Current Therapeutic Research, Vol. 11,
   June, 1960.

2. Lenahan, J. G., Fry, S., and Phillips, G. E.: "Use of the
   Activated Partial Thromboplastin Time in the Control of
   Heparin Administration", Clin. Chem., Vol. 12, 1966.

3. Hirsh, J., O'Sullivan, E. F., Gallus, A. S., and Martin, M.:
   "The Activated Partial Thromboplastin Time in the Control of
   Heparin Treatment", Aust. Ann. Med., 4:334-337, 1970.

4. Stuart, R. K. and Michel, A.: "Monitoring Heparin Therapy
   with the Activated Partial Thromboplastin Time", Canad. Med.
   Assoc. J., Vol. 104, 1971.

Whole Blood PTT (Continued):

INTERPRETATION:

A Lee-White of 20-40 minutes corresponds to a Whole Blood PTT of
66-117 seconds. The Whole Blood PTT should be prolonged to two to
two and one-half times the Control for adequate Heparin Anticoagu-
lation. See Lee-White Interpretation on page 56.

There has been general agreement for some time that the Lee-White
Coagulation Time has very poor reproducibility and is extremely time
consuming.

Several new tests can be used to monitor heparin therapy that have
proved much more satisfactory. These include the Activated Clotting
Time, Recalcification Time, and the Activated Partial Thromboplastin
Time. The Whole Blood Activated Partial Thromboplastin Time is a
substitute for the Lee-White.

The Partial Thromboplastin Time, especially performed on the Fibrometer, is more accurate than the Lee-White Clotting Time because it
eliminates variations in surface activation, phospholipid release
from platelets, temperature, and endpoint detection. For monitoring
heparin therapy, whole blood is preferable to plasma because platelet
have anti-heparin activity which should affect the determination.

The Whole Blood PTT has a reproducibility of $\pm$ 2% at normal levels
and $\pm$ 3% at therapeutic levels. Reproducibility of Lee-Whites is
$\pm$ 30%.

PERIODIC ACID-SCHIFF STAIN (PAS)

PRINCIPLE: Periodic Acid acts as an oxidizing agent which causes breakage of C - C bonds. A typical type of chemical reaction is the conversion of CHOH - CHOH to CHO · CHO which is a dialdehyde. Dialdehydes can be detected by utilization of Schiff's stain to form a red color.

SPECIMEN: Air dried blood or bone marrow smears.

REAGENTS:

1. Periodic Acid Solution
   Dissolve 5 gm. of periodic acid crystals in 500 ml. distilled water. This solution is stable for 3 months in a dark brown bottle.

2. Schiff's Reagent
   Can be purchased commercially. It may be prepared by dissolving 5 gm. of basic fuchsin in 500 ml. of hot distilled water. Filter the solution when cool and saturate it with sulfur dioxide gas by bubbling for 1 hour. Extract with activated charcoal and filter. The solution is stable for 3 months in a dark brown bottle.

3. Formalin-Ethanol Fixative
   Mix 10 ml. of 40% Formaldehyde with 90 ml. of absolute ethanol. Keep solution refrigerated.

4. Sodium Metabisulfite Solution
   Prepare solution by adding 10 gm. of sodium metabisulfite to 2 liters of distilled water.

5. Harris Hematoxylin
   Purchased commercially through Ortho Pharmaceutical Corp., Raritan, New Jersey.

PROCEDURE:

1. Fix air dried blood or bone marrow smears for 5 minutes in Formalin-Ethanol fixative.

2. Wash smears with tap water and place in Periodic Acid solution for 10 minutes and wash again.

PAS Stain (Continued):

3. Place smears in Schiff stain for 30 minutes.

4. Rinse in sodium metabisulfite solution for 2 minutes three times.

5. Wash with tap water for 10 minutes and counterstain with Harris Hematoxylin for 15 minutes.

RESULTS: PAS Positive cells will stain pink to red while PAS negative cells do not stain pink or red.

REFERENCE: Wislocki, G., Rheingold, J. and Dempsey, E.: "The Occurrence of the Periodic Acid-Schiff Reaction in Various Normal Cells of Blood and Connective Tissue". Blood 4:562, 1949.

INTERPRETATION:

The PAS stain identifies the presence of glycoprotein, mucoprotein, and muco and polysaccarides. Mature myeloid cells are strongly positive with all myeloid cells showing some reaction in all stages. Platelets and megakaryocytes stain prominently with PAS. Monocytes and lymphocytes contain a few PAS positive granules. Red blood cells and normoblasts are negative. Eosinophilic granules do not stain but the background is pink. Increased PAS staining is found in acute and chronic lymphocytic leukemia, Sezary syndrome, and Hodgkin's disease lymphocytes. The atypical lymphocytes of infectious mononucleosis also have increased PAS activity.

The normal normoblast is negative, but the malignant megaloid normoblast in Di Guglielmo's disease exhibits a positive reaction which is also found in anemia of ineffective erythropoiesis, thalassemia, and acquired hemolytic anemia.

PEROXIDASE REACTION
(Graham-Knoll)

PRINCIPLE: The enzyme peroxidase is present in the granules of myeloid cells. Its acts on hydrogen peroxide, liberating oxygen. The
liberated oxygen oxidizes benzidine to a brown compound. Therefore,
any structure containing peroxidase stains brown by this reaction.

REAGENTS:

1. 10% alcoholic formalin
   40% (full strength) formaldehyde   10 ml.
   95% ethanol   90 ml.

2. Peroxidase Reagent
   PREPARE FRESH JUST PRIOR TO USING. Use enough benzidine to
   cover the point of a knife (approximately 30 mg.). This is dissolved in 6.0 ml. of 95% ethanol. 4.0 ml. of distilled water
   are added plus 0.02 ml. of 3% hydrogen peroxide. The hydrogen
   peroxide must be fresh.

PROCEDURE:

1. Fix smears exactly 30 seconds in alcoholic formalin. Rinse with
   tap water and air dry.

2. Flood the slide with peroxidase reagent and leave on for 5 minutes. Rinse thoroughly with tap water and dry.

3. Counterstain with dilute Giemsa for 5 minutes.

COMMENTS:

1. The peroxidase reaction becomes gradually weaker when slides are
   more than one day old. Best results are obtained by using fresh
   smears and fresh hydrogen peroxide.

2. The amount of hydrogen peroxide added must be carefully measured.
   If too much hydrogen peroxide is used, the enzyme is destroyed
   before oxygen can be liberated. If not enough hydrogen peroxide
   is added or if the solution is old, the reaction will be weak or
   negative.

3. Control slides with a high percentage of myeloid cells should be
   included with each test. Negative controls should be made from

Peroxidase Reaction (Continued):

slides with a low percentage of myeloid cells. Peroxidase positive cells should approximate the number of myeloid cells seen on a differential.

REFERENCES:

1. Miale, John B.: LABORATORY MEDICINE HEMATOLOGY, 4th. Ed., C. V. Mosby Co., St. Louis, pg. 1210, 1972.

2. Kaplow, L. S.: "Myeloperoxidase Stain Utilizing Benzidine Dihydrochloride". Blood 26:215, 1965.

INTERPRETATION:

The peroxidase stain is positive in cells of the myeloid and monocytic series. The myeloblast is negative but the other cells in the myeloid series exhibit peroxidase activity. Eosinophils are positive in contrast to a negative reaction for basophils. Lymphocytes do not exhibit peroxidase activity.

6 - PHOSPHOGLUCONIC DEHYDROGENASE ASSAY

PRINCIPLE: 6-PGD in the presence of TPN converts 6-PG to pentose phosphate with the reduction of TPN to TPNH. The formation of TPNH is followed spectrophotometrically.

SPECIMEN: 5.0 ml. whole blood collected in EDTA and centrifuged.

REAGENTS:

1. <u>0.5 M. Tris</u>, pH 8.2
   Purchased commercially from Sigma Chemical Company. Adjust pH with 10 N. and 1.0 N. HCl.

2. <u>0.05 M. MgCl$_2$</u>

3. <u>0.05 M. 6-PG</u>
   Purchased from Sigma Chemical Company as sodium salt.

4. <u>0.05 M. TPN</u>
   Purchased from Sigma Chemical Company as sodium salt.

COMMENTS ON PROCEDURE:

1. Blood may be stored as whole blood refrigerated for a maximum of 48 hours.

2. pH of reagents must be within $\pm$ 0.05.

3. All enzyme reagents must be weighed quickly as they tend to be hydroscopic.

4. Working solutions of reagents (except buffers) should be kept frozen when not in use.

5. Keep reagents in ice bucket when using - NOT AT ROOM TEMPERATURE!

PROCEDURE:

A. <u>Preparation of Hemolysate</u>
   1. 5.0 ml. whole blood collected in EDTA and centrifuged; remove plasma and buffy coat.

   2. Wash <u>ONCE</u> using 5.0 ml. cold normal saline and after centrifuging remove supernatant.

263

6 - Phosphogluconic Dehydrogenase Assay (Continued):

3. Remove 0.2 ml. packed RBC and place in a pyrex test tube. Freeze-thaw twice using dry ice-acetone mixture. Do <u>NOT</u> allow the temperature of the hemolysate to exceed 10 to 15°C.

4. Add 10 ml. distilled water to the hemolysate, swirl and refrigerate for 15 minutes.

5. Determine the hemoglobin concentration in gm%. and then dilute the hemolysate with distilled water to give a final hemoglobin concentration of 0.20 gm%.

B. <u>Test</u>
Use 3.0 ml. Beckman cuvettes.

	Blank	1 Control	2 Patient
Tris, 0.5 M. pH 8.2	0.5	0.5	0.5
MgCl$_2$ 0.05 M.	0.6	0.6	0.6
6-PG 0.05 M.	0.0	0.2	0.2
Hemolysate, 0.2 gm%. Control	0.5	0.5	0.0
Hemolysate, 0.2 gm%. Patient	0.0	0.0	0.5
Distilled Water, ml.	1.3	1.1	1.1

Mix contents well and take a base reading at 340 nm. Add with shaking at zero time:

TPN 0.05 M.	0.1	0.1	0.1

O.D. Readings taken at 30 seconds
5 minutes
10 minutes
15 minutes
30 minutes

C. <u>Calculations</u>

Measure the difference in O.D. reading between 30 seconds and 30 minutes. There will be an increase in O.D. and it should be linear. Activity is calculated by multiplying ΔO.D. x 2900 and is expressed as micromoles substrate converted per hour per 10" RBC.

NORMAL VALUES: 400 - 975 um/hr./10" RBC

6 - Phosphogluconic Dehydrogenase Assay (Continued):

REFERENCE: Marks, P. A.: "6-Phosphogluconate Dehydrogenase: Clinical Aspects". In W. A. Wood (Ed.) METHODS IN ENZYMOLOGY, Vol. IX, Chapter on Enzymes of Carbohydrate Metabolism, Academic Press, pg. 141, 1966.

INTERPRETATION:

6-Phosphogluconate dehydrogenase (6-PGD) deficiency relates to the pentose phosphate pathway. Such deficient individuals may have minimal hemolysis. An assay for this enzyme is based on the reduction of NADP in the presence of excess 6-phosphogluconate.

PLASMA PROTAMINE PARACOAGULATION

PRINCIPLE: Protamine permits the release of soluble fibrin monomer from the complex with fibrin degradation products. The monomer polymerizes to become visible insoluble fibrin strands.

SPECIMEN: Citrated plasma (9 parts blood, 1 part 3.8% sodium citrate

REAGENTS:

1. 1.0% Protamine Sulfate

2. Imidazole Buffer, pH 7.35 $\pm$ 0.05
   6.8 gm. imidazole
   16.7 gm. sodium chloride
   372 ml. 0.1 M. HCl
   Dilute to 2 liters and check pH.

SOURCES OF ERROR:

1. Tubes should be kept at 37°C. and not allowed to cool before reading.

2. Hemolysis or tissue fluid in specimen will give false positive results.

PROCEDURE:

1. Make serial dilutions of 1% protamine sulfate:
   1:5, 1:10, 1:20, 1:40
   Warm to 37°C.

2. Pipette 0.2 ml. patient's plasma in 4 tubes labelled for the dilutions above. Warm to 37°C.

3. Add 0.2 ml. of dilutions to plasma; mix gently, and incubate 30 minutes at 37°C.

4. To 0.2 ml. normal plasma add 0.2 ml. of 1:5 dilution.

5. To 0.2 ml. positive control, add 0.2 ml. of 1:10 dilution. Mix and incubate controls.

Plasma Protamine Paracoagulation (Continued):

6. Remove tubes one at a time and look for fibrin threads, gel, or feathery precipitate. Opalescence and granular precipitate is read as negative.

NORMAL VALUES: Negative Test.
Report positive in the highest dilution with fibrin threads.

POSITIVE CONTROL:

Plasma containing fibrin monomers may be made by adding enough thrombin to normal plasma to give a final concentration of 0.02 NIH units of thrombin/ml. of plasma. Incubate at 37°C. for 30 minutes. Centrifuge to remove fibrin threads formed. This may be stored for a brief time, usually about 2 weeks, until it loses activity in the freezer.

REFERENCES:

1. Seaman, Arthur J.: "The Plasma Protamine Paracoagulation Test". Arch. Int. Med. 125:1016, 1970.

2. Sanfelippo, Michael J., Stevens, David J., Koenig, Robert R.: "Protamine Sulfate Test for Fibrin Monomers". Am. J. Clin. Path. 56:166-173, 1971.

INTERPRETATION:

The main value of the PPP Test is to detect soluble fibrin monomer present in the plasma associated with disseminated intravascular coagulation. A titer above 1:5 with decrease in platelets, intrinsic and extrinsic factors, and fibrinogen is suggestive of DIC.

A false positive PPP Test may occur in other conditions associated with bleeding and clotting, such as post-operative state, idiopathic thrombocytopenic purpura, bleeding gastrointestinal lesions, menstruation, phlebothrombosis, and pulmonary embolism.

PLATELET ADHESION

PRINCIPLE: The decrease in platelet count which occurs when blood is passed through a standard glass bead column at a standard flow rate is determined. This decrease is due to the adhesive ability and aggregation of normal platelets.

REAGENTS AND EQUIPMENT:

1. Infusion Pump

2. Glass Bead Column

3. EDTA Tubes

4. Plastic Tubing

5. Syringes, 10 cc.

6. Needles, 20 Gauge

7. Platelet Counting Reagents and Equipment

SPECIMEN: 10 ml. blood.

PROCEDURE:

1. Draw about 10 ml. blood into a plastic syringe without a tourniquet and without introducing bubbles.

2. Place 3 to 4 ml. into an EDTA tube for a control.

3. Immediately attach the syringe to the infusion pump which has been set to deliver 5.8 ml./minute.

4. Attach the bead column with a short adaptor of plastic tubing to the syringe tip.

5. Turn the infusion pump on and collect 4.0 ml. of blood into an EDTA Tube labeled "Test". It is important to collect 4.0 ml. since variation of more than 0.5 ml. changes the number of platelets which are retained.

Platelet Adhesion (Continued):

6. Do platelet counts on test and control bloods and calculate the percentage which was retained in the bead column.

7. CALCULATIONS:

Control Platelets - Test Platelets = Platelets Retained.

$$\frac{\text{Platelets Retained}}{\text{Control Platelets}} \times 100 = \% \text{ Platelet Adhesion.}$$

NORMAL VALUES: Each Laboratory must Establish a Normal Range with the Equipment Used.

REFERENCES:

1. Helem, A. J.: "Platelet Adhesiveness in von Willebrand's Disease". Scand. J. Haemat. 7:374-382, 1970.

2. Rossi, E. C.: "A Study of Platelet Retention by Glass Bead Columns". Brit. J. of Haematology 23:47-57, 1972.

3. Zacharski, L. R.: "A Standardized Test of Platelet Adhesiveness". Amer. J. Clin. Path. 58:422-427, 1972.

4. Williams, W. J.: HEMATOLOGY McGraw-Hill Co., New York, pgs. 1414-1415, 1972.

INTERPRETATION:

Platelet adhesion is decreased in patients with von Willebrand's disease and in acquired functional platelet disorders, such as in uremia or excessive sensitivity to various drugs, most commonly aspirin. Platelet adhesiveness is decreased by aspirin, and the test should not be made within 1 week after taking aspirin. An increased sensitivity to aspirin may be demonstrated by making the test before and 4 hours after taking 10 grains of aspirin.

PLATELET ADHESIVE TEST (IN VIVO)

PRINCIPLE: A small incision is made on the forearm. Serial platelet counts in the exuded blood decrease rapidly to low levels since platelets adhere to the surface of the incised tissue.

SPECIMEN:

1. Venous platelet count from 5.0 ml. of anticoagulated antecubital vein blood.

2. Capillary platelet counts from incised volar arm at 1, 3, and 5 minutes.

REAGENTS AND EQUIPMENT:

1. Blood Pressure Cuff

2. Alcohol, 70%

3. Bard-Parker Blade, No. 11

PROCEDURE:

1. Clean an area on the volar surface of the forearm with 70 percent alcohol.

2. Place a blood pressure cuff on the upper arm and inflate to 40 mm. of mercury.

3. Make a 5.0 mm. deep incision with a No. 11 Bard-Parker Blade.

4. Perform three serial platelet counts on the exuding blood at 2 minute intervals.

5. Gently wipe the wound with dry gauze before each collection to insure a fresh blood sample.

6. CALCULATIONS:

   a). Average the three capillary platelet counts.

   b). Adhesive Platelet Count = Venous Platelet Count - Average
       Capillary Platelet Count

Platelet Adhesive Test (Continued):

c). Adhesive Platelet Count = Venous Platelet Count - Average
Capillary Platelet Count

d). Platelet Adhesiveness = $\dfrac{\text{Adhesive Platelet Count}}{\text{Venous Platelet Count}}$ x 100

REFERENCE: Owen, C., Jr., Bowie, E., Didisheim, P., and Thompson, J.,
Jr.: THE DIAGNOSIS OF BLEEDING DISORDERS, Little, Brown
and Company, Boston, pg. 80, 1969.

INTERPRETATION:

The normal range of platelet adhesiveness is 15 to 45 percent. Abnormal platelet function is induced by drugs such as aspirin or hereditary conditions such as von Willebrand's disease or Glanzmann's
thrombasthenia. An elevated IgM, as is found in Waldenstrom's Macroglobulinemia or multiple myeloma may cause decreased platelet adhesiveness by coating the platelets.

PLATELET AGGREGATION

PRINCIPLE: Platelets clump or aggregate if adenosine diphosphate (ADP) is added to platelet rich plasma (citrated). This procedure measures platelet function.

SPECIMEN: Patient's platelet rich plasma collected in 3.2 to 4.0% citrate and normal control platelet rich plasma.

REAGENTS AND EQUIPMENT:

1. Beckman Spectrophotometer

2. Adenosine Diphosphate (ADP)
   100 to 1000 mg./ml.

3. Small Plastic Tubes (2)

PROCEDURE:

1. Obtain patient's platelet rich plasma (citrated) in a small plastic test tube. Mix venous blood with 0.1 ml. volume of 3.2 to 4.0% sodium citrate.

2. Centrifuge at 250 x G for 10 minutes.

3. Record the optical density on the Beckman Spectrophotometer.

4. At 37°C., add ADP. The concentration should be 100 to 1000 mg. per ml. Add a volume of 0.1 to 0.2 the volume of platelet rich plasma.

5. Record the decrease in optical density as the platelets aggregate.

6. Perform the same procedure on the control platelet rich plasma.

REFERENCE: Mustard, J. F., Negardt, B., Rowsell, H. and MacMilan, R.
"Effect of Adenine Nucleotides on Platelet Aggregation and Clotting Time". J. Lab. Clin. Med. 64:548, 1964.

Platelet Aggregation (Continued):

INTERPRETATION AND RESULTS:

Platelets which are functionally abnormal will not aggregate. The process of aggregation is dependent on:

1. The Platelet Count
2. Capacity to aggregate
3. Calcium

In addition to ADP, thrombin, collagen or epinephrine may also be utilized to aggregate platelets.

Two waves of aggregation occur at 37°C. with epinephrine and ADP. At room temperature a single wave occurs. At 37°C. the second wave is due to ADP released from the platelets.

Various platelet abnormalities are characterized by decreased release of ADP. It is important that patients do not take aspirin or other anti-inflammatory drugs for approximately one week prior to the platelet aggregation test since these drugs interfere with platelet function.

PLATELET AGGREGATION
(Aggregometer Method)

PRINCIPLE: When an aggregating agent is added to platelet-rich plasma the shape change and aggregation of platelets causes a decrease in optical density of the plasma.

COLLECTION AND PREPARATION OF SPECIMEN: Blood is obtained by clean venipuncture. Nine volumes of blood is added to one volume of 3.8% trisodium citrate. Centrifuge at room temperature for 10 to 15 minutes at 200-220 g's. $[g = 11.28 \times 10^{-6} \times$ radius of centrifuge head in cm. x (speed in rpm)$^2]$. Plastic pipettes are used to transfer plasma to plastic tubes. The remaining blood is centrifuged to obtain platelet-poor plasma at about 1500 g's for 30 minutes. Keep plasma at room temperature until it is to be tested. Complete test within 3 hours.

EQUIPMENT AND REAGENTS:

1. Plastic or Siliconized Tubes

2. Plastic or Siliconized Pipettes

3. Aggregometer

4. Aggregating Reagents
   A. Adenosine Diphosphate
      Dilute with distilled water to 40 micromoles/ml. Store in 1.0 ml. aliquots at -60°C. Stable about 6 months.

   B. Collagen
      Determine potency of each lot of collagen and dilute so that 0.05 ml. will give optimal aggregation with normal plasma. Store at -60°C. in 1.0 ml. aliquots.

   C. Epinephrine
      Dilute to 100 micromoles/ml. with Tris saline buffer, pH 7.4. Freeze in 1.0 ml. aliquots at -20°C.

   D. Thrombin, Bovine or Human
      Dilute to 3 units/ml. in Tris Buffer, pH 7.4. Store in 1.0 ml aliquots at -20°C.

5. Tris Buffer, pH 7.4
   Adjust pH with HCl. About 16 ml./100 ml. is usually needed.

274

Platelet Aggregation - Aggregometer Method (Continued):

6. Control
Obtain normal donor, draw blood, and process in same manner as patient plasma.

PROCEDURE:

1. Warm 1.0 ml. aliquot of plasma as needed to 37°C. for 5 minutes in siliconized glass cuvette.

2. Place in cell compartment of aggregometer and maintain temperature at 37°C. while testing.

3. Determine 100% transmittance with patient's platelet-poor plasma.

4. Place patient's prewarmed platelet-rich plasma in aggregometer.

5. Adjust sensitivity to read 0 - 10%.

6. After stirring 2 minutes add 0.05 ml. of aggregating agent.

7. Record continuously.

8. Run in duplicate.

9. Rate and amount of aggregation is obtained from recorder tracing.

10. ADP and epinephrine should give double waves of aggregation.

11. Collagen and thrombin give single waves.

REFERENCES:

1. Michal, F.: "Measurement of Platelet Aggregation and Shape Change". Advances in Exper. Med. & Biol. 34:257-262, 1972.

2. Born, G. V. R.: "Aggregation of Blood Platelets by Adenosine and its Reversal". Nature 194:927, 1962.

3. Weiss, Harvey, J. L.: "Platelet Aggregation" in HEMATOLOGY ed. by William Williams, et. al., McGraw-Hill, New York, pgs. 1415-1417, 1972.

4. Cronberg, S.: "Evaluation of Platelet Aggregation". Coagulation 3:39, 1970.

Platelet Aggregation - Aggregometer Method (Continued):

INTERPRETATION:

See Interpretation Section of Platelet Aggregation on page 273.

AUTOANALYZER PLATELETS

PRINCIPLE: A whole blood sample is diluted with a 2.0 M. urea solution to hemolyze the RBC and the final dilution is pumped to the Autoanalyzer cell counter. The cell counter utilizes a dark-field microscopic light scattering principle to detect cells passing through the flow cell viewing area. To determine the count, the frequency at which the detected cells pass through the viewing area is converted to a voltage of direct proportion. The recorder plots the changing voltage level on the chart paper, resulting in individual curves.

EQUIPMENT: See Technicon Operating Manual for assembly and maintenance of Sampler, Pump II, manifold, cell counter and recorder.

REAGENTS:

1. 2.0 M. Urea
    Commercially prepared.

2. Cell Counter Wash Solution, 0.2 N. NaOH

3. Sample Wash Solution
    1 liter distilled water plus 0.5 ml. Brij-35 Wetting Agent
    (Technicon).

4. Platelet Standard
    Human platelet standard; store at room temperature.

5. Whole Blood Controls
    Those bloods within normal range, chosen and held over from
    previous day.

POINTS TO REMEMBER: Daily (Before Operation)

1. Check ink supply.
2. Check that all waste lines are positioned in waste receptacles
    (especially in sink).
3. Check reagent supply.
4. Check Brij - water supply.
5. Check for uniform bubble pattern.
6. With urea only in lines, check to see that pattern on cell counter-
    screen is not wider than 2 grid-widths.

Autoanalyzer Platelets (Continued):

OPERATION:

1. Timer switch in OFF position and wash-time knob pointing to grey area.

2. Turn on power to cell counter. (Warm up 30 minutes.)

3. Turn recorder-instrument on.

4. With left side stationary, stretch manifold to position right side in designated hole (1, 2, or 3) on the manifold posts. Once manifold is positioned, be <u>sure</u> the <u>metal side-rails</u> are on the manifold posts <u>under the manifold bars</u>!

5. Secure platen.

6. Turn proportioning pump on and immediately --

7. Turn stop-cock to urea reagent.

8. Shake urea filter to rid line of air.

9. Wait for consistent bubble pattern throughout system.

10. Turn Chart-drive on, and wait for baseline to maintain zero position. If baseline does <u>not</u> go to zero in 5 minutes, adjust with "ZERO ADJUST" knob in top of cell counter. DO NOT TOUCH ANY OTHER KNOBS IN THIS COMPARTMENT.

11. Begin sampling with two Isoton washes.

12. Follow with 3 <u>well-mixed</u> Standards.

13. Then follow with one Isoton wash.

14. Begin running whole blood checks. (Whole blood checks should be between 150,000 and 350,000.)

15. Begin patient bloods.

16. <u>WITH ALL SAMPLES</u>:
    a). Do not set up more than six cups ahead (this includes washes)
    b). Wash between every <u>five</u> consecutive bloods.
    c). With a wash before it, run a Standard or whole blood Control every 10 to 15 patient bloods. If the Controls rise or fall

Autoanalyzer Platelets (Continued):

> more than 15,000, RESET STANDARD!
>
> d). When making dilutions to rerun high counts, DO NOT make the dilution more than 1 to 2 cups before it will be sampled, since these cups settle exceptionally fast!

17. The recorder is always 2 specimens behand the sampler.

18. <u>Standards</u> (3):
   a). The <u>first</u> standard to record: Observe and set sensitivity to phase value; start wash-timer cycle, and turn to "40" position simultaneously, just as the peak begins to fall. If unable to start as first peak falls, start cycle on next peak.
   b). The sensitivity may be adjusted on <u>second</u> standard also.
   c). The <u>third</u> standard is <u>not</u> to be adjusted! If more adjustments are needed run more standards.

NOTE: Before reporting out any platelets BE SURE that all the whole blood Controls are within a 2 Standard Deviation range from the previous day's results. If <u>all</u> the Controls have dropped or risen, consider resetting the machine.

TO END A.M. RUN:

1. Turn Chart-drive off.

2. Run 3 Isoton washes to clear lines.

3. With lines cleared: Return sampling probe to wash-well and turn Sampler power off.

4. When wash-timer is in any grey zone; turn "40" setting to off position.

5. Turn cell counter power off.

6. Turn recorder instrument power off.

7. Turn proportioning pump off.

8. Important: Turn reagent stopcock to off position and <u>then</u> remove platen and release <u>right</u> side of manifold.

9. Clean work area (especially empty waste container).

Autoanalyzer Platelets (Continued):

TO END P.M. RUN:

1. Finish sampling with 3 Isoton washes.

2. Stop sampling probe power when probe returns to wash-well, and return mixing paddles to up position.

3. Turn chart-drive off.

4. Turn recorder instrument off.

5. IMPORTANT:
   With wash cycle still on, changing only the large wash tube (small tube to remain in Brij-water at all times):
   a). Run Brij-water for 10 minutes
   b). Run NaOH for 5 minutes
   c). Then run Brij-water again for a mininum of 5 minutes.

6. When wash-timer returns to any part of the grey area, turn "40" setting to off position.

7. Turn proportioning pump off.

8. Turn stop-cock arrow to off position.

9. Remove platen and right side of manifold.

10. Check again to make sure that all switches are in off positions.

11. Close recorder door and cover manifold tray with a towel.

12. Clean up area and flush out sink.

RECORDING IN PLATELET BOOK:

1. Standard
   When beginning days run, record both the value at which you set the Standard and the value gotten by phase. Record value of Standard each time one is run.

2. Checks
   Be sure the phase count on the checks is recorded in the book. (In so far as possible, choose whole blood checks that have been counted by phase.)

Autoanalyzer Platelets (Continued):

3. Label peaks from your "scratch sheet" and record only final results in the permanent record book.

4. It is the responsibility of the platelet person to see that platelet counts are corrected as necessary:
   a). All platelet counts of 100,000 or lower must have WBC subtracted.
   b). All WBC of 20,000 or higher must be subtracted from the platelet count. Person running the Coulter S should notice whether specimens with WBC or 20,000 or higher have platelets ordered, and inform platelet person about high WBC.

5. In general, any one lot of Standard should be set at the same value from day to day, although the phase count may vary up or down. Change setting for the lot only as difficulties arise with checks.

MAINTENANCE

1. Daily

   Flow-Cell
   Observe and focus to achieve narrowest baseline on cell counter screen (cell counter must be ON, and urea running through).

   Tubing and Fittings
   Check for leaks. Check to see that platen is clean and dry. Check ink supply.

   Bubble Pattern
   Observe closely before and after sampling begins.

   Wash-Timer Valve
   Check for any leaks or white precipitate.

2. Weekly
   Remove and clean wash-well.
   Wash reagent filters under tap water.
   Oil mixer paddles.
   Clean metal tubing connectors with a wire.
   Add ink once a week.

3. Monthly
   Remove sample probe and clean.
   Clean air filters under running water at END of day's run.

282

Autoanalyzer Platelets (Continued):

Clean wash-timer valve and replace (clean more often if precipitate begins to accumulate).
Change manifold tubing.

4. Every 3 Months
General lubrication.
Replace large reagent filter.
Check lamp for blackening; clear dust.

NORMAL VALUES: 150,000 - 350,000 cu. mm.

REFERENCE: Technicon Operating Instruction Manual

INTERPRETATION:

See Interpretation of Coulter Counter Platelets on page 285 and
Phase Contrast Platelets on page 287 in addition to the following.

Platelet values may be read directly from the chart paper. Readings
greater than 650,000 cu. mm. should be rediluted 1:2. Samples following a high reading should be rerun to check for platelet carryover.

Low platelet counts (less than 100,000 cu. mm.) should be preceded by
a wash cup and run in duplicate. WBC correction should be done for
the low platelet counts (less than 100,000 cu. mm.) and for bloods
with an uncorrected WBC of greater than 20,000 cu. mm.

Fresh smear evaluations should accompany each machine count. Any dis-
crepancy should be checked manually.

PLATELETS ON COULTER COUNTER

PRINCIPLE: Platelet counts are done on platelet-rich plasma which is obtained by sedimenting red cells. The count is done on a Coulter Model B which has a lower and upper threshhold control. The lower control eliminates counting debris and electrical interference. The upper control prevents counting larger cells as red cells and white cells. The RBC's seem to be surrounded by a fixed amount of platelet-free plasma. During sedimentation, the red cell will carry this platelet-free plasma with them, leaving a relatively higher concentration of platelets in the supernatant. The mechanism by which the red cells retain the platelet-free zone of plasma around them is not clear; however, it may be related to the known negative charges on red cells as well as platelets.

SPECIMEN: EDTA tube of blood.

EQUIPMENT AND REAGENTS:

1. Coulter Model B with two position monometer (0.1 and 0.5) and a 70 mu. aperture.

2. Normal Saline, 0.85%

3. Tygon Tubing, 1/8 inch internal diameter

4. Capillary Pipettes, 2 Microliter and 4 Microliter

5. Autodilutor

COMMENTS ON PROCEDURE:

1. Digital readout should read between 5.0 and 10 on Coulter, additional dilutions are frequently necessary for this.

2. Two phase counts must be done each morning to check the Coulter.

3. Slide estimations must be done on all Coulter platelets. Incompatibilities are checked by phase.

4. Counts below 50,000 must be done by phase.

5. Patients with giant platelets must be done by phase.

Platelets - Coulter Counter (Continued):

6. Background count must be less than 40.

7. Patients with high ESR may not settle sufficiently and must be done by phase.

COULTER SETTINGS:

> AMP ¼   Lower Threshhold   5
> ACS ¼   Upper Threshhold 50 (Separate

Controls Under Cover

> Gain Control   50
> Matching Set L 64

PROCEDURE:

1. Fill tygon tubing with well mixed whole blood using a Pasteur pipette, avoiding bubbles.

2. Approximately 10 - 15 minutes are required to settle the RBC's sufficiently for the platelets to be removed. When a sufficient amount of plasma-platelet suspension is available, pipette (by capillary action) 2 microliters into each of three vials containing 12 ml. saline to make a 1:6000 dilution. The red cells should not be allowed to settle more than 1/3 the length of the tygon tubing before the pipetting is done. After pipetting each specimen, carefully rinse pipette 2 to 3 times with the saline in cup. One microcap pipette may be used for each patient. Cap vials and mix well.

3. If six specimens are being run simultaneously, count the first vial of each sample as soon as possible to determine the dilution necessary for an accurate count on that particular patient. If the Coulter count is below 5.0, immediately pipette 4 microliters of plasma-platelet suspension into 12 ml. of saline for a 1:3000 dilution. If this is below 3.0, do platelet count by phase microscopy. If the original 1:6000 dilution records a count of 10, add 6.0 ml. of saline to each vial to make a 1:9000 dilution.

4. Count each vial twice. Results should not differ by more than 0.1 (100 particles). Record the results of three vials in the appropriate column.

Platelets - Coulter Counter (Continued):

5. CALCULATIONS:

The calculations are adapted from those used on the Coulter Model A for WBC. The dilution factor is derived from the 1:500 dilution, i.e., the 1:3000 dilution has a factor of 6 (6 x 500 = 3000). The constant "5" is derived from the fact that the total volume counted is 0.1 ml. rather than 0.5 as in WBC. The corrected plasma factor is used because during sedimentations, the RBC trap some plasma which is free of platelets. This makes an excess of platelets in supernatant plasma. This is read from the chart using the patient's PCV. The 10 is to correct for the sampling - 2 microliters as compared to 20 microliters used in white counts.

Coulter count x dilution factor x 5 x corrected plasma volume x 10 = Whole blood platelet count.

EXAMPLES:

a. 4 microliters in 12 ml. saline 1:3000
Coulter count x 5 x 6 x corrected plasma volume x 10
= platelet count

b. 2 microliters in 12 ml. saline 1:6000
Coulter count x 5 x 12 x corrected plasma volume x 10
= platelet count

c. 2 microliters in 24 ml. saline 1:12,000
Coulter count x 5 x 24 x corrected plasma volume x 10
= platelet count

NORMAL VALUES: 150,000 - 350,000/mm^3

REFERENCE: Bull, B., Schniederman, L., and Brecker, G.: <u>Am. J. Clin. Path.</u>, Vol. 44, December, 1965.

INTERPRETATION:

See Interpretation Section of Phase Contrast Enumeration of Blood Platelets on page 287.

PHASE CONTRAST ENUMERATION OF BLOOD PLATELETS

PRINCIPLE: The optical properties of the phase system are such that materials with different densities appear to differ from each other in the intensity and shade of light transmitted through them.

SPECIMEN: An EDTA lavender top tube of whole blood.

EQUIPMENT AND REAGENTS:

1. 1% Ammonium Oxalate (W/V)
   Store in refrigerator and filter before use.

2. Special Thin Flat Bottom Counting Chamber

3. No. 1 Glass Cover Slips

4. RBC Diluting Pipettes

5. B-D Vacutainer Tubes (versenate) #3204 Q

6. Microscope
   Equipped with a long distance working condenser and a 43X phase objective.

COMMENTS:

1. Platelets are round dark bodies sometimes showing dendritic processes. Dirt particles are refractile. RBC will appear as ghost cells.

2. If the platelets are clumped together the count should be rediluted

3. Platelets must be pipetted immediately but the pipettes may be stored in the refrigerator for not more than 8 hours.

4. Because of the adhesive quality of about 1/3 of the platelets, finger stick platelets counts should be discouraged.

PROCEDURE:

1. Draw 5.0 ml. in a lavender top.

2. Triplicate red blood cell pipettes are filled to the 1 mark with blood and diluted to the 101 mark with 1% ammonium oxalate.

286

Phase Contrast - Platelets (Continued):

3. Shake two pipettes for five minutes and fill chamber. Fill one side of chamber with each pipette.

4. Cover the counting chamber with a Petri dish containing a moistened filter paper and let stand for 15 minutes.

5. Each side should be counted by a different technologist.

6. The total RBC area is counted (25 small squares). The total number of platelets x 1,000 will give the whole blood platelet count per cu. mm. If the number of cells in the area is less than 100, the WBC area is counted until one has a minimum of 150 cells or has counted 5 large squares. In this case divide the count by the number of large squares counted and then multiply by 1,000.

7. The two sides of a chamber must agree within 2 M, where M is the square root of the mean.
   FOR EXAMPLE:
   If 80 cells were counted on one side of the chamber and 120 on the other, this would constitute the maximum variation tolerable as:

$$\text{MEAN} = 100$$
$$M = 10$$
$$2M = \pm 20$$
$$100 \pm 20 = 80 \text{ and } 120$$

If the two sides of the chamber do not agree, the pipettes must be reshaken and the chamber recounted. If there is still lack of agreement in these or if clumps are present, the third pipette is counted.

NORMAL VALUES: 150,000 - 350,000

REFERENCE: Brecker, G., Cronkite, E.: "Morphology and Enumeration of Human Blood Platelets". J. Appl. Physiol. 3:365, 1950.

INTERPRETATION:

It is important to determine the total platelet count in the evaluation of the coagulation system. Venous blood should be obtained for platelet counts since fingertip or heel stick blood has lower counts from platelets adhering to the wound.

Phase Contrast - Platelets (Continued):

Decrease in the platelet count or thrombocytopenia may be due to:

1. Bone marrow failure with decrease in megakaryocytes, drugs, chemotherapeutic agents, or irradiation may be etiologic factors.

2. Replacement of the bone marrow by metastatic malignancy, leukemia, or lymphoma.

3. Splenomegaly with platelet sequestration.

4. Immune destruction secondary to drugs, antibody or idiopathic thrombocytopenic purpura.

5. Various hematologic or infectious disorders, such as pernicious anemia, paroxysmal nocturnal hemoglobinuria or viral diseases.

Severe thrombocytopenia is accompanied by an increased bleeding time and poor clot retraction.

An increase in the platelet count or thrombocytosis occurs in:

1. Myeloproliferative syndrome, including Polycythemia Rubra Vera.

2. Following splenectomy.

3. Associated with utilization of adrenal cortical steroids. Thus, the acute stress reaction associated with trauma or after surgery will increase the platelet count.

4. Acute hemorrhage.

5. Iron deficiency anemia.

6. Various epithelial malignancies. An important cause for the tendency of venous thrombosis in malignancy is thrombocytosis and increase in the blood fibrinogen.

^{51}CHROMIUM PLATELET SURVIVAL TEST

PRINCIPLE: Platelet survival is determined by this procedure, utilizing a ^{51} Cr radioactive label. Normal platelet survival with this test is approximately 10 days.

SPECIMEN: 500 ml. of whole blood collected in a blood bank donor unit in ACD donor bag.

REAGENTS AND EQUIPMENT:

1. 500 ml. ACD Blood Bank Donor Set

2. 300 ml. Transfer Packs

3. 0.15 M. Citric Acid (filtered and autoclaved)

4. $Na^{51}CrO_4$
   Specific activity 0.5 uc/mg. preferred

5. NaCl, 5.0%

6. EDTA, 5.0%

7. Normal Saline

8. Ammonium Oxalate, 1.0%

9. Plastic or Siliconized Test Tubes and Syringes

PROCEDURE:

1. Labelling of Platelets
   a). 500 ml. of whole blood is collected in a standard ACD bag. Centrifuge at 1,200 rpm at 10°C. for 15 minutes.

   b). The supernatant platelet-rich plasma is collected in a 300 ml. transfer pack and centrifuged at 1,500 rpm for 5 minutes to remove remaining erythrocytes.

   c). The supernatant is transferred to a fresh transfer pack and 0.15 M. citric acid is added under sterile conditions to lower the pH to 6.4. The acidified platelet-rich plasma is then centrifuged at 2,300 rpm for 15 minutes.

289

[51]Chromium Platelet Survival Test (Continued):

d). The supernatant plasma is transferred to a fresh transfer pack. 10 ml. of plasma should remain with the platelet button.

e). The platelets are resuspended in the remaining plasma.

f). 250 - 350 microcuries of NaCr[51] are added.

g). A 20 to 30 minute incubation at room temperature is necessary for adequate labeling of the platelets.

h). All but 50 to 75 ml. of the supernatant plasma is returned to the platelet concentrate and centrifuged at 2,300 rpm for 15 minutes.

i). The supernatant plasma is discarded and 10 ml. of remaining plasma is floated over the platelet button and discarded.

j). The platelet button is resuspended in 30 to 50 ml. of the remaining plasma and is drawn up in a plastic 50 ml. syringe.

k). Record volume and inject intravenously.

l). One ml. is saved for determining platelet radioactivity.

2. Concentration of Platelets for Determining Radioactivity
   a). 10 ml. of blood is collected with a plastic syringe and anti-coagulated with 0.3 ml. of 5 percent EDTA in a plastic tube.

   b). The tube is filled with normal saline and centrifuged at 1,500 rpm for 7 minutes at 20°C.

   c). The supernatant platelet-rich plasma is removed and placed in another tube and the procedure repeated. 95 percent of the platelets are thus removed.

   d). The platelet-rich plasma is centrifuged at 3,500 rpm for 30 minutes and the supernatant is discarded.

   e). The platelet button is washed with 1 percent ammonium oxalate (at 3,500 rpm for 30 minutes) and resuspended in 2.0 ml. of oxalate for counting in the scintillation counter.

51Chromium Platelet Survival Test (Continued):

3. Determination of Platelet Activity

a). Platelet radioactivity is determined by obtaining a 0.3 ml. aliquot of the original platelet suspension.

b). Suspend it in oxalate to hemolyze red blood cells present.

c). Centrifuge at 3,500 rpm for 30 minutes.

d). The supernatant contains the red blood cells and plasma radioactivity.

e). The platelet button, resuspended in 2.0 ml. of oxalate can be used to calculate the total platelet radioactivity injected.

f). The percent recovery of platelets may be calculated by estimating the patients blood volume.

g). Survival is usually plotted as a percent of the recovery. During the initial 6 hours, draw frequent samples.

NORMAL VALUES: Normal platelet survival time is approximately 10 days. Any cause for platelet destruction will give a shortened survival.

REFERENCE: Cohen, P., Gardner, F. & Barnett, G.: "Reclassification of The Thrombocytopenias by the 51Cr Labeling Method for Platelet Lifespan". New Eng. J. Med. 264:1294, 1961.

INTERPRETATION:

Normal recovery of 51Cr labeled platelets is 50 - 70 percent at 2 to 4 hours. If the recovery is lower than normal, rapid destruction of platelets has occurred or splenic sequestration is present. An excessive recovery indicates splenectomy.

The normal platelet survival time is approximately 10 days. Any cause for platelet destruction will give a shortened survival.

QUALITATIVE URINARY PORPHOBILINOGEN

PRINCIPLE: Porphobilinogen reacts with Ehrlich's aldehyde reagent to form a red compound, porphobilinogen aldehyde, which is soluble in aqueous solutions but not in n-butyl alcohol. Urobilinogen reacts with Ehrlich's reagent also but is readily extracted by butyl alcohol.

SPECIMEN: Urine sample must be a freshly voided specimen as porphobilinogen is unstable.

REAGENTS:

1. Modified Ehrlich's Reagent
   0.7 gm. paradimethylaminobenzaldehyde
   150.0 ml. concentrated HCl
   100.0 ml. distilled water. Store in a brown bottle.

2. Sodium Acetate, saturated aqueous solution

3. N-Butyl Alcohol

PROCEDURE:

1. To 2.5 ml. urine, add 2.5 ml. Ehrlich's reagent and mix.

2. Add 5.0 ml. saturated sodium acetate. Shake vigorously.

3. Add 5.0 to 10 ml. n-butyl alcohol and mix.

4. Examine the lower aqueous layer for red color of porphobilinogen aldehyde.

5. The aldehyde compound of urobilinogen will be extracted by the n-butyl alcohol while the insoluble porphobilinogen will remain in the lower aqueous layer.

6. Report: Negative, trace, or positive.

NORMAL VALUE: Normal Porphobilinogen is a Negative Reading.

Qualitative Urinary Porphobilinogen

REFERENCE: Schwartz, S., et. al.: METHODS OF BIOCHEMICAL ANALYSIS
Vol. 8, Interscience Publishers, New York, pg. 221,
1960.

INTERPRETATION:

Porphobilinogen is a monopyrrole formed by condensation of two molecules of delta-amino-levulinic acid. Porphobilinogen is colorless
and converts to a red porphobilin and uroporphyrin after excretion.
Urinary excretion of porphobilinogen is greatly increased in acute
intermittent porphyria. These individuals exhibit acute abdominal
pain and neurologic symptoms or peripheral neuropathy. When the
patient is asymptomatic, the test for porphobilinogen may be negative.

Patients with Porphyria Cutanea Tardea may excrete porphobilinogen
occasionally.

PORPHYRINS

PRINCIPLE: Most porphyrins give a bright red fluorescence in ultra-violet light. This characteristic and the different solubilities of coproporphyrins and uroporphyrins allow extraction and qualitative separation in this screening test.

SPECIMEN: 25 ml. of urine that has been protected from light. Specimen may be stored in the refrigerator.

REAGENTS:

1. Glacial Acetic Acid

2. Ether

3. HCl, 5%

COMMENTS ON PROCEDURE: Small amounts of coproporphyrins are present in normal urine. Uroporphyrins are not normally present in urine.

PROCEDURE:

1. In a separatory funnel, place 25 ml. of urine.

2. Add 10 ml. of glacial acetic acid and shake.

3. Extract this mixture twice with 25 ml. portions of ether and combine the extractions.

4. Wash the combined ether extracts with 10 ml. of 5% HCl.

5. Examine the urine residue after extractions, the HCl washings, and the washed ether extract under ultraviolet light.

NORMAL VALUES: Uroporphyrins: 10 - 30 micrograms/day
                Coproporphrins: Up to 160 micrograms/day

REFERENCE: Miale, John B.: LABORATORY MEDICINE AND HEMATOLOGY,
            4th Ed., Mosby Co., pg. 1218, 1972.

INTERPRETATION:

A red fluorescence in the washings or extract is evidence of coproporphyrins. A red fluorescence in the urinary residue is evidence
294

Porphyrins (Continued):

of uroporphyrins.

Porphyrins are tetrapyrrole pigments which are precursors of the hemoglobins and cytochromes. Porphyrins exist in two isomeric forms: Types I and III, mainly coproporphyrin and uroporphyrin.

Uroporphyrins are tetrapyroles formed as a by product of heme synthesis. Its excretion is greatly increased in acute porphyrias and may be increased in lead poisoning, cirrhosis of liver and hemochromatosis. Normal urinary uroporphyrin levels are 10 to 30 micrograms per day.

Coproporphyrin excretion in the urine up to 160 micrograms per day is normal. Diseases associated with elevated excretion are listed below.

Coproporphyrins I and III are extracted from urine with ethyl ether. Type I is increased in vitamin deficiency (Pellagra) in acute hepatitis, obstructive jaundice, and in acute porphyria. Type III is increased in toxic states such as lead poisoning, after salvarsan, quinine, and sulfonamide therapy, in acute poliomyelitis, and in acute intermittent porphyria, and in alcoholic cirrhosis.

Uroporphyrins I and III are left in urine after ether extraction, but are extracted with ethyl acetate. Type I is increased in acute porphyria and type III is increased in acute intermittent porphyria, both in greater quantities than coproporphyrins.

All of the above porphyrins are distinguished by their solubilities in organic solvents, their absorption spectra, and by the melting points of the crystalline materials.

1. Porphyria Erythropoietica
   Increase in urine of Uroporphyrin and Type I Coproporphyrin.

2. Acute Intermittent Porphyria
   Increased excretion of Coproporphyrin and Uroporphyrin similar to Uroporphyrin I.

3. Porphyria Cutanea Tarda
   Uroporphyrins and Coproporphyrins are present in increased levels in the urine.

PROTHROMBIN TIME QUICK

PRINCIPLE: This is a clotting time obtained when tissue thromboplastin and calcium are added in excess to citrated plasma.

SPECIMEN: Whole blood drawn in proportion of part 3.8% sodium citrate anticoagulant to 9 parts blood (full blue top Vacutainer Tube).

REAGENTS AND EQUIPMENT:

1. Tissue Thromboplastin and calcium mixture (Hyland Dried Thromboplastin) is used.

2. Control Plasmas (Hyland 100% Control and Hyland 20% Control)

3. Fibrometer

4. 37°C. Heat Block

5. Fibrometer Tips

SOURCES OF ERROR:

1. Dilution with anticoagulant: The 9:1 ratio of blood to anticoagulant is critical, and underfilled and overfilled tubes will give erroneous results.

2. Temperature: The temperature should be 37°C. $\pm$ 0.5. Air conditioning and/or drafts can cause temperature problems.

3. pH: pH should be 7.2 $\pm$ 0.3. The distilled water used to reconstitute Dried Thromboplastin and controls should be no lower than 6.0.

4. The test should be run within 2 hours after being drawn. If this is impossible, it may be stored at 4°C. for up to 4 hours or frozen overnight.

PROCEDURE:

1. Reconstitute Thromboplastin and controls according to manufacturer instructions.

2. Place plasma to be tested and controls in a 37°C. heat block for 5 minutes. (Do not warm longer than 10 minutes.)

296

Prothrombin Time Quick (Continued):

3. Place 0.2 ml. Thromboplastin in plastic cups of fibrometer and allow to warm 5 minutes.

4. Simultaneously add 0.1 ml. plasma and start timer. Tests should be done in duplicate and results should be $\pm$ 0.5 seconds.

NORMAL VALUES: 60 - 100%.

REFERENCES:

1. Quick, A. J.: HEMORRHAGIC DISEASES, Philadelphia, Lea & Febiger, 1957.

2. Wintrobe, M. M.: CLINICAL HEMATOLOGY, Philadelphia, Lea & Febiger, 1956.

3. Tocantins, L. M.: THE COAGULATION OF BLOOD, New York, Grune & Stratton, 1955.

PROTHROMBIN CURVE:

1. Using one lot number of Thromboplastin and 100% Control, reconstitute enough, following directions on label, to run complete test. (3 vials of 20 determination of Thromboplastin and six of 100% Controls usually are enough.) Pool the reagents and keep Control in an ice bath.

2. Make dilutions following chart below and run prothrombin times on them. The prothrombin times should be run immediately as they are unstable when diluted.

Percent	Plasma	Imidazole Buffer
80	.40	.10
70	.35	.15
60	.30	.20
50	.25	.25
40	.20	.30
30	.15	.35
20	.10	.40
10	.05	.45

3. Plot the curve on regular graph paper, the percent (%) on the X axis and seconds on the Y axis.

Prothrombin Time Quick (Continued):

INTERPRETATION:

The prothrombin and proconvertin may be prolonged in liver disease, disseminated intravascular coagulation, with consumption of the extrir sic system factors or by the utilization of coumadin. The Quick Prothrombin Time is a measure of the extrinsic system. It is utilized to follow the course of coumadin therapy as is the P and P Test. See Interpretation of the P and P Test on page 301.

PROTHROMBIN AND PROCONVERTIN

PRINCIPLE: This is a one-stage prothrombin time done on diluted plasma in which a constant source of proaccelerin and fibrinogen is provided through the use of prothrombin-free beef plasma.

SPECIMEN: A full blue top Vacutainer or blood drawn in 3.8% sodium citrate in proportioned 1 part anticoagulant to 9 parts blood.

EQUIPMENT AND REAGENTS:

1. Simplastin A, tissue thromboplastin containing optimal amounts of Factor V, fibrinogen, calcium, and sodium chloride.

2. Control Plasmas
   (Verify Normal, Verify I, and Verify II)

3. Fibrometer System

4. 37°C. Waterbath

COMMENTS ON PROCEDURE:

1. Because of the instability of proaccelerin in plasma, this is a particularly good test for specimens which cannot be run immediately.

2. Fibrinogen is added so that there will still be a firm clot in a plasma which is diluted 10-fold.

3. The dilution reduces the effect of clotting inhibitors and varying citrate concentrations.

4. Factor V does not occur normally in tissue thromboplastin extracts and is highly unstable. For this reason, Simplastin A should be used within one working day and not frozen after being reconstituted. It should be returned to refrigerator after being reconstituted.

PROCEDURE:

1. Reconstitute Verify and Simplastin A following manufacturer's instructions. Prewarm 0.9 ml. distilled water at least 5 minutes.

Prothrombin and Proconvertin (Continued):

2. Place 0.2 ml. Simplastin A in fibrometer cup, and allow to warm 3 to 5 minutes. DO NOT use reagent warmed more than 15 minutes.

3. Prepare a 1:10 dilution of plasma to be tested by adding 0.1 ml. plasma to 0.9 ml. prewarmed distilled water. Run within 2 minutes

4. Add 0.1 ml. diluted plasma to Simplastin A, and start timer. Tests should be run in duplicate and check within $\pm$ 0.5 seconds (or 1%).

5. Run controls: Verify Normal, Verify I, and Verify II diluted 1:10 with distilled water.

P and P CURVE:

1. Using one lot number of Simplastin A and Verify Normal, reconstitute enough (following instructions on label) to run complete curves (3 vials of 20 determination Simplastin A and 6 of Verify Normal usually are enough).

2. Make dilutions as follows, and run immediately as the dilutions are unstable.

Percent	Plasma	Imidazole Buffer	Plasma-Buffer Dilution	Prewarmed Distilled Water
80	0.40	0.10	0.1	0.9
70	0.35	0.15	0.1	0.9
60	0.30	0.20	0.1	0.9
50	0.25	0.25	0.1	0.9
40	0.20	0.30	0.1	0.9
30	0.15	0.35	0.1	0.9
20	0.10	0.40	0.1	0.9
10	0.05	0.45	0.1	0.9

Use log - log graph paper.

3. The times are plotted on the Y axis and seconds on the X axis. This is a straight line curve.

NORMAL VALUES: 60 - 140%.

REFERENCES:

1. Biggs, R. and MacFarlane, R. G.: HUMAN BLOOD COAGULATION AND ITS DISORDERS, 3rd Edition, pp. 385-388, 1962.

Prothrombin and Proconvertin (Continued):

2. Sussman, L. N., Cohen, I. B., and Gittler, R.: J. Amer. Med. Assoc. 156:702, 1954.

3. Ware, A. G. and Stragnell, R.: Am. J. Clin. Path. 22:791, 1952.

INTERPRETATION:

The P and P may be prolonged in liver disease, disseminated intravascular coagulation, with consumption of the extrinsic system factors or by the utilization of coumadin. The P and P is an assay of Factors II, VII, and X since V is added in the determination. When coumadin is utilized, the desired range to be achieved is that between 10 - 20%. If the P and P is below 10%, it indicates excessive utilization of coumadin and vitamin K should be employed to return the P and P to the 10 - 20% range.

PYRUVATE KINASE

PRINCIPLE: Under the controlled conditions of enzymatic reactions (sample size, substrate concentration, time, temperature, pH, ionic strength, and various salt concentrations), pyruvate kinase catalyzes the conversion of phosphoenolpyruvate to pyruvate, which is further converted to lactate, as shown in the following reaction:

$$ADP \quad + \quad PEP \xrightleftharpoons{PK} ATP \quad + \quad Pyruvate$$

| Adenosine Diphosphate | Phosphoenol- Pyruvate | Adenosine Triphosphate |

$$Pyruvate \quad + \quad DPNH \quad + \quad H^+ \xrightarrow{LDH} Lactate \quad + \quad DPN^+$$

The decrease in absorbance of DPNH due to its oxidation to DPN^+ is a direct measurement of the concentration of pyruvic kinase.

One of the metabolic abnormalities of the red cell associated with hemolytic disease is due to pyruvic kinase deficiency. The determination of this enzyme is of utmost value in cases of hemolytic anemia.

SPECIMEN: 1.0 ml. of fresh serum, free from hemolysis and 0.2 ml. of blood for hemolysate.

REAGENTS AND EQUIPMENT: (Biochemica Test Combination U.V. Method, Cat. No. 15985 TPAB)

1. Buffer (Bottle No. 1)
   0.16 M. Triethanolamine buffer, pH 7.5; 0.12 M. KCl; 0.021 M. $MgSO_4$; 0.0013 M. Ethylene Diamine Tetraacetate

2. Stock NADH (Bottle No. 2)
   0.006 M. NADH; 0.0325 M. Phosphenolpyruvate

3. LDH (Bottle No. 3)
   0.5 mg. LDH/ml.

4. ADP (Bottle No. 4)
   0.1 M. Adenosine Diphosphate

5. Saline
   0.9 gm. Sodium Chloride, A. R. in 100 ml. of deionized water.

Pyruvate Kinase (Continued):

6. Spectrophotometer, Gilford 300N, 340 nm.
This instrument is used to analyze one sample at a time. The change in absorbance per minute is read from the Data Lister printout. The linearity of the reaction is visually monitored on the strip chart recorder. The thermocuvette is set at 25°C.

COMMENTS:

1. Solutions No.'s 1 and 3 are stable for a year at room temperature.

2. Solutions No.'s 2 and 4 are stable for three weeks at refrigerator temperatures.

3. Make dilutions with optical density differences above 0.600/10 minutes.

PROCEDURE:

A. Hemolysate
1. Determine the number of erythrocytes/ml. of blood.

2. Wash 0.20 ml. of blood 3 times with 2.0 ml. of physiological saline each.

3. After each wash, centrifuge for 10 minutes at 3000 rpm.

4. Suspend washed and centrifuged erythrocytes in 2.0 ml. of deionized water.

5. Allow to stand for 15 minutes in the refrigerator.

6. Centrifuge. Use supernatant for determination of enzyme activity.

B. Enzyme Activity
1. Using disposable culture tubes (12 x 75 mm.), set up 2 tubes, Blank and Test, for serum and also 2 tubes, Blank and Test, for hemolysate.

2. To the serum tubes (Blank and Test), add 2.5 ml. of buffer, 0.10 ml. of NADH-PEP, 0.5 ml. of serum, and 0.05 ml. of LDH.

3. To the hemolysate tubes (Blank and Test), add 2.0 ml. of buffer, 0.9 ml. of deionized water, 0.1 ml. of NADH-PEP, 0.1 ml. of hemolysate and 0.05 ml. of LDH.

Pyruvate Kinase (Continued):

4. Mix and incubate all tubes in a 25°C. waterbath for 5 minutes.

5. Set the machine to zero with deionized water. Aspirate the serum Blank and measure the optical density (S) E_1. Aspirate the hemolysate Blank and measure the optical density (H) E_1. Take another reading after 10 minutes (S) E_2 and (H) E_2.

6. To the serum Test and Hemolysate Test, add 0.1 ml. of adenosine diphosphate.

7. Mix and obtain optical density of both serum (S) E_3 and hemolysate (H) E_3. Take another reading after 10 minutes (S) E_4 and (H) E_4.

8. To obtain $\Delta A/10$ minutes, subtract optical density difference $(E_1 - E_2)$, from optical density difference $(E_3 - E_4)$ for both serum and hemolysate.

9. CALCULATIONS:

A. Serum

$$I.U. = \frac{\Delta A/10 \text{ Min.}}{\epsilon \times d} \times 10^6 \times \frac{TV}{SV} \times \frac{1}{Time}$$

ϵ = Molar Extinction Coefficient of NADH at 340 nm.
   = 6.22×10^3 Liter/Mole x cm.
d = Diameter of the cuvette in cm.
   = 1.0 cm.
TV = Total Volume
   = 3.25 ml.
SV = Sample Volume
   = 0.5 ml.
T = Time
   = 10 Minutes

10^6 converts Moles/Liter into micromoles/liter
   1 I.U./Liter = 1 mU/ml.

$$I.U. = \frac{\Delta A/10 \text{ min.}}{6.22 \times 10^3} \times 10^6 \times \frac{3.25}{0.50} \times \frac{1}{10}$$

$$I.U. = \Delta A/10 \text{ minutes} \times 104.5$$

$$\Delta A/10 \text{ minutes} \times 104.5 = mU/ml. \text{ of serum.}$$

Pyruvate Kinase (Continued):

B. Hemolysate

Calculated the same way as for the serum.

$\Delta A/10$ minutes x 5486 = mU/number of erythrocytes in 1.0 ml. of blood.

Report results in I.U. at 25°C.

NORMAL VALUES: Normal Values compiled by BMC at 25°C.

Serum   Up to 26 mU/ml. of serum.
Erythrocytes   60 - 220 mU/10^9 erythrocytes.

REFERENCES:

1. Tanaka, K. R., Valentine, W. N., and Miwa, S.: Blood, 19:267, 1962.

2. Bergmeyer, H. U.: METHODS OF ENZYMATIC ANALYSIS, 2nd. Ed., Academic Press, New York, pg. 573, 1965.

INTERPRETATION:

One of the important enzyme deficiencies of the anaerobic glycolytic pathway causing hemolytic anemia is a deficiency of pyruvate kinase (PK). The most common cause next to G-6-PD deficiency of congenital and nonspherocytic hemolytic anemia is PK deficiency. Individuals with heterozygous deficiency may have two to three times the levels found in the homozygous type. The red cells may appear bizarre with marked acanthrocytosis. Splenectomy affords some relief in this condition. Lack of the enzyme causes an inhibition of glycolysis with poor ATP synthesis. Individuals with PK deficiency have a prominent increase in the 2,3-diphosphoglycerate levels of the red cell. If total organic phosphate is present in high amounts in red cells, the possibility of PK deficiency should be considered. In diagnosis of the deficiency, the chemistry is related to the conversion of phosphoenolpyruvate to pyruvate in the presence of ATP. This reaction is catalyzed by PK in red cell homogenates. The white blood cells should be removed since PK activity is present in the white cells and will give false results.

Another simple assay measures the disappearance of phosphoenolpyruvate; a third test is a screening test which shows that the PK reaction, in

Pyruvate Kinase (Continued):

the absence of a buffer, is accompanied by a displacement of pH toward an alkaline one. A color indicator is used. Another screening test is a fluorescent one similar to that for G-6-PD deficiency. A decrease in fluorescence during the pyruvate kinase reaction occurs because NADH fluoresces and NAD does not.

RETICULOCYTE COUNTS

PRINCIPLE: Reticulocytes are immature erythrocytes representing a stage of development between a normoblast and an adult cell. They are non-nucleated cells which still retain some basophilic substance that appears as a reticulum when exposed to vital stains.

SPECIMEN: One lavendar top tube (EDTA) or capillary blood.

EQUIPMENT AND REAGENTS:

1. New Methylene Blue N Solution
   (Commercially prepared Harleco Product Brecher Formula)

2. 75 x 100 mm. test tubes

3. Pasteur Pipettes

4. Capillary Tubes

5. Slides

PROCEDURE:

1. Using a pasteur pipette, place two drops of dye solution in the test tube. Add four capillary tubes of blood.

2. Mix well and let stand for 10 minutes. Do not leave capillary tubes in test tube during incubation period.

3. Mix again and with the capillary tube place small drop of mixture on slide and smear. Make four smears.

4. Two technologists each count the number of reticulocytes per 500 erythrocytes on different slides.

5. Add the results of the two counts and divide by 10. This equals the percent reticulocytes. They must agree within two means.

6. If the total number of reticulocytes per cu. mm. is desired, an erythrocyte count is done and multiply the results by the total number of reticulocytes counted, then divide by 1,000.

308

Reticulocytes (Continued):

NORMAL VALUES: Adults 0.5 to 1.5%. Normal values at birth range
from 2.5 to 6.5%, falling to the adult level by the
end of the second week.

REFERENCES:

1. Miale, John B.: LABORATORY MEDICINE HEMATOLOGY 4th. Ed.,
   C. V. Mosby Co., St. Louis, pg. 1204, 1972.

2. Wintrobe, M.: CLINICAL HEMATOLOGY 6th. Ed., Lea & Febiger,
   Phil., pg. 67-73, 1967.

INTERPRETATION:

The degree of reticulocytosis is proportional to erythropoietic
activity. Increased activity with higher reticulocyte counts may be
found after acute hemorrhage, hemolytic anemias, and treatment with
hemopoietic substances. A low reticulocyte count means decreased
erythropoiesis. When pernicious anemia is treated successful therapy results in a rise in the reticulocyte count. If the reticulocyte
count does not rise, an associated iron deficiency may be present.
A higher reticulocyte count occurs when the anemia is more severe.
The reticulocyte count is low characteristically in the anemias
associated with ineffective erythropoiesis, aplastic anemia and
di Guglielmo's disease.

SCHILLING TEST

PRINCIPLE: This test is designed to detect the malabsorption of vitamin B_{12} secondary to pernicious anemia or in patients with malabsorption due to small intestinal disease.

SPECIMEN: 24 hour urine collection for 2 days.

MATERIALS AND EQUIPMENT:

1. Vitamin B_{12}, 1000 micrograms/ml.

2. ^{57} or ^{60}Cobalt, Radioactive, Vitamin B_{12}

3. Scintillation Counter

PROCEDURE:

1. Patient should be fasting. Void urine in a.m. and discard.

2. Patient drinks 24 ml. radioactive vitamin B_{12} in water (1.0 uc. with 5 umg. diluted into 25 ml. water.

3. Inject I. M. 1000 ug. vitamin B_{12} which is a flushing or saturating dose.

4. Collect 24 hour urine specimen.

5. Inject I. M. 1000 ug. vitamin B_{12} as a second flushing dose.

6. Collect a second 24 hour urine specimen.

7. Remove a 15 ml. aliquot from each 24 hour urine specimen.

8. Count the radioactivity of each aliquot in a scintillation counter.

9. CALCULATION:

$$\text{Percent Radioactivity Absorbed} = \frac{\frac{\text{Counts/Min./ml.}}{\text{Urine}} \times \frac{\text{Urine}}{\text{Vol.}} \times \frac{\text{Dil. Factor}}{\text{Urine}}}{\frac{\text{Total Counts}}{\text{Administered}} \times 100}$$

$$\frac{\text{Total Counts}}{\text{Administered}} = \frac{\text{Counts/Min./ml.}}{\text{Diluted Sample}} \times 24 \times \frac{\text{Dilution}}{\text{Factor}}$$

309

Schilling Test (Continued):

COMMENTS:

1. False positive tests result if renal insufficiency is present and the radioactive B_{12} cannot be excreted.

2. Pernicious anemia may be distinguished from malabsorption due to small intestinal disease by administering intrinsic factor with the oral radioactive vitamin B_{12}. The B_{12} malabsorption in pernicious anemia is corrected by the intrinsic factor.

NORMAL VALUES: When a 1 microgram dose of labeled vitamin B_{12} is utilized, normal individuals excrete 7 percent or more of the administered radioactivity in the first 24 hours. A greater amount is excreted with a smaller dose.

REFERENCE: Schilling, R. F.: "Intrinsic Factor Studies in the Effect of Gastric Juice on the Urinary Excretion of Radioactivity after the Oral Administration of Radio-Active Vitamin B_{12}". J. Lab. Clin. Med. 42:860, 1953.

INTERPRETATION:

The test detects malabsorption of B_{12} due to a lack of intrinsic factor. One should repeat the test after giving commercial intrinsic factor. If the test is corrected, the patient has intrinsic factor deficiency. If not, he has malabsorption due to small intestinal disease.

The test is especially helpful in determining the presence of B_{12} malabsorption in a patient who has been treated and has no evidence of B_{12} deficiency. The test should not be performed in a patient with renal failure since the radioactive B_{12} will not be excreted into the urine.

SIA WATER TEST
FOR
MACROGLOBULINS

PRINCIPLE: Various serum globulins especially macroglobulins, have a lower solubility when the electrolyte concentration of serum is lowered by water dilution.

SPECIMEN: 1.0 ml. of serum.

REAGENTS: Distilled water.

PROCEDURE:

Add 2 drops of serum to a test tube containing distilled water.

NORMAL VALUES: No cloud or precipitate formation.

REFERENCE: Waldenstrom, J.: "Pathological Globulins and Protein Synthesis", Exp. Med. & Surg. 12:187, 1954.

INTERPRETATION:

If a macroglobulin is present in the serum, a heavy cloudy precipitate forms in the test tube. Globulins other than macroglobulins may give a cloudy precipitate. Furthermore, some sera containing a large amount of macroglobulin may not cause a precipitate, and a small amount of macroglobulin in the serum may give a false negative test.

AUTOMATED DITHIONITE TEST
FOR
RAPID HEMOGLOBIN S AND NON-S SICKLING HEMOGLOBINOPATHIES

PRINCIPLE: Automated adaptations of dithionite and urea-dithionite tube tests are accurate, reliable, inexpensive methods for detecting hemoglobin S. The dithionite reagent consists of potassium phosphate, sodium dithionite, and saponin. When S hemoglobin contacts this reagent, the red cells lyse, and the hemoglobin deoxygenates and sickles, forming a hydrophobic-bond-dependent nematic liquid crystal system that is manifested as turbidity. The resulting AutoAnalyzer curve is strikingly and diagnostically different from that produced by hemoglobin A in the same reagent. Specificity of the automated dithionite test may be enhanced by use of the automated urea-dithionite test, which consists of a specimen set of two aliquots: one traverses a dithionite line, the other a urea-dithionite line. A comparison of transmittance in the two lines yields typical diagnostic curves because the urea disperses the sickling, with a consequently increased transmittance over that of the dithionite aliquot. Methods are discussed for recognizing non-S sickling hemoglobins and a few other rare hemoglobinopathies.

SPECIMEN: 2.0 ml. blood collected in EDTA.

REAGENTS AND EQUIPMENT:

1. Components are standard AutoAnalyzer modules (Technicon Instruments Corp., Tarrytown, N. Y. 10591).

2. Stock Buffer
   1.18 M. KH_2PO_4 and 1.615 M. K_2HPO_4. Add 160.48 gm. of KH_2PO_4 and 281.88 gm. K_2HPO_4 in a 1000 ml. volumetric flask to which 800 ml. of distilled water is added. Dissolve and dilute to volume.

3. Dithionite Working Solution
   To a 1 liter volumetric flask add 800 ml. of the Stock Buffer. Add 20 gm. of $Na_2S_2O_4$ and mix until dissolved. Add 60 ml. of Saponin solution "Zaponin" (Coulter Diagnostics, Inc., Hialeah, Fla. 33010) and sufficient distilled water to make one liter.

Automated Dithionite Test (Continued):

PROCEDURE:

A. Automated Dithionite Test
1. Assemble the manifold.   (Fig. 1.)

2. Place reagent lines 4 and 6 in dithionite working solution. Place the saline lines into the saline. Start pump and allow 10 minutes to fill the system with reagents.

3. Adjust the baselines on both recorders to 95% transmittance.

4. Fill one or two cups with 0.5 to 2.0 ml. of normal blood (collected in EDTA). Fill 20 cups with the unknowns. After the 20th cup place one cup of saline, one or two cups of normal blood and 20 cups of unknowns. This loading pattern should be maintained throughout; it is easier to label the peaks if they are in sets of 20.

5. Start mixers and samplers.

6. After all specimens have passed through the system, remove the charts and label the peaks. The "positive" specimens will have a 15 to 20% (or more) lower transmittance than those specimens that are normal by this procedure. The presence of hemoglobins other than hemoglobin-S in the "positive" specimens should be determined by an electrophoretic pattern.

7. When all specimens have been screened, rinse the system with 1.0 N. NaOH (plus 20 ml. of "Tergitol NPX" per liter) for 15 minutes, then with distilled water for 15 to 20 minutes.

B. Automated Urea-dithionite Test
1. Assemble the manifold and the other Technicon modules. (Fig. 2)

2. The dithionite working solution is the same as described above.

3. Take one-half of the reagent from Step 2 (dithionite working solution) and add sufficient urea to make a 2 Mol/Liter solution.

4. Place all reagent lines in appropriate reagents. Start pump. Allow 10 minutes for the system to fill with reagents.

314

Automated Dithionite Test (Continued):

5. Adjust the baseline of the dithionite line (without urea) to 90% transmittance on the chart paper. Adjust the urea-dithionite line to 70% transmittance.

6. Fill three or four cups with 0.5 to 2.0 ml. of well-mixed normal blood (collected in EDTA). Fill 20 cups with the unknowns. After the unknowns, place a cup of saline, one or two cups of a normal blood, and 20 cups of unknowns. Maintain this loading pattern throughout.

7. Start the mixer and the sampler. Adjust colorimeters so that the peaks in each set of 2 curves of the first 4 specimens are of equal percent transmittance.

8. After all the specimens have passed through the system, remove the chart and label the peaks. The "positive" specimens in the dithionite line (without urea) will have peaks that are lower by 15 to 20% (or more) transmittance than the peak of the corresponding urea-dithionite line. For example, a positive may read 10% transmittance on the dithionite line and 30% transmittance on the urea-dithionite line. This pattern of "positive" specimens will only occur with hemoglobin-S and hemoglobin-C (Harlem) (a structural variant of hemoglobin-S). The peaks of both lines will have a lower transmittance if the specimen is a non-S sickling hemoglobin.

9. After the run is completed, rinse the system with 1.0 N. NaOH (plus 20 ml. of Tergitol NPX per liter) for 15 minutes, then rinse the system with distilled water for 15 to 20 minutes.

REFERENCES:

1. Nalbandian, R. M., et al.: "Dithionite Tube Test-a Rapid, Inexpensive Technique for the Detection of Hemoglobin S and Non-S Sickling Hemoglobin", Clin. Chem. 17:1028, 1971.

2. Davidsohn I., and Henry, J. B., Eds.: CLINICAL DIAGNOSIS BY LABORATORY METHODS, 14th Ed., W. B. Saunders Co., Phil., pg. 235, 1969.

3. Nichols, B. M., Nalbandian, R. M., Henry, R. L., Wolf, P. L., and Camp, Jr., F. R.: "Murayama Test for Hemoglobin S: Simplification in Technique". Clin. Chem. 17:1059, 1971.

Automated Dithionite Test (Continued):

4. Henry, R. L., et al.: "An Automated Screening Method for the Specific Detection of Homozygous and Heterozygous S Hemoglobin". U.S. Army Med. Res. Lab. Rep. No. 898 (17 Sept. 1970), Fort Knox, Ky.

5. Bookchin, R. M., et al.: "Hemoglobin C Harlem: A Sickling Varient containing Amino Acid Substitutions in Two Residues of the Beta-Polypeptide Chain". Biochem. Biophys. Res. Commun. 23:122, 1966.

6. Bookchin, R. M., Nagel, R. L., and Ranney, H. M.: "Structure and Properties of Hemoglobin C Harlem, a Human Hemoglobin Varient with Amino Acid Substitutions in 2 Residues of the Beta-Polypeptide Chain". J. Biol. Chem. 242:248, 1968.

7. Konotey-Ahulu, F. I. D., et al.: "Haemoglobin Korle-Bu (β73 Aspartic Acid→Asparagine)." J. Med. Genet. 5:107, 1968.

8. Pierce, L. E., Rath, C. E., and McCoy, K.: A New Hemoglobin Variant with Sickling Properties". New Eng. J. Med. 268:862, 1963.

9. Gerald, P. S. and Rath, C. E.: "Hb C Georgetown: First Abnormal Hemoglobin due to Two Different Mutations in the Same Gene". J. Clin. Invest. 45:1012, 1966.

10. Lie-Injo, L. E.: "Haemoglobin 'Bart's' and the Sickling Phenomenon". Nature 191:1314, 1961.

11. Lie-Injo, L. E.: "Alpha-chain Thalassemia and Hydrops Fetalis in Malaya: Report of Five Cases". Blood 20:581, 1962.

12. Schwartz, I. R., et al.: "Sickling of Erythrocytes with I-A Electrophoretic Hemoglobin Pattern". Fed. Proc. 16:115, 1957.

13. Atwater, J., et al.: "Sickling of Erythrocytes in a Patient with Thalassemia-Hemoglobin-I Disease". New Eng. J. Med. 263:1215, 1960.

14. Carrell, R. W. and Lehmann, H.: "The Unstable Haemoglobin Haemolytic Anaemias". Semin. Hematol. 6:116, 1969.

15. Sathiapalan, R. and Robinson, M. G.: "Hereditary Haemolytic Anaemia due to an Abnormal Haemoglobin (Haemoglobin King's County)". Brit. J. Haematol. 85:579, 1968.

Automated Dithionite Test (Continued):

16. Dherte, P., et al.: "Stanleyville I and II. Two New Variants of Adult Hemoglobin". Brit. Med. J. 2:282, 1959.

17. Kraus, A. P., et al: "Hemoglobin Memphis/S, a New Variant of Sickle Cell Anemia". Trans. Ass. Amer. Physicians 80:297, 1967.

18. Kraus, L. M., et al.: "Characterization of 23GluNH2 in Hemoglobin Memphis. Hemoglobin Memphis/S, a New Variant of Molecular Disease". Biochemistry 5:3701, 1966.

INTERPRETATION:

With the automated dithionite test, it is possible to screen 120 hemoglobin specimens per hour at a reagent cost of approximately 2 to 4 cents each. With the automated urea dithionite test, the results are more specific but the rate is half that of the automated dithionite test. Thus, about 60 determinations per hour are performed at about 4 to 8 cents per set. Both of these automated methods have proven to be highly reliable in extended field trials in both military and civilian populations.

These automated tests have a molecular basis. The reagents consist of potassium phosphate, sodium dithionite, and saponin. When sickling red cells are introduced into such a solution, they lyse immediately, the hemoglobin deoxygenates, the beta globin chains of each hemoglobin tetramer are displaced laterally, complementarity of steric fit between interacting hemoglobin tetramers is achieved in accordance with the Murayama hypothesis for the molecular mechanism of sickling, a nematic liquid system is formed, and in the presence of hemoglobin S or non-S sickling hemoglobins the system becomes turbid. On addition of urea, those nematic liquid systems dependent on hydrophobic bonds are dispersed, wheras others will persist. Thus, on theoretical grounds this simple test, coupled with molecular insights and electrophoresis of all positive specimens, promises to yield an impressive quantity of information on hemoglobinopathies that, at present, are overlooked.

From previous studies by Henry et al., it was shown that when a specimen of hemoglobin S is divided and moves in phase along two channels, one with an appropriate reducing reagent and the other with urea in addition to the same quantities of reducing agent, the transmittance of the liquid in the line carrying the urea will be significantly greater than that of the contents of the other line. Briefly, the

Automated Dithionite Test (Continued):

turbidity produced by the sickled or nematic liquid crystal system of hemoglobin S in the dithionite-reagent line is dispersed in the urea-dithionite-reagent line by the urea, which breaks the hydrophobic bonds essential to sickling; hence the clearing and the gain in trans-mittance when the specimen is hemoglobin S in the urea-dithionite line.

PREDICTIONS. This simple observation can be put to good use in the diagnosis not only of hemoglobin S but also rare non-S sickling hemoglobins and, perhaps, other hemoglobinopathies as specified below.

HEMOGLOBIN C (HARLEM). This sickling hemoglobin is a structural var-iant of hemoglobin S because it is produced by a homologous crossing over of hemoglobins S and Korle-Bu. Hence, the submolecular lesion in hemoglobin C (Harlem) is identical in part with hemoglobin S. Thus, sickling is mediated by hydrophobic bonding, and this hemoglobin should give a positive dithionite test and become clear in a urea-dithionite system.

HEMOGLOBIN C (GEORGETOWN). This sickling hemoglobin forms a nematic liquid crystal system mediated by electrovalent bonding, according to Murayama et al. Hence, this hemoglobin should form a nematic liquid crystal system that is stable in dithionite as well as in urea-dithi-onite systems.

HEMOGLOBIN BART'S. This sickling hemoglobin found most often at birth in association with alpha thalassemia, is a homogeneous tetra-mer of gamma globin chains. It has already been shown to sickle under conditions similar to the dithionite test.

HEMOGLOBIN I. This sickling hemoglobin is an alpha globin chain abnormality, and sickles by a molecular mechanism distinctly differ-ent from that of hemoglobin S. The dithionite test was negative on the one specimen tested.

HEMOGLOBIN H. This Heinz-body forming hemoglobinopathy, under condi-tions similar to the Itano solubility test has been reported to give a positive reaction. Hence, in the dithionite test it may also give a positive test, possibly along with other Heinz-body forming hemo-globinopathies.

HEMOGLOBIN KING'S COUNTY AND STANLEYVILLE II. In both of these rare nonsickling hemoglobinopathies, the hemoglobins are known to have low solubilities, approaching that of hemoglobin S. The reactions of these hemoglobins in the dithionite test systems would be of interest.

Automated Dithionite Test (Continued):

HEMOGLOBIN ALEXANDRA. This rare sickling hemoglobinopathy has not been sufficiently characterized to make possible a prediction about its reaction in the dithionite test system.

HEMOGLOBIN MEMPHIS/S. This sickling hemoglobinopathy is composed of two genetic errors, one involving the beta globin chain (S) and the other involving the alpha globin chain (Memphis). Hence, Memphis hemoglobinopathies will give a negative dithionite test but when presenting with beta S globin chains, as in Memphis/S, they may be expected to give a positive dithionite test.

To obtain the greatest accuracy in the diagnosis not only of hemoglobin S, but with little effort in diagnosis of other rare hemoglobinopathies including non-S sickling ones-all hemoglobin specimens producing a positive dithionite or urea-dithionite tests should be studied additionally by electrophoresis.

Although the automated urea-dithionite greatly increases the specificity of the automated dithionite test, reagent cost per specimen increases to about 4 to 8 cents per set and the rate of determinations is slowed to 60 per hour. Even the positive specimens by the automated urea-dithionite test must be studied by electrophoresis to differentiate specimens of hemoglobin S from its rare structural variant, hemoglobin C (Harlem), a "non-S" sickling hemoglobin.

When the chemistry of the dithionite test is coupled with the ever-expanding fund of molecular information on hemoglobinopathies, specificity and accuracy of detection of both hemoglobin S and non-S sickling hemoglobins will be forth-coming.

Automated Dithionite Test (Continued):

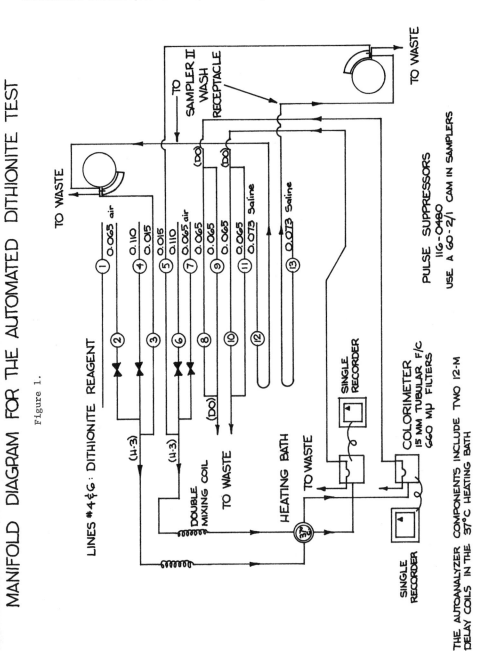

MANIFOLD DIAGRAM FOR THE AUTOMATED DITHIONITE TEST

Figure 1.

320

Automated Dithionite Test (Continued):

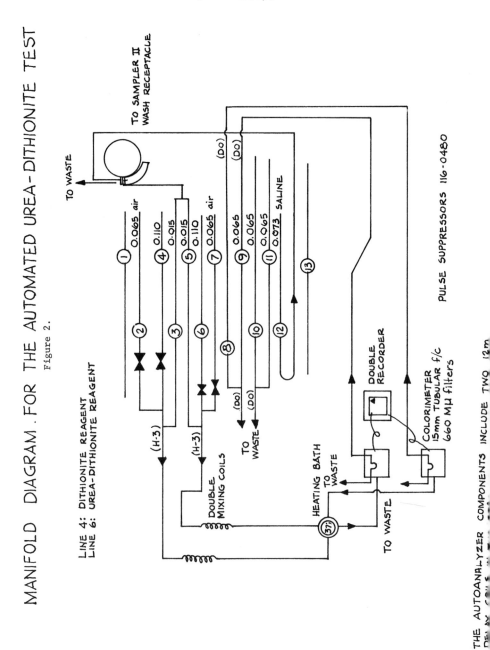

MANIFOLD DIAGRAM . FOR THE AUTOMATED UREA-DITHIONITE TEST

Figure 2.

DITHIONITE TUBE TEST
A RAPID TECHNIQUE FOR
THE DETECTION OF HEMOGLOBIN S AND NON-S SICKLING HEMOGLOBIN

PRINCIPLE: An inexpensive, rapid, convenient screening tube test
for the detection of hemoglobin S and non-S sickling hemoglobins has
been developed, which has a molecular basis. The reagents consist
of potassium phosphate, sodium dithionite, and saponin. When sickling
red cells are introduced into such a solution, the red cells lyse
immediately, the hemoglobin deoxygenates, the beta globin chains of
each hemoglobin tetramer are displaced laterally, complementarity of
steric fit between interacting hemoglobin tetramers is achieved in
accordance with the recently modified Murayama hypothesis for the
molecular mechanism of sickling, a nematic liquid crystal system is
formed, and in the presence of hemoglobin S or non-S sickling hemoglobins, the system becomes turbid. On addition of urea, those nematic liquid crystal systems dependent upon hydrophobic bonds are
dispersed.

SPECIMEN: 20 microliters of blood collected in EDTA.

EQUIPMENT AND REAGENTS:

1. Stock Buffer
   KH_2PO_4 (1.18 Mol/L.) and K_2HPO_4 (1.615 Mol/L.). Place about
   800 ml. of distilled water in a 1 liter volumetric flask. Add
   160.48 gm. of KH_2PO_4 and 281.88 gm. of K_2HPO_4. Dissolve and
   dilute to one liter.

2. Working Buffer
   To a 1 liter volumetric flask, add 800 ml. of the stock buffer.
   Add 20 gm. of $Na_2S_2O_4$ and mix until dissolved. Add 60 ml. of
   saponin solution ("Zaponin", Coulter Electronics, Inc., Hialeah,
   Fla. 33010) and sufficient distilled water to make one liter.

3. Test Tubes, 12 x 75 mm.

4. Urea

5. Pipettes, 20 microliters

6. Lined Reader Scale

7. Timer

321

Dithionite Tube Test (Continued):

PROCEDURE:

1. Pipet 2.0 ml. of dithionite working solution into a 12 x 75 mm.
   test tube. To this add 20 microliters of well-mixed whole blood
   (collected in EDTA).

2. Mix by inverting the tube and allow to set at room temperature
   for 5 to 6 minutes.

3. After 5 minutes hold the tube 3.0 cm. from a lined reader scale.
   A positive test will be represented by a turbid solution. A
   negative test is represented by a clear, transparent solution.

4. When the dithionite tube test is positive the urea-dithionite
   tube test must be done to determine if the abnormal hemoglobin
   detected is hemoglobin S or some other hemoglobinopathy. Also,
   all positive dithionite test specimens must be electrophoresed.
   A positive dithionite tube test means that the specimen may be
   among one of the following hemoglobinopathies: S, C (Harlem),
   C (Georgetown), Bart's, and possibly Alexandra.

5. Strict adherence to the techniques set forth will ensure consistent results. Test tubes measuring 12 x 75 mm. must be used.
   If 10 x 75 mm. tubes are used, a false negative could result,
   particularly if the patient is anemic.

6. Urea-dithionite tube test. To the working solution (above), add
   sufficient urea to make a 2 mol/liter solution with respect to
   urea.

7. Pipet 2.0 ml. of urea-dithionite solution into a 12 x 75 mm.
   test tube.

8. Add 20 microliters of whole blood (collected in EDTA). Mix by
   inverting the tube.

9. Allow to set at room temperature for 5 minutes, then hold the
   tube 3.0 cm. from a lined reader scale or printed material. If
   the urea-dithionite solution is transparent (ruled lines are
   visible) but the same specimen gave a positive dithionite tube
   test, the hemoglobin present is either hemoglobin S or hemoglobin
   C (Harlem). If the urea-dithionite solution remains turbid and
   the dithionite tube test was positive, the presence of a non-S
   sickling hemoglobin is indicated - such as hemoglobin C (Georgetown), Bart's, or perhaps Alexandra. For structural reasons,

Dithionite Tube Test (Continued):

hemoglobin I (also a non-S sickling hemoglobin) will be negative.

10. The dithionite reagent remains stable under refrigeration at 4°C.
for at least one month. Urea should be added just before use if
the urea-dithionite solution is to be used.

REFERENCES:

1. Davidsohn, I., and Henry, J. B., Eds.: CLINICAL DIAGNOSIS
BY LABORATORY METHODS 14th. Ed., W. B. Saunders, Co., Phil.,
Pa., pg. 235, 1969.

2. Nalbandian, R. M., et al.: "The Murayama Test. Evidence
for the Modified Murayama Hypothesis for the Molecular Mechanism of Sickling". U.S. Army Med. Res. Lab. Rept. No. 893
(17 Sept. 1970), Ft. Knox, Ky.

3. Nalbandian, R. M., Henry, R. I., Nichols, B. M., Camp, F. R.,
Jr., and Wolf, P. L.: "Molecular Basis for a Simple, Specific Test for S Hemoglobin: The Murayama Test". Clin. Chem.
16:945, 1970.

4. Itano, H. A.: "Solubilities of Naturally-Occurring Mixtures
of Human Hemoglobin". Arch. Biochem. Biophys. 47:148, 1953.

5. Itano, H. A. and Pauling, L.: "A Rapid Diagnostic Test for
Sickle Cell Anemia". Blood 4:66, 1949.

6. Perutz, M. F. and Mitchison, J. M.: "State of Hemoglobin in
Sickle-Cell Anemia". Nature 166:677, 1950.

7. Muirhead, H. and Perutz, M. F.: "Structure of Hemoglobin.
A Three-Dimensional Fourier Synthesis of Reduced Human Hemoglobin at 5.5 A Resolution". Nature 199:633, 1963.

INTERPRETATION:

Diggs proposed the "Sickledex" test as "specific for hemoglobin S,"
without disclosing the reagents, chemical reactions, or principle.
Nalbandian et al. concluded that the Sickledex test was based on the
Itano solubility test. This indicated that phosphate buffer and
sodium dithionite were the essential reagents, along with a lytic
agent that was subsequently identified as saponin. Two recent papers
also hint that the Sickledex test is in fact based on the Itano

Dithionite Tube Test (Continued):

solubility test.

Itano and Pauling introduced the use of sodium dithionite in phosphate
buffered solutions as a sickling test for hemoglobin S. Harris later
described spindle-shaped liquid crystals (nematic tactoids), 1μm to
15μm long, in deoxygenated hemolysates of S hemoglobin. Shortly
thereafter, Perutz demonstrated that deoxygenated hemoglobin S has a
uniquely low solubility. Itano used these observations to develop
his solubility test (using potassium phosphate and sodium dithionite)
to identify hemoglobin S and to differentiate it from hemoglobins A,
C, D, and F. By 1963, Muirhead and Perutz had shown that there is a
configurational molecular change in oxygen-transporting hemoglobins
(homogeneous tetrameric hemoglobins such as Bart's and H do not transport oxygen) such that on oxygenation the beta globin chains are displaced laterally about 0.7 nm. with reference to the central molecular
axis of symmetry. On oxygenation, the beta globin chains are displaced centrally the same distance. These beta globin chain shifts
relative to oxygenation are equally true of hemoglobin S; that is,
beta S globin chains undergo displacements identical with tose of
beta A globin chains. In 1966 Murayama published his hypothesis for
the molecular mechanism of sickling in hemoglobin S. His recently
modified concept shows that the hydrophobic bonds essential to the
molecular event of sickling are actually intertetrameric. The Murayama test was predicated on the simple visual detection of the existence of the implicated hydrophobic bands.

Consequently, an aqueous system consisting of appropriate concentratio
of sodium phosphate, sodium dithionite, and saponin is a most appropriate reagent solution for selectively detecting hemoglobin S. When
hemoglobin S is introduced into such a system, the intact red cells
lyse immediately, the hemoglobin S tetramers are deoxygenated by the
sodium dithionite, the beta S globin chains are displaced laterally
about 0.7 nm. in each hemoglobin tetramer, and hemoglobin S tetramer
tetramer interaction proceeds in accordance with the Murayama hypothesis so that first microfilament, then microcable, and, ultimately,
nematic liquid crystal systems are formed. One of the properties of
a nematic liquid crystal system is that it will disperse transmitted
light. Hence, when hemoglobin S is present, lines on a lined reader
scale are obscured. In contrast, with hemoglobin A the lines can be
clearly seen through the transparent solution.

All dithionite tube test specimens read as positive may be due to
both hemoglobin S and non-S sickling hemoglobins. All hemoglobins
positive to dithionite tube tests must be electrophoresed, because

Dithionite Tube Test (Continued):

the dithionite tube test is a screening procedure.

If, in a screening procedure, specificity is preferred to speed, the dithionite tube test can be made more specific by additional manipulation. Specimens producing positive dithionite tube test results can be reexamined in the presence of urea, according to the method described for the urea-dithionite tube test, which makes the test more specific. In the presence of urea, under conditions of the dithionite tube test, hemoglobin S will be converted to a negative test from a prior positive test because urea will break the hydrophobic bonds essential to the sickling event (the maintenance of the nematic liquid crystal system producing the turbidity) and thus transmittance will be enhanced. On the other hand, non-S sickling hemoglobins should remain positive (turbid) in the presence of urea, because the molecular mechanism of sickling is not mediated by the hydrophobic bonds. Thus, the urea-dithionite tube test should discriminate for two categories: hemoglobin S, or its structural variant C (Harlem), and non-S sickling hemoglobins. However, by using a variation of the Itano Solubility test, Heller and Yakulis reported that hemoglobin H gave a positive test. Hence, perhaps other rare Heinz-body forming hemoglobins may be detected by this test.

We emphasize that this dithionite tube test and the urea-dithionite tube test are suitable for the determination of hemoglobin S as described above in specimens collected in EDTA, sodium citrate, or heparin, and from sites remote from the laboratory where it is processed. That is to say, mailing at ambient temperatures does not adversely affect the test results.

SICKLE CELL PREPARATION

PRINCIPLE: This hereditary familial form of chronic hemolytic anemia is distinguished morphologically by the presence of peculiar sickle-shaped and oat-shaped red corpuscles, as well as signs of excessive blood destruction and active blood formation.

An erythrocyte containing hemoglobin S and a few other rare abnormal hemoglobins will undergo bizarre shape changes when oxygen tension or pH is reduced. Sodium metabisulfite acts as a reducing agent in this procedure.

SPECIMEN: Capillary blood or EDTA tube.

REAGENTS AND EQUIPMENT:

1. Slide and coverslip

2. Sodium Metabisulfite

3. Vaseline

PROCEDURE:

1. Dilute 0.2 gm. sodium metabisulfite to 10 ml. with distilled water.

2. Draw blood up to the 1 mark and dilute up to 11 with sodium metabisulfite in a white cell pipette.

3. Place a drop on a slide and coverslip, sealing with vaseline.

4. Examine under low power immediately, at 2 hours, and at 24 hours.

5. Report as positive or negative.

REFERENCES:

1. Wintrobe, M.: CLINICAL HEMATOLOGY 6th. Ed., Lea & Febiger, Phil., pg. 699-703, 1967.

2. Miale, John B.: LABORATORY MEDICINE HEMATOLOGY 4th. Ed., C. V. Mosby Co., St. Louis, pg. 855, 1972.

Sickle Cell Preparation (Continued):

INTERPRETATION:

The Metabisulfite Test is a nonspecific test for detection of sickling. The reagent is a reducing agent which with the vaseline sealing of the area under the coverslip, results in a low oxygen tension. Thus, erythrocytes containing hemoglobin S and those listed in the following table will sickle. This test is gradually being replaced by the Dithionite Test since the Dithionite Test is able to identify the condition more readily than the Metabisulfite Test.

HEMOGLOBINOPATHIES MANIFESTING SICKLED ERYTHROCYTES

Human Origin	Nonhuman Origin
S	Deer
C (Harlem)	Sheep
C (Georgetown)	Goat
I	Mongoose
Bart's	Racoon
Alexandra	Hamster
Memphis/S	Squirrel

A SIMPLE, SPECIFIC TEST FOR S HEMOGLOBIN:
THE MURAYAMA TEST

PRINCIPLE: The Murayama test, a new, specific test for S hemoglobin, is based on the molecular mechanism of sickling for S hemoglobin proposed by Murayama. The test depends on a feature of molecular structure: hydrophobic bonds formed between interacting tetramers by the No. 6 valine, which is substituted for glutamic acid near the N-terminal end of each βS globin chain. Existence of these particular hydrophobic bonds is manifested in deoxygenated, concentrated hemolysates by reversible sol-gel transformations at 0° and 37^oC. In such systems, demonstration of reversible, temperature-dependent sol-gel transformations (a negative temperature coefficient of gelation) is specific for S hemoglobin or the S structural variant, hemoglobin C (Harlem). The test is simple, has clear endpoints, will detect both homozygous and heterozygous S hemoglobin, and is specific. A practica approach is suggested to the precise identification of S and non-S sickling hemoglobins in the diagnostic laboratory. The close agreement between Murayama's hypothesis for sickling in S hemoglobin and our results with 29 cases of S hemoglobin and 37 controls further support his views.

SPECIMEN: 2.0 ml. blood collected in EDTA.

REAGENTS AND EQUIPMENT:

1. Physiological Saline

2. Distilled Water

3. Toluene

4. Solid CO_2

5. Centrifuge Tube, 12 ml.

6. Centrifuge

7. Erlenmeyer Flask

8. Test Tube and Rubber Stopper (10 x 75 mm.)

9. Needles, 20 Gauge and 22 Gauge

10. Waterbath, 37^oC.

328

The Murayama Test (Continued):

11. <u>Ice Water or Ice Bath</u>

PROCEDURE:

1. Place 2.0 ml. of blood specimen, originally collected in EDTA ("Vacutainer," Becton, Dickinson & Co., Rutherford, N. J.), in a glass test tube.

2. Wash the cells three times with physiological saline, centrifuging at 3000 rpm for 15 minutes between washings.

3. After the last washing, decant the saline, and add distilled water equivalent to one-fourth the volume of packed erythrocytes.

4. Add 1 drop of toluene.

5. Centrifuge at 3000 rpm for 15 minutes and decant the supernatant hemolysate. (This step eliminates erythrocyte stromata.)

6. The concentrated hemolysate must now be deoxygenated by preparing a rubber stopper (to fit a 10 x 75 mm. tube) and piercing it with a 20 and 22 gauge needle. (Do not use a larger tube.)

7. Connect the 20 gauge needle with rubber hosing to an Erlenmeyer flask containing solid CO_2, so that CO_2 flows continuously over the surface of the hemolysate during the remaining steps. (Avoid formation of bubbles. Air-hemoglobin interfaces denature hemoglobin.)

8. Insert the rubber stopper with its needles into a 10 x 75 mm. test tube containing 0.5 ml. of hemolysate from Step 6. (In Step 7, hemoglobin is deoxygenated.)

9. Place the tube in a waterbath at 37°C. $\pm$ 1°C. Gently tilt the tube. (Do not allow formation of bubbles. To deoxygenate the hemolysate, CO_2 needs merely to pass over the surface of the hemolysate, not through it.) Observe for 10 minutes before interpreting test as negative. Most positive tests will be evident within 5 minutes.

10. When gel is formed, place the tube into ice water. Gently tilt the tube to observe whether the gel becomes liquid at 0°C. Again, avoid bubble formation.

The Murayama Test (Continued):

11. To demonstrate REVERSIBILITY of negative temperature coefficient of gelation, repeat steps 9 and 10 two or three times. Do not disconnect hosing.

REFERENCES:

1. Schneider, R. G., Alperin, J. B., Lehmann, H.: "Sickling Tests: Pitfalls in Performance and Interpretation". J. Amer. Med. Assoc. 202:419, 1967.

2. Isaacs, R.: "Sickling: A Property of all Red Blood Cells". Science 112:716, 1950.

3. Murayama, M.: "Molecular Mechanism of Red Cell 'Sickling'". Science 153:145, 1966.

4. Murayama, M.: "Structure of Sickle Cell Hemoglobin and Molecular Mechanism of the Sickling Phenomenon". Clin. Chem. 14:578, 1967.

5. Bookchin, R. M., Nagel, R. L., and Ranney, H. M.: "Structure and Properties of Hemoglobin C Harlem, a Human Hemoglobin Variant with Amino Acid Substitutions in Two Residues of the β-Polypeptide Chain". J. Biol. Chem. 242:248, 1967.

6. Bookchin, R. M., Davis, R. P., and Ranney, H. M.: "Clinical Features of Hemoglobin C-Harlem, a New Sickling Hemoglobin Variant". Ann. Intern. Med. 68:8, 1968.

7. Harris, J. W.: "Studies on the Destruction of Red Blood Cells VIII. Molecular Orientation in Sickle Cell Hemoglobin Solutions". Proc. Soc. Exp. Biol. Med. 75:197, 1950.

8. Singer, L., and Singer, L.: "Studies on Abnormal Hemoglobins. VII. The Gelling Phenomenon of Sickle Cell Hemoglobin: Its Biologic and Diagnostic Significance". Blood 7:1008, 1953.

9. Charache, S. and Conley, C. L.: "Rate of Sickling of Red Cells during Deoxygenation of Blood from Persons with Various Sickling Disorders". Blood 24:25, 1964.

10. Bertles, J. F., Rabinowatz, R., and Dobler, J.: "Hemoglobin Interaction: Modification of Solid Phase Composition in the Sickling Phenomenon". Science 169:375, 1970.

The Murayama Test (Continued):

11. Loh, W. P.: "A New Solubility Test for Rapid Detection of Hemoglobin S." J. Ind. Med. Assoc. 61:1651, 1968.

12. Itano, H. A.: "Solubilities of Naturally-occurring Mixtures of Human Hemoglobins". Arch. Biochem. Biophys. 47:148, 1953.

INTERPRETATION:

Only S hemoglobin or hemoglobin C (Harlem), a structural variant, gives a positive Murayama test. Hemoglobin C (Georgetown) (a non-S sickling hemoglobin) gels at 37°C. and remains gelled at 0°C. Hemoglobin A and other nonsickling hemoglobins will not gel at either 37°C. or 0°C.

It is important to realize that the hemolysate must be concentrated to achieve consistently reliable results with the Murayama test. Thus, strict adherence to technique as recorded in this paper is essential. Harris showed that when the concentration of S hemoglobin in hemolysate systems is less than 10%, no gelling occurs. We suggest that the test should not be attempted when S hemoglobin is less than 15% of the concentrated hemolysates. The technique of this test will concentrate the S hemoglobin content of the blood far more than 10% of the final hemolysate. Hemolysates with S hemoglobin concentrations as low as 10% will gel because hemoglobins A and C, but not F, interact with S hemoglobin to decrease the amount of S hemoglobin required to produce gelling - i.e. sickling. Hemoglobin D (Punjab) also interacts in a similar manner with S hemoglobin. Recently, Bertles et al. confirmed the interaction of hemoglobins S and A.

All specimens were collected as whole blood in EDTA (Vacutainer) and were processed in one laboratory by one group of investigators. Mailing sterile specimens at ambient temperatures without freezing did not adversely affect the validity of the test results. In fact, specimens received by mail and kept at refrigerator temperatures for as long as 2.5 months gave repeatedly consistent, positive results with the Murayama test. No blood specimens were taken from individuals who had received blood transfusions during the preceding four months.

Given the above insights into the molecular pathology of S hemoglobin, we believe that the precise identification of S hemoglobin requires a three-stage procedure in the routine hospital laboratory: the Sickledex test, the Murayama test, and hemoglobin electrophoresis at pH 8.6. Theoretically, the Sickledex test should detect both non-S and S sickling hemoglobins, as well as other hemoglobinopathies with low

The Murayama Test (Continued):

solubilities in the deoxygenated state. Thus, a positive Sickledex
test indicates a hemoglobin of unusually low solubility in the deoxygenated state; it may be either an S or other hemoglobin. Hemoglobin
testing "positive" with the Sickledex test in the first stage of the
determination should be segregated into two groups in the second
stage by the Murayama test: non-S sickling hemoglobins and S sicklin
hemoglobins (either S or C (Harlem)). The distinction between hemoglobin S and C (Harlem), a structural variant of hemoglobin S, is
easily made in the third stage by hemoglobin electrophoresis at pH 8.
Such a diagnostic approach will assure correct identification of S
hemoglobin and disclose non-S sickling hemoglobins.

MURAYAMA TEST FOR HEMOGLOBIN S:
SIMPLIFICATION IN TECHNIQUE
(A Modification of Original Test)

PRINCIPLE: An improved technique is reported for the Murayama test, which is a simple and specific test for S hemoglobin. Moisturized N_2 is used optimally and several steps are eliminated in the part of the test in which concentrated hemolysates are prepared by use of a dense sucrose solution. Each test, which took 1 hour can now be done in 20 minutes with equal reliability and accuracy.

SPECIMEN: 2.0 ml. blood collected in EDTA.

REAGENTS AND EQUIPMENT:

1. Saline Solution (10 gm./Liter)

2. Sucrose Solution
   300 gm. of sucrose diluted to liter with Tris buffer, 0.01 M.
   Keep refrigerated at 3 to 5°C.

3. Distilled Water

4. Toluene

5. Pure Nitrogen Gas

6. Centrifuge Tube, 12 ml.

7. Centrifuge

8. Test Tube and Rubber Stopper (10 x 75 mm.)

9. Needles, 20 Gauge and 22 Gauge

10. Waterbath, 37°C.

PROCEDURE:

A. Preparation of the Hemolysate
   1. Collect the 2.0 ml. blood in an EDTA-containing "Vacutainer" (Becton, Dickinson & Co., Rutherford, N. J. 07070).

Murayama Test - Modification (Continued):

2. Dilute the blood with an equal volume of saline solution and mix.

3. Place 5.0 ml. of cold sucrose solution in a 12 ml. centrifuge tube.

4. Layer 5.0 ml. of the diluted blood on top of the sucrose solution. Centrifuge for 10 minutes at 2300 g.

5. Decant the sucrose-plasma layers. Rinse the sides of the tube with a small amount of distilled water to remove all the sucrose, and decant the water.

6. Add a quantity of distilled water equivalent to one-fourth the volume of packed erythrocytes. Mix well by inversion by hand.

7. Add one drop of toluene (to dissolve the erythrocyte stromata and mix gently by inversion by hand.

8. Centrifuge at 2300 g for 10 minutes. Decant the supernatant fluid. The concentrated hemolysate must now be deoxygenated, by using solid CO_2 or by the following technique.

B. Deoxygenation
1. Pierce a rubber stopper (to fit a 10 x 75 mm. tube) with a 20 gauge and with a 22 gauge needle (do not use a larger tube).

2. Prepare a gas moisturizing bottle. Connect the inlet of the bottle to a tank of pure N_2 (with gauges to reduce the flow to 2 or 2.5 liters per minute). Connect the outlet to the 20 gauge needle. The N_2 must be moisturized (bubble through water with a gas deflector) to prevent drying of the hemolysate.

3. Insert the rubber stopper, with its needles, into a 10 x 75 mm test tube containing 0.5 ml. of the hemolysate from the last step of the hemolysate preparation.

4. Place the tube in a waterbath at 37°C. Gently tilt the tube from time to time. (Do not allow bubbles to form; the N_2 needs only to pass over the surface of the hemolysate, not through it.) Observe the hemolysate for 10 minutes before concluding that the test is negative. Most S hemoglobin

Murayama Test - Modification (Continued):

systems give a gel within 5 minutes. When a gel forms, the
tube should be inverted to demonstrate the fact.

5. If a gel forms, place the tube into an ice water bath. Tilt
   · the tube gently to observe if the gel becomes a liquid at
   0^oC. Avoid bubble formation. The gel-sol transformation at
   0^oC. and 37^oC. should be repeated several times to demonstrate
   the negative temperature coefficient of gelation. Do not
   disconnect the N_2 or CO_2 tubing in these deoxygenating steps
   at any time.

COMMENTS ON PROCEDURE:

1. The hemoglobin concentration of the hemolysate must be 17 gm.
   per 10 ml. or greater. This is important. It is advisable to
   do a hemoglobin determination on the hemolysate.

2. If a larger volume of hemolysate is desired, the erythrocyte and
   water mixture (Step A-6) may be frozen to obtain complete lysis.
   Such freezing does not affect the results of the Murayama test.

3. The concentration of the sucrose solution must be as described,
   and it must be used while still cold to achieve good separation
   of plasma and erythrocytes.

REFERENCES:

1. Nalbandian, R. M., Henry, R. L., Nichols, B. M., Camp, Jr., F. R.,
   and Wolf, P. L.: "Molecular Basis for a Simple, Specific Test for
   S Hemoglobin: The Murayama Test". Clin. Chem. 16:945, 1970.

2. Murayama, M.: "Structure of Sickle Cell Hemoglobin and Molecular
   Mechanism of the Sickling Phenomenon". Clin. Chem. 13:578, 1967.

3. Murayama, M.: "Molecular Mechanism of Red Cell 'Sickling'".
   Science 153:145, 1966.

4. Scott, R. B.: "Rapid Technic for Preparation of Hemoglobin
   Solutions for Electrophoresis". Amer. J. Clin. Path. 54:78, 1970.

INTERPRETATION:

The Murayama test, a new specific test for hemoglobin S based on the
molecular mechanism of sickling for S hemoglobin, as proposed by Murayama, has been previously reported. The test is a simple visual

Murayama Test - Modification (Continued):

method for the detection of implicated hydrophobic bonds within deoxygenated S hemoglobin hemolysates. Murayama has published his
original conception of the molecular events involved in sickling of
S hemoglobin, but has recently provided a modified hypothesis.

This modification is a significant simplification of the technique of
the Murayama test, which makes it possible to perform the test in one
third the time with equal reliability and accuracy.

This modification of the technique of Murayama test has two advantag-
eous results: the method is simplified because several steps are
eliminated and the performance time per test is decreased from 1 hour
to 20 minutes. This technical improvement is achieved principally
by preparing the concentrated hemolysates by a variation of the method
of Scott. Another improvement is related to the optional use of
moistened nitrogen instead of solid carbon dioxide for deoxygenation
of the hemolysate as a matter of increased convenience to some
laboratories.

SIDEROCYTES

PRINCIPLE: Siderocytes are erythrocytes containing granules of iron. The granules give a positive Prussian Blue reaction. They sometimes appear in a Wright's stain as faint bluish granules (Pappenheimer Bodies). Only on occasion is a siderocyte found in normal blood, but a large number is present in the hemoglobinopathies, in lead poisoning, and after splenectomy.

EQUIPMENT AND REAGENTS:

1. 2% Potassium Ferrocyanide
   Place 2.0 gm. potassium ferrocyanide in a 100 ml. volumetric flask and dilute to volume with distilled water.

2. 1% HCl
   Measure 1.0 ml. of concentrated HCl into a 100 ml. volumetric flask and dilute to volume with distilled water.

3. Approximate 0.2% Aqueous Safranin Solution

4. Coplin Staining Jars

PROCEDURE:

1. Fix blood smear in methyl alcohol for 2 minutes and air dry.

2. Stain for 10 minutes in a freshly mixed solution of 75 ml. 1% HCl and 25 ml. 2% potassium ferrocyanide.

3. Wash with water.

4. Counterstain 1 minute with the 0.2% Safranin stain.

5. Wash with water and let air dry.

6. Examine for blue-green granules.

7. Always run a control; a positive bone marrow may be used for a control.

REFERENCE: Miale, John B.: LABORATORY MEDICINE HEMATOLOGY, 4th Ed. C. V. Mosby Co., St. Louis, pg. 1214, 1972.

337

Siderocytes (Continued):

INTERPRETATION:

Siderotic granules can be found in developing normoblasts, in some
of the reticulocytes, and in a small number of adult erythrocytes.
They represent intraerythrocytic iron not yet incorporated into hemoglobin. They are found in large numbers when hemoglobin synthesis
is impaired, and are absent in iron deficiency states. They also
appear in large numbers after splenectomy in hemoglobinopathies and
in lead poisoning. It is not known whether the absence of the spleen
retards iron utilization, or whether the spleen normally removes
siderotic granules from the erythrocytes or otherwise disposes of
them.

SUCROSE TEST FOR PAROXYSMAL NOCTURNAL HEMOGLOBINURIA

PRINCIPLE: This determination is a confirmatory test for PNH. It demonstrates that the erythrocytes of a PNH will hemolyze in buffered sucrose solution.

SPECIMEN: 10 ml. of anticoagulated (citrate or oxalated) whole blood from patient and from an ABO compatible control.

REAGENTS:

1. Buffer
   a. 5 mM $NaH_2PO_4 \cdot H_2O$
      690 mg. per liter of distilled water.
   b. 5 mM $Na_2HPO_4 \cdot H_2O$
      135 mg./100 ml. distilled water.
      Mix 910 ml. of Solution A and 90 ml. of Solution B for buffer.

2. Sucrose Hemolysis Mixture
   10 ml. buffer
   924 mg. sucrose (0.27 M. sucrose)
      Adjust pH to 6.1 with 0.75 N. NaOH or 0.75 N. HCl.
      Prepare a fresh mixture weekly.

3. 0.75 N. NaOH
   3.0 gm. NaOH/100 ml. distilled water.

4. 0.75 N. HCl
   6.25 ml. of 12 N. HCl/100 ml. distilled water.

PROCEDURE:

1. Obtain defibrinated anticoagulated blood from patient and from an ABO compatible control.

2. Wash cells 3 times with 0.85% saline, filling the 10 x 75 mm. test tubes each time and centrifuging at 1000 rpm for 1 minute.

3. Prepare a 50% washed cell suspension of patient's cells and control cells in saline.

4. Add to each of two 10 x 75 mm. test tubes.
   a. 0.85 ml. sucrose mixture
   b. 0.05 ml. unacidified ABO group-compatible fresh normal defibrinated serum or plasma that was collected in oxalate or citrate.

339

Sucrose Test for PNH (Continued):

    c. 0.1 ml. of the 50% solution of patient's red cells are added to Tube 1 and a similar suspension of control cells to Tube 2.

5. Incubate 30 minutes at 37°C.

6. Invert tube several times, then centrifuge 2000 rpm for 1 minute.

7. Examine supernatant for hemolysis.

NORMAL VALUES: Minimal or Trace Degree of Hemolysis

REFERENCE: Hartmann, R. C. and Jenkins, D. E.: "The 'Sugar-Water' Test for PNH". New Eng. J. Med. 275:155, 1966.

INTERPRETATION:

A positive test for paroxysmal nocturnal hemoglobinuria is when the buffered sucrose solution causes more than 10 percent hemolysis in the PNH erythrocytes. The control cells should show only a minimal or trace degree of hemolysis. The amount of hemolysis may be determined by spectrophotometry of the supernatant.

SUDAN BLACK B LIPID STAIN

PRINCIPLE: The granules of myeloid cells are sudanophilic and can also be stained for peroxidase. An advantage of the Sudan Black B Stain is that smears do not have to be fresh.

SPECIMEN: Peripheral Blood Smears.

REAGENTS:

1. Buffer Solution
   Mix a solution of 0.6 gm. of pure phenol in 30 ml. of absolute ethyl alcohol with a solution of 0.3 gm. of $Na_2HPO_4 \cdot 12H_2O$ in 100 ml. of distilled water.

2. Stock Sudan Black B Solution
   To 100 ml. of absolute ethyl alcohol add 0.3 gm. of Sudan Black B Stain.

3. Working Stain Solution
   The staining solution is prepared by mixing 60 ml. of Sudan Black B solution with 40 ml. of buffer.

4. Giemsa's Stain
   Used as a counterstain.

5. Formalin, 40%

PROCEDURE:

1. Obtain air-dried peripheral blood smears and fix them in 40% Formalin vapor.

2. Stain the fixed peripheral blood smears in Sudan Black B Stain for 30 minutes.

3. Wash in absolute ethyl alcohol.

4. Counterstain with Giemsa's stain.

REFERENCE: Lillie, R. D. and Burtner, H. J.: "Stable Sudanophilia of Human Neutrophil Leukocytes, in Relation to Peroxidase and Oxidase". J. Histochem. Cytochem. 1:8, 1953.

Sudan Black B Lipid Stain (Continued):

NORMAL VALUES AND INTERPRETATION:

The myeloid cell series especially exhibits positive Sudan staining.
Promyelocytes contain minimal sudanophilic granules with increasing
number of granules in more mature cells such as the polymorphonuclear
neutrophil. Monocytes contain only a few sudanophilic granules
while eosinophils contain many granules. Lymphocytes and normoblasts
are not sudanophilic.

The main purpose of the stain is to identify myeloblasts in acute
myelogenous leukemia which are sudanophilic, from lymphoblasts in
acute lymphocytic leukemia which are negative. Monoblasts in acute
monocytic leukemia are minimally sudanophilic.

THROMBIN HEMOLYSIN TEST
FOR
PAROXYSMAL NOCTURNAL HEMOGLOBINURIA

PRINCIPLE: This procedure is a specific one for paroxysmal nocturnal hemoglobinuria. Increased hemolysis occurs when thrombin is added to an acidified PNH red blood cell suspension.

SPECIMEN: Defibrinated blood from patient, about 20 to 25 ml. and defibrinated blood from control SAME ABO AS PATIENT.

REAGENTS AND EQUIPMENT:

1. HCl, 0.2 N.

2. HCl, 0.3 N.

3. Thrombin,
   Prepare when needed. USE FRESH ONLY.

PREPARATION OF CELLS:

Prepare cells by washing three times with normal saline. Make a 50% suspension of part of the cells leaving about 1.0 ml. of packed cells for Thrombin Test.

PROCEDURE:

Tube	1	2	3	4	5	6	7
			Heat 56°C. 30 Min.				
	-	-		-	-	-	-
0.5 ml. serum	P	P	N	N	N	P	P
0.05 ml. 0.2 N HCl	0	+	+	0	+	0	+
			Mix Well				
0.05 ml. 50% cells	P	P	P	P	P	N	N

Incubate 37°C. for 1 hour
Centrifuge 1000 rpm for 2 minutes
Read supernatant for hemolysis and if necessary
Quantitate with Benzidine Plasma Hemoglobin

Results:	±	+	±	±	+	Control	Control

Thrombin Hemolysin Test for PNH (Continued):

THROMBIN TEST

Tube	1	2	3	4	5	6	7	8
2.0 ml. serum	N		P		P		N	
0.1 ml. 0.3 N HCl	+		+		+		+	
0.2 ml. Packed cells	P		P		N		N	

Mix well and transfer
1.0 ml. from Tube 1 to Tube 2
1.0 ml. from Tube 3 to Tube 4
1.0 ml. from Tube 5 to Tube 6
1.0 ml. from Tube 7 to Tube 8

50 Units Thrombin in Tris Buffer	0	+	0	+	0	+	0	+

Incubate all tubes at 37°C. for 15 minutes
Centrifuge lightly and read for hemolysis
if necessary, quantitate hemolysis using
Benzidine Hemoglobin.

Results: ±   +   ±   + Control Control Control Contr

REFERENCE: Crosby, W. H.: "Paroxysmal Nocturnal Hemoglobinuria A Specific Test for the Disease Based on the Ability of Thrombin to Activate Hemolytic Factor". Blood 5:843, 1950.

INTERPRETATION AND RESULTS:

The Thrombin Hemolysin Test was proposed by Crosby who found that when Bovine thrombin was added to acidified serum hemolysis was enhanced. Thrombin may act as a proteolytic enzyme. The addition of thrombin has not given consistent enhancement to the acidified serum test.

THROMBIN TIME

PRINCIPLE: Thrombin is diluted with $CaCl_2$ until it gives a clotting
time of 12 to 16 seconds with fresh normal plasma. The clotting
time of the patient is compared to the time of the fresh normal plasma.

SPECIMEN: Collect blood in acid citrate (1 part acid citrate to
9 parts blood). Spin and remove plasma. DO NOT FREEZE!

REAGENTS AND EQUIPMENT:

1. Thrombin
   Dilute vials of 5000 units with 5.0 cc. of 0.025 M. $CaCl_2$.
   Aliquot 0.1 ml. amounts into 10 cc. plastic tubes. Store in
   freezer. When needed, thaw and add 9.9 ml. of 0.025 M. $CaCl_2$ to
   give 10 units/ml.

2. Fresh Normal Control

3. 0.025 M. $CaCl_2$

4. Fibrometer and 0.3 ml. Probe

5. Acid Citrate
   2 parts 0.1 M. citric acid to 3 parts 0.1 M. Na_3 citrate.

COMMENTS ON PROCEDURE:

1. Thrombin adsorbs on glass and loses activity rapidly. All dilutions must be made in plastic.

2. The final dilution of thrombin is not stable, and the test must
   be run rapidly after this dilution is made.

PROCEDURE:

1. Pipette 0.7 ml. of 0.025 M. $CaCl_2$ into a plastic tube. Warm in
   heat block.

2. Warm fresh normal plasma and patient's plasma for 3 minutes in
   37°C. heat block.

3. To the $CaCl_2$ add (with plastic tip) 0.3 ml. of thrombin. Mix
   gently. Run at once. Thrombin is not stable at this dilution.

Thrombin Time (Continued):

4. Aliquot 0.2 ml. plasma samples into fibrometer cups.

5. Add 0.1 ml. thrombin, starting the timer.

6. Normal fresh plasma should be between 12 - 16 seconds. If the normal plasma does not fall within this range, redilute thrombin so that it does.

7. If the patient's thrombin time exceeds the normal range, repeat the test on a 1:2 mixture of patient's plasma and normal plasma.

8. Report the thrombin time of patient and normal plasma (and thrombin time corrected with normal plasma if this was done).

NORMAL VALUES: 12 - 16 Seconds.

PROTAMINE CORRECTION:

When it becomes necessary to neutralize heparin activity with protamine, the laboratory may be required to evaluate the amount of protamine needed.

ADDITIONAL REAGENTS AND EQUIPMENT:

1. Protamine Sulfate, 1.0%

2. Imidazole Buffer
   6.8 gm. imidazole
   16.7 gm. sodium chloride
   372 ml. 0.1 M. HC1
      Dilute to 2 liters and adjust pH to 7.35 $\pm$ 0.05.

3. 0.4 ml. Probe
   For Fibrometer.

PROCEDURE:

1. Run thrombin time on normal control and on patient.

2. Dilute 1.0% protamine to 0.4 mg./ml. (0.4 ml. with 9.6 ml. buffer).

3. To fibrometer cup, add 0.2 ml. patient's plasma and 0.1 ml. of diluted protamine.

4. Add, with timer on, 0.1 ml. of thrombin.

Thrombin Time (Continued):

5. If this does not correct the thrombin time to normal, more concentrated solutions of thrombin should be used.

REPORT: The amount of protamine necessary to correct patient's plasma to normal (as above, 0.04 mg. of protamine/0.2 ml. plasma).

REFERENCES:

1. Sirridge, M. S.: LABORATORY EVALUATION OF HEMOSTASIS, Lea & Febiger, pp. 132-135, 1967.

2. Hardisty, R. M. and Ingram, G. I. C.: BLEEDING DISORDERS INVESTIGATION AND MANAGEMENT, F. A. Davis Co., pp. 285-318, 1966.

INTERPRETATION:

If the patient's Thrombin Time is significantly longer than the Control, this suggests a deficiency of fibrinogen or the presence of a substance inhibitory to the thrombin-fibrinogen reaction.

If the 1:1 mixture of patient and control plasma gives a clotting time which approximates the diluted control plasma, deficiency is more likely.

Fibrinogen deficiency occurs in severe hepatic disease, disseminated intravascular coagulation, or fibrinolysis. See Interpretation of Semiquantitative Fibrinogen on page 89.

URINARY DELTA-AMINOLEVULINIC ACID
(ALA)

PRINCIPLE: The quantity of lead in blood and the quantity of ALA (delta-aminolevulinic acid) in urine are the most reliable indices of lead poisoning. The effect of increased lead exposure is the declining ability of the body to adequately convert ALA, by the enzymatic action of ALA dehydrase, to porphobilinogen, as shown in the following mechanism:

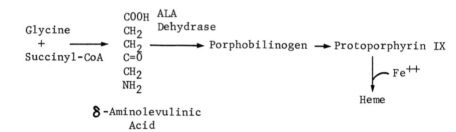

$$\begin{array}{c} \text{Glycine} \\ + \\ \text{Succinyl-CoA} \end{array} \longrightarrow \begin{array}{l} COOH \\ CH_2 \\ CH_2 \\ C=O \\ CH_2 \\ NH_2 \end{array} \xrightarrow{\text{ALA Dehydrase}} \text{Porphobilinogen} \longrightarrow \text{Protoporphyrin IX} \searrow Fe^{++}$$

δ-Aminolevulinic Acid

Heme

Since the function of ALA dehdrase is hampered, its substrate (ALA) increases and is excreted in the urine. No other heavy metal is known to affect this enzyme.

The method is a rapid, sensitive, and simplified determination using the Bio-Rad prefilled, disposable ion-exchange chromatography columns.

In order to isolate the ALA from the urine, the urine sample must first be passed through an anionic ion-exchange resin which permits both ALA and urea to pass through while porphobilinogen is retained on the resin. The effluent passing through the anionic resin must then be passed through a cationic ion-exchange resin which retains ALA while allowing urea to pass through. The ALA which has been retained on the cationic resin can then be eluted and collected for analysis.

After elution from the column, ALA is condensed with acetylacetone to form a pyrrole, 2-methyl-3-acetyl-4-(3-propionic acid) pyrrole. This pyrrole then reacts with Ehrlich's Reagent (p-dimethylamino-benzaldehyde) in acid solution to produce a cherry-red complex which can be measured spectrophotometrically.

Delta-Aminolevulinic Acid (Continued):

SPECIMEN: Only 0.5 ml. of a random urine sample is required for
testing. It is advisable not to use the first voided morning
specimen, late evening specimens after 8:00 p. m., or specimens
obtained following excessive fluid intake. Add 0.1 ml. of concentrated glacial acetic acid to every 10 ml. of urine to keep the pH
below 6.0. The urinary ALA content of samples stored in a dark
refrigerator will remain constant up to 4 months, while frozen
samples will remain constant up to a year.

REAGENTS AND EQUIPMENT:

1. Sodium Acetate 1.0 M.
   Weigh out 82 gm. of anhydrous sodium acetate into a liter volumetric flask. Dissolve and bring to volume with deionized
   water.

2. Stock Standard 100 micrograms ALA/ ml.
   Delta-Aminolevulinic Acid Hydrochloride (Calbiochem) M. W.
   167.6 is used to prepare the solution. Weigh out 12.8 mg. of
   ALA · HCl into a 100 ml. volumetric flask. Dissolve and dilute
   to volume with deionized water. This standard has a concentration of 100 micrograms ALA/ml. Solution is stable under
   refrigeration.

3. Working Standard of ALA, 0.2 mg./100 ml.
   2.0 ml. of Stock Standard is diluted to 100 ml. with deionized
   water.

4. Perchloric Acid, 70 - 72%
   Available from J. T. Baker Chemical Company.

5. Acetylacetone, 2,4-pentanedione
   Obtained from Eastman Organic Chemicals, Rochester, N. Y.

6. p-Dimethylaminobenzaldehyde Acid Solution
   10 gm. of reagent grade p-dimethylaminobenzaldehyde (DMAB) is
   dissolved in 420 ml. of reagent grade glacial acetic acid.
   Solution is stored in an amber bottle in the refrigerator.

7. Fresh Ehrlich's Reagent
   To every 100 ml. of acid DMAB, add 19 ml. of 72% perchloric
   acid. Reagent is stable up to six hours. Prepare only the
   amount needed for the determination.

Delta-Aminolevulinic Acid (Continued):

8. Chromatography Columns
   Available in 20 ALA Column Units complete with reagents and
   Standard from Bio-Rad Laboratories.

9. Gilford Spectrophotometer 300 N.
   Equipped with an aspiration cuvette.

CALIBRATION CURVE: (To be set up with each determination)

1. Using culture tubes with screw caps, (20 x 150 mm.), aliquots
   of Working Standard are pipetted in the following manner:

Volume of Standard	Concentration of ALA	Corresponding Mg%. of ALA for 0.5 ml. of Urine
0.5 ml.	0.1 mg./100 ml.	0.2 mg./100 ml.
1.0 ml.	0.2 mg./100 ml.	0.4 mg./100 ml.
2.0 ml.	0.4 mg./100 ml.	0.8 mg./100 ml.
3.0 ml.	0.6 mg./100 ml.	1.2 mg./100 ml.
5.0 ml.	1.0 mg./100 ml.	2.0 mg./100 ml.

2. Dilute each of the Standards to 7.0 ml. with 1.0 M. NaAc.

3. BLANK - 7.0 ml. of 1.0 M. NaAc.

4. Add 0.2 ml. of acetylacetone to each tube and mix.

5. Place tubes in a boiling water bath for 10 minutes, remove,
   and cool to room temperature.

6. Add 7.0 ml. of fresh Ehrlich's Reagent to each tube, mix, and
   let stand for 15 minutes. The ALA colored product reaches a
   maximum in 6 - 15 minutes, and then remains stable for at
   least 15 minutes.

7. Using the Reagent Blank, set the Gilford Spectrophotometer to
   zero at 553 nm. and read the absorbance of the Standards.

8. Prepare a standard curve by plotting concentration of standards
   in Mg%. versus absorbance.

PROCEDURE:

1. Preparation of the Column
   Use one blue tinted column and one clear column for each
   sample to be run. Shake each column vigorously until all the

Delta-Aminolevulinic Acid (Continued):

resin is resuspended. Allow the resin to settle in each
column. First remove the cap of the clear column and then
snap off the tip and place in rack. Then remove the cap of
the blue tinted column and then snap off the tip, placing the
blue tinted column "piggy-back fashion" into the clear column.
This two column set is referred to as the column unit. Each
urine sample requires one column unit for the determination of
ALA.

2. To each column unit, add 10 ml. of distilled water and allow
   to drain through both columns into the drain tray.

3. Pipette 0.5 ml. of random urine sample into the top of the
   column unit.
   CONTROL - 0.5 ml. of Supplemental Urine Control (Available
             from Hyland Laboratories.
   STANDARD RECOVERY - 0.1 ml. of Stock Standard corresponding
             to 2.0 mg%. ALA.

4. Wash three times with 30 ml. of deionized water, 10 ml. at a
   time. It is important that all column units are completely
   drained of the previous water wash before applying the next
   aliquot of water to the column unit. This prevents the column
   from overflowing.

5. Discard the blue tinted column, and place the clear column into
   a culture tube.

6. Elute with 7.0 ml. of 1.0 M. Sodium Acetate. Allow all of
   the sodium acetate to drain completely.

7. BLANK - 7.0 ml. of 1.0 M. Sodium Acetate.

8. Add 0.2 ml. of acetylacetone to each tube and mix.

9. Place tubes in a boiling water bath for 10 minutes, remove
   and cool to room temperature.

10. Add 7.0 ml. of fresh Ehrlich's Reagent to each tube, mix,
    and let stand for 15 minutes.

11. Read the absorbance of the colored product against the Reagent
    Blank on the Gilford Spectrophotometer 300 N at 553 nm.

352

Delta-Aminolevulinic Acid (Continued):

12. Read off Concentration of Delta-Aminolevulinic Acid in mg%.
    from the Standard Curve.

NORMAL VALUES: Children and Adults 0.00 - 0.54 mg%.

REFERENCES:

1. Mauzerell, D., and Granick, S.:   J. Biol. Chem., 219:435,
       1956.

2. Davis, J., and Andelman, S.:   Arch. Environ. Health, Vol. 15,
       1967.

3. Bio-Rad ALA Instruction Manual.

INTERPRETATION:

ALA is synthesized from glycine and succinyl-coenzyme A.   Urinary
excretion of ALA is greatly increased in lead poisoning. The major
reason for the increased ALA in the urine in lead poisoning is the
lack of conversion of ALA to porphobilinogen because of the inhibition of ALA dehydrase by lead.

ALA urinary excretion is also found in acute intermittent porphyria
and has been found to be slightly increased in acute hepatitis,
carcinoma of the liver and Porphyria Cutanea Tardea.

URINARY MYOGLOBIN
(Qualitative)

PRINCIPLE: Myoglobin is a respiratory pigment found in muscle cells and is functionally and structurally related to hemoglobin. It consists of a single polypeptide chain and an iron-porphyrin-heme group, while hemoglobin has four such peptide chains and four heme groups. The primary function of myoglobin is oxygen storage.

The molecular weight of myoglobin (16,700) is one-fourth that of hemoglobin and, unlike hemoglobin, myoglobin is not bound significantly by plasma proteins. These two factors account for a low renal threshhold for myoglobin and its rapid excretion in the urine.

SPECIMEN: 5.0 ml. of urine from a random collection. The specimen should be fresh. A fresh morning voiding or a voiding just after exercise is preferred.

REAGENTS:

1. <u>Ammonium Sulfate</u> $(NH_4)_2SO_4$

2. <u>Sulfosalicylic Acid</u>, 3.0%

COMMENTS ON PROCEDURE:

1. Urine containing myoglobin will have a reddish-tinge when fresh, which gradually turns black on standing.

2. First test the urine for protein with sulfosalicylic acid. If the pigment is precipitated, it is protein-bound and therefore not myoglobin. If the pigment persists in the supernatant it may be myoglobin or hemoglobin.

3. The heat and acetic acid test for protein does not precipitate either myoglobin or hemoglobin and should not be used in this instance.

PROCEDURE:

1. Dissolve 2.8 gm. of ammonium sulfate in 5.0 ml. of urine, mix well, and centrifuge. Compare the color of the supernatant fluid to that of the untreated urine sample. If the pigmentation persists in the supernatant, then myoglobin (or metmyoglobin) is

353

Urinary Myoglobin (Continued):

present. If the pigmentation has been precipitated or removed
from the supernatant, then hemoglobin is present.

2. This presumptive differential test can be confirmed by spectrophotometric scan or the myoglobin identified by electrophoresis
(myoglobin migrates only half the distance of hemoglobin).
Immunologic identification is also reliable.

NORMAL VALUES: Negative Urine

REFERENCES:

1. Henry, R. B.: CLINICAL CHEMISTRY: PRINCIPLES AND TECHNIQUES,
   Hoeber, pg. 733, 1964.

2. Blondheim, S. H., Lathrop, D., and Zabrinskie: J. Lab. Clin.
   Med., 60:31, 1962.

3. Sahuburger, A. B.: BIOCHEMISTRY, pg. 116 - 117, 1970.

4. Davidsohn, I. and Henry, J.: TODD-SANFORD: CLINICAL DIAGNOSIS
   BY LABORATORY METHODS, 14th Ed., pg. 68, 1969.

INTERPRETATION:

Myoglobinuria results from necrosis of skeletal or cardiac muscle.
Patients complain of painful skeletal muscle weakness. The urine is
dark and the Benzidine test is positive with the absence of RBC's in
the urine. Myoglobin is toxic to renal tubules and acute tubular
necrosis occurs with renal failure.

The commonest cause for myoglobin to be present in the urine is
skeletal muscle necrosis. Some common etiologies are crush injury,
alcoholic myopathy, extensive burns, electric shock, viral influenza
myositis, and dermatomyositis.

Acute myocardial infarction may be diagnosed by the presence of
cardiac muscle myoglobin in the urine.

URINE UROBILINOGEN
(Rapid Two Hour Test)

PRINCIPLE: Urobilinogen, along with other aldehyde-reacting substances found in urine, reacts with Ehrlich's Aldehyde Reagent to
produce a red color, the intensity of which is proportional to the
amount of pigment present.

SPECIMEN: There is a greater quantity of urobilinogen excreted in
the urine during the afterncon and evening than during the morning.
In order to make the test more quantitative, the total urine excreted during a two hour period in the afternoon should be used (preferably 1:00 p.m. to 3:00 p.m.). No preservative is used, and the test
should be run as soon as possible, since urobilinogen is unstable.

REAGENTS AND EQUIPMENT:

1. Sodium Acetate, a saturated aqueous solution
   Approximately 1100 gm. of sodium acetate containing 3 molecules
   of water of crystallization is added to 800 ml. of deionized
   water (0.8 ml. water dissolves 1.0 gm. of sodium acetate). The
   mixture is heated to approximately 60°C. When the solution
   cools, there should be a large excess of crystals. (DO NOT
   PIPETTE FROM THIS BOTTLE.)

2. Ehrlich's Aldehyde Reagent, Watson's modification
   Dissolve 0.7 gm. of paradimethylaminobenzaldehyde in a mixture
   of 150 ml. concentrated HCl and 100 ml. deionized water. The
   reagent is stable if stored in a brown bottle. (DO NOT PIPETTE
   FROM THIS BOTTLE.)

3. Stock Standard, Phenol Red (LaMotte Chemical Co., Chestertown, Md.)
   Dissolve 22 mg. Phenol red (pH 6.8 - 8.5; Code 2411-C), in 100 ml.
   of 0.05%. NaOH. Store in a brown polyehtylene bottle. (DO NOT
   PIPETTE FROM THIS BOTTLE.)

4. Working Standard
   Dilute the stock standard 1:100 with 0.05% NaOH to make a
   0.22 mg%. solution, which is equivalent in color to 0.35 mg%.
   urobilinogen. Store in a brown polyethylene bottle. (DO NOT
   PIPETTE FROM THIS BOTTLE.)

5. Beckman DU Spectrophotometer
   The working standard must first be read on the Beckman DU before
   proceeding with the unknowns at a wavelength of 562 nm. against
   a 0.05% NaOH Blank, and should have an O.D. of .385 ± .002.

355

356

Urine Urobilinogen (Continued):

COMMENTS ON PROCEDURE:

1. The determination of urobilinogen with aldehyde reagent is not specific for urobilinogen. Other aldehyde-reacting chromogens, notably indols, are excreted in the urine. Abnormal porphyrins may also add to the color development.

2. The greatest source of error is inadequate mixing of the urine and reagent during each step of the procedure.

PROCEDURE:

1. Measure and record volume of urine

2. If a known positive is available it should be used as a control and run like patient specimen.

3. Two tubes should be set up for each unknown, standard, and control when available.

   A. UNKNOWN

      1). Patient Blank:
          Combine 2.5 ml. Ehrlich's and 5.0 ml. sodium acetate and mix well. Add 2.5 ml. of urine and mix.
          NOTE: There should not be any pink to purple color development in the blank.

      2). Patient Test:
          To 2.5 ml. of urine, add 2.5 ml. of Ehrlich's Reagent. Mix well for 15 seconds, then immediately add 5.0 ml. of sodium acetate, and mix thoroughly.
          NOTE: Sodium acetate stops the color reaction of Ehrlich's Reagent and also develops the color complex formed.

          If the urine is cloudy or precipitated upon adding Ehrlich's, repeat the test on a bile-free filtrate (equal amounts of urine and 10% BaCl filtered), and multiply calculations x 2.

   B. STANDARD
      1). Blank:
          Deionized water.

Urine Urobilinogen (Continued):

    2). Standard:
       0.35 mg%. urobilinogen standard.

4. Read unknowns, standard, and control (when available) against
their respective blanks on the Beckman DU at 562 nm.

5. CALCULATIONS:

$$\frac{O.D. \ Unk.}{O.D. \ Std.} \times 0.35 \ (Conc. \ of \ Std.) \times \frac{10 \ (Vol. \ Final \ Sol.)}{2.5 \ (Vol. \ Urine \ used)}$$

= Ehrlich units/100 ml. Urine

$$\frac{O.D. \ Unk.}{O.D. \ Standard} \times 1.4 = Ehrlich \ units/100 \ ml. \ Urine$$

$$\frac{1.4}{100} = .014 \ (Factor) \quad THUS:$$

$$\frac{O.D. \ Unk.}{O.D. \ Std.} \times 0.014 \times vol. \ of \ Urine = Ehrlich \ units/2 \ hours.$$

NOTE: Report Ehrlich units/2 hours.

NORMAL VALUES: 0.3 - 1.0 Ehrlich Units/2 Hours

REFERENCES:

1. Davidsohn and Wells: TODD-SANFORD CLINICAL DIAGNOSIS BY
LABORATORY METHODS, 13th Ed., Saunders, pg. 548 - 550,
1963.

2. Henry, R. B.: CLINICAL CHEMISTRY: PRINCIPLES AND TECHNIQUES,
Hoeber, pg. 611 - 613, 1964.

INTERPRETATION:

The total urinary excretion of urobilinogen is 3 Ehrlich Units. A
diurnal excretion of 1.5 Ehrlich Units exists during a 2 hour period
from 1:00 to 3:00 p. m. Urobilinogen is colorless while urobilin
is amber in color.

An increase in urinary urobilinogen occurs in hemolytic anemia
because of increased production of unconjugated and conjugated

Urine Urobilinogen (Continued):

bilirubin. Conjugated bilirubin is converted to stercobilinogen (urobilinogen) in the colon by the action of E. coli. Hepatic disease also results in an increase in urinary urobilinogen because with liver disease, the urobilinogen remains in the blood stream instead of being removed from the enterohepatic circulation by the hepatic cell.

Decreased urinary urobilinogen occurs in intra or extrahepatic obstructive jaundice because conjugated bilirubin does not reach the colon for conversion by E. coli, or when E. coli function is negated by broad spectrum antibiotic usage or severe diarrhea.

SERUM VISCOSITY

PRINCIPLE: This procedure utilizes a viscosometer to determine increase in the blood viscosity in patients with macroglobulinemia.

SPECIMEN: 5.0 ml. serum, patient and control.

EQUIPMENT AND REAGENTS:

1. Oswald-Cannon Viscosometer

2. Stopwatch

3. Distilled Water

COMMENTS ON PROCEDURE

1. Volumes of water, normal serum and patient's serum must all be the same.

2. The minimum volume is 4.0 ml.

3. If timing area of viscosometer is not completely submerged and at 37°C., let sample rewarm to 37°C. before repeating timing.

4. Gently blow on smaller glass opening to rid column and sera of bubbles.

5. Water, normal serum and most patient samples should run ± 1 second or closer. Samples taking 10 or 12 minutes or longer do not check well so run 3 or 4 times and average.

6. Convert all time to seconds and average each sample time.

7. Acid clean viscosometer when through.

8. The use of #272 and 229 are not interchangeable.

PROCEDURE:

1. Read "Comments on Procedure".

2. Must have at least 5.0 ml. of serum.

360

Serum Viscosity (Continued):

3. Warm Oswald-Cannon Viscosometer, patient serum, normal pooled serum and distilled water to 37°C.

4. Volumetrically place 5.0 ml. of sample in viscosometer.

5. By means of rubber bulb and tubing pump sample partially into the uppermost reservoir.

6. Using a stopwatch, time sample descent between two lines.

7. Repeat timing 2 to 3 times or until good checks are gotten.

8. Clean viscosometer by drawing:
   a). Haemo-Sol through 2 times
   b). Tap water 4 times
   c). Distilled water 4 times
   d). Acetone 1 time
   e). Suction air through until dry

9. Reheat to 37°C. and run next sample.

10. CALCULATIONS:

1. $\dfrac{\text{Time in seconds normal serum}}{\text{Time in seconds distilled water}}$ = No. of times water

2. $\dfrac{\text{Time in seconds patient serum}}{\text{Time in seconds normal serum}}$ = No. of times normal serum

3. Report number of times normal serum

4. Report number x water

NORMAL VALUES: The Viscosity of Serum compared to distilled water is approximately 1.5 with a range of 1.2 to 1.8.

REFERENCE: Fahey, J., Barth, W., Solomon, A.: "The Syndrome of Serum Hyperviscosity". J. Amer. Med. Assoc. 192:464, 1965.

Serum Viscosity (Continued):

INTERPRETATION:

The viscosity of serum increases with an increase in concentration of immunoglobulin especially IgM. The diseases associated with hyperviscosity are thus, Waldenstrom's macroglobulinemia, multiple myeloma, and certain lymphomas. An elevated serum viscosity is associated with vaso-occlusive signs and symptoms, and may be relieved by chemotherapy of the above conditions or plasmaphoresis.

SERUM VITAMIN B_{12} ESTIMATION
USING LACTOBACILLUS LEICHMANNII

PRINCIPLE: Vitamin B_{12} is determined utilizing the following microbiological procedure. The determination of serum vitamin B_{12} is
essential when a macrocytic megaloblastic anemia is present.

SPECIMEN:

1. Serum samples arriving at the laboratory should be labelled and
   then placed in the deep freeze without delay, that is 30 minutes
   of receipt. They should not be unfrozen until time of assay.

2. If sample consists of clotted blood, the clot should be "rimmed"
   with a sterile, acid-washed rod. (A previously unused, sterile
   wooden applicator stick is also satisfactory.)

3. The tube is then centrifuged for 5 minutes at "3/4 speed", and
   the supernatant serum aspirated (using previously unused, capillary pipette, or an acid-washed standard pipette).

4. This serum is placed in a sterile, acid-washed glass container
   (or disposable container), is labelled, and promptly placed in
   deep freeze.
   NOTE: Cap or plug for container must also be sterile, and
   should either be acid-washed, or washed twelve times in tap
   water, and rinsed three times in distilled water.

5. Record if serum sample is hemolyzed.

REAGENTS USED IN ASSAY:

1. 0.1% NaCN
   In a 100 ml. volumetric flask, dissolve 0.1 gm. NaCN and dilute
   to volume with distilled water.

2. Acetate Buffer, pH 4.5
   400 ml. distilled water is placed in a 1 liter volumetric flask,
   to which is added 22.8 ml. glacial acetic acid and 160 ml. 1.0 N.
   NaOH. The solutions are mixed and then diluted up to volume
   with distilled water and mixed again.

3. Cyanocobalamine (Vitamin B_{12})
   Fresh Stock Solution is made up every six months and stored in
   the refrigerator.

Serum B_{12} Assay (Continued):

4. B_{12} Medium (Difco #0457-15)
    Make up desired quantity each time using 8.5 gm. in 120 ml. of distilled water.

    NOTE: All equipment (including stirrers) used in the preparation of these reagents must be acid-washed, or very thoroughly washed (12 times in tap water, and then rinsed three times in distilled water).

GENERAL COMMENTS: This is a microbiological assay and is dependent upon meticulous attention to detail for results to be meaningful.

1. Trace contamination with B_{12} will completely nullify the significance of the assay, and thus ALL equipment must be acid-washed or extremely thoroughly cleaned, washed 12 times in tap water and rinsed 3 times with distilled water.

2. Bacterial contamination is a problem that is dealt with by autoclaving. However, delays between the various steps of the assay will reduce the reliability of this technique. If any delay becomes necessary, it should always be timed to occur after an autoclaving and before the solutions are handled again.

3. Handling of the initial serum specimens should be minimal, and once deep frozen they should not be thawed out until time of assay.

4. Certain phases of the assay procedures are dependent upon very accurate pipette measurement. These are marked with an asterisk, "*".

PREPARATION OF BACTERIA FOR B_{12} ASSAYS:

A. Initial Preparation and Subsequent Maintenance of Culture

    1. The initial basic cultures are prepared by rehydrating the lyophilized organisms, Lactobacillus leichmannii.

        These organisms are placed in tubes containing the appropriate Difco Culture Broth and are then incubated at 37°C. for 48 hours.

Serum B$_{12}$ Assay (Continued):

These basic cultures are used for the first subcultures, and then are stored in the refrigerator for possible use if difficulties arise with subsequent cultures.

2. Fresh agar stabs must be prepared every 2 weeks for Lacto-bacillus leichmannii.

Using overnight broth culture, plunge flamed stab wire into culture and then down into 10 ml. of agar in one stab. Set up 2 agar cultures.

Incubate at 37°C. for at least 48 hours, and then store in refrigerator.

NOTE: Retain previously used stab for 2 further weeks.

B. Subcultures

1. Flame wire loop and place it down side of agar culture tube to cool it. Then place wire loop into the middle of the bacterial growth.

2. Put wire loop into 10 ml. of inoculum broth in a 40 ml. test tube and agitate. Set up 2 tubes.

3. Plug the broth tube with cottonwool and incubate at 37°C. overnight.

C. Harvesting Bacteria

1. Centrifuge the broth culture for 15 minutes at 2,000 rpm. in the cold.

2. Pour off the broth leaving a pellet of bacteria.

3. Add sterile, distilled water to the 35 ml. mark and mix the bacterial pellet into this using a sterile, cottonwool plug-ged pipette.

4. Centrifuge for 15 minutes at 2,000 rpm in the cold and decant the water.

5. Add 5.0 ml. of sterile distilled water using a sterile pipet-te and resuspend the bacteria.

Serum B_{12} Assay (Continued):

6. Take 0.2 ml. of this suspension and add it to 20 ml. of sterile distilled water. Thoroughly mix this dilute suspension by means of a sterile, cottonwool plugged pipette.

7. Add *one drop of this dilute suspension into each assay tube (except the blank for each specimen) using a sterile cottonwool plugged Pasteur pipette.

D. Media and Equipment

1. Every 2 weeks prepare fresh "Difco" broth and agar for Lactobacillus leichmannii (light brown). These should be autoclaved in 40 ml. test tubes (150 x 20 mm.) in 10 ml. amounts using cottonwool plugs.

   Special medium for the actual assay of B_{12} is also provided by Difco, but this should be made up freshly for each assay.

   Instructions on how to make up these preparations will be found on the label of the various media bottles. The particular Difco Code Numbers are as follows:

   Lactobacillus leichmannii

   Broth   0320-15
   Agar   0319-15
   Medium   0457-15

2. All equipment used for bacterial preparation must be sterile, and when broth or agar stabs are inoculated, the mouths of the tubes should be flamed.

3. The wire loops and wire stabs used for the culture should be labelled and kept in a glass jar.

4. Always have a spare vial of lyophilized Lactobacillus leichmannii stored in the refrigerator. (Can be obtained from: The American Type Culture Company, 12301 Parklawn Drive, Rockville, Maryland 20852)

5. Checking Bacteria
   Every 4 weeks send spare broth culture tube (from sub-culture routine) to a Bacteriology Laboratory for a check on culture purity.

Serum B_{12} Assay (Continued):

AUTOCLAVE ROUTINE:

1. Check "Shut Out" Valve — open (counter-clockwise).

2. Check "By-Pass" Valve — closed (clockwise).

3. Liquid load selection (Drying time = 0).

4. Time selection adjusted.

5. Set temperature timing device.

6. Set pressure in "jacket" of autoclave (on left hand pressure dial) for the level required for particular run.

A. First Autoclave (5 lbs./square inch) - 108°C./20 Minutes

   1. Set indicator at 220° F. (105°C.) - timing for 20 minutes.

   2. Set pressure in jacket at 10 lbs. pressure (use Pressure-reducing Valve).

   3. Close door - bring pressure inside chamber to 4 lbs./square inch in 1 minute - then adjust to 5 lbs./square inch in both chambers (using Pressure-reducing Valve).

   4. When 20 minutes completed and cooling starts, slowly reduce pressure in chamber by very gradually turning "By Pass" Valve counterclockwise ¼ to ½ turn.

                   Pressure down   1 minute 5 lbs. - 4 lbs.
                   in 5 minutes   1 minute 4 lbs. - 3 lbs.
                   by gradual   1 minute 3 lbs. - 2½ lbs.
                   reduction   1 minute 2½ lbs.- 2 lbs.
                                    1 minute 2 lbs. - 1½ lbs.
                        Machine now turns off.

B. Second Autoclave (10 lbs./square inch) - 115°C./6 Minutes

   1. Set indicator at 230°F. - (110°C.) - timing for 6 minutes.

   2. Set pressure in jacket at 15 lbs. pressure (use Pressure-reducing Valve).

Serum B_{12} Assay (Continued):

3. Close door - bring pressure inside chamber to 9 lbs./square inch in 1 minute - then adjust to 10 lbs./square inch in both chambers (using Pressure-reducing Valve).

4. When 6 minutes are completed and cooling starts, slowly reduce pressure in chamber by very gradually turning "By Pass" Valve counterclockwise ¼ to ½ turn.

Pressure down	1 minute	10 lbs.	- 7 lbs.
in 5 minutes	1 minute	7 lbs.	- 5 lbs.
by gradual	1 minute	5 lbs.	- 3½ lbs.
reduction	1 minute	3½ lbs.	- 2½ lbs.
	1 minute	2½ lbs.	- 1½ lbs.

Machine now turns off.

PROCEDURE:

1. Prepare growth of **Lactobacillus leichmannii** in broth the night before using (See "Bacterial Preparation").

2. Using 40 ml. graduated centrifuge tubes and take,

   2.0 ml.* serum (bulb pipette)
   Total = 20 ml.   0.4 ml. of 0.1% NaCN (1.0 ml. pipette)
   1.0 ml. Na Acetate buffer (10 ml. pipette)
   16.6 ml. Distilled water
   Plug tubes with cottonwool.

3. Autoclave at 5 lbs. pressure for 20 minutes at 220°F. (See Autoclave Protocol).

4. Cool tubes.

5. While tubes are cooling, prepare B_{12} Standard Curve. B_{12} Standard Stock Solution consists of:

   a). 1 ampule Vitamin B_{12} (cyanocobalamine) 1,000 ugm./ml.
   b). Dilute this in 200 ml. distilled water (5 ugm./ml.)
   c). Take 1.0 ml. of this and add to 100 ml. water in volumetric flask. This gives a stock solution of 50 mugm./ml.

   It should be stored in the refrigerator (4°C.) for weekly use.

Serum B_{12} Assay (Continued):

B_{12} Standard Curve

Solution "A" 0.5 ml. Stock Solution + 9.5 ml. distilled water
             (2.5 mugm./ml.)
Solution "B" 0.5 ml. of Solution "A" + 9.5 ml. distilled water
             (0.125 mugm./ml.)
Solution "C" 2.0 ml. of Solution "A" + 8.0 ml. distilled water
             (0.5 mugm./ml.)

6. Make 1:25 dilution of 0.1% NaCN by putting 2.0 ml. of 0.1% NaCN
   into 48 ml. of distilled water.

7.

Row No.	1	2	3	4	5	6	7
1:25 Dil. NaCN	1.0	1.0	1.0	1.0	1.0	1.0	1.0
*Solution "B"	0	0.1	0.2	0.4	0.8	0	0
*Solution "C"	0	0	0	0	0	0.4	0.8
Distilled water	1.0	0.9	0.8	0.6	0.2	0.6	0.2

Final Amount

B_{12}

mugm.	0	.0125	.025	.05	0.1	0.2	0.4
(or in uugm.	0	12.5	25	50	100	200	400

This gives a total volume of 2.0 ml. in each tube. The tubes
must be set up in quadruplicate. Cover temporarily with parafilm

8. Now take autoclaved (and cooled) tubes from Step No. 4 and cen-
   trifuge at 2,000 rpm for 10 minutes.
   NOTE: Cover with parafilm having removed cotton plugs first.
   Pour off the supernatant fluid into clean tubes.

9. Using supernatant fluid, prepare unknowns for assay:

   1st Row: 1.0 ml.* supernatant + 1.0 ml. of 1:50 dil. 0.1% NaCN.
            (1.0 ml. of 0.1% NaCN + 49 ml. water)

   2nd Row: 2.0 ml.* supernatant

   Both rows should be done in quadruplicate.

10. Add 3.0 ml. of Difco B_{12} Medium to each assay tube - both Stan-
    dard and unknowns. Cap and autoclave at 10 lbs. for 6 minutes.
    (Using caps that have been rendered B_{12}-free by thorough wash-
    ing; twelve times in tap water and three times in distilled
    water.)

Serum B_{12} Assay (Continued):

11. After tubes have cooled, place one* drop of <u>Lactobacillus leichmannii</u> inoculum in 3 of the 4 tubes of each serum dilution, the fourth tube being set aside as a blank. (This must be done with a sterile Pasteur Pipette, taking care to avoid contamination and only inoculating with one drop).

12. Cap all tubes and incubate for 18 hours at 37°C. (including the blanks).

13. If growth is excessive, it may be necessary to add 2.0 ml. of distilled water to each tube with an automatic syringe before reading.

14. Shake all tubes well before transferring fluid to cuvettes. Read at 600 nm. in a spectrophotometer.

    Read each dilution against its own blank which must be used to zero the instrument.

15. Plot Standard Curve on arithmetic graph paper, using spectrophotometric growth densities against the known amount of B_{12} per tube. (See Example of Standard Curve).

16. CALCULATIONS:

    Calculate the amount of B_{12} in the unknown serum samples by reading directly from the Standard Curve (utilizing the mean value of the 3 Spectrophotometric readings on the 3 tubes of each dilution). Each serum sample will have 3 readings at dilutions of 1 in 10 (Row No. 1) and dilutions of 1 in 5 (Row No. 2).

	Mean of 3 Photometer Readings	EXAMPLE B_{12} (uugm./ml.)	Dilution	Actual B_{12} Value (uugm./ml.)	Final Average
Row "1"	46	24.5	1:10	245	250 uugm. per ml.
Row "2"	88	51.1	1:5	255.5	

NORMAL VALUES: 150 - 1,500 uugm./ml. (i.e. pg./ml.)

REFERENCES:

1. Spray, G. H.: "An Improved Method for the Rapid Estimation of Vitamin B_{12} In Serum", <u>Clin. Sci.</u>, 14:661, 1955.

Serum B_{12} Assay (Continued):

2. Spray, G. H.: "The Estimation and Significance of the Level of Vitamin B_{12} in Serum", J. Postgrad. Med., 38:35, 1962.

3. Spray, G. H. and Witts, L. J.: "Results of Three Years Experience with Microbiological Assay of Vitamin B_{12} in Serum", Brit. Med. Journal, 1:295, 1958.

INTERPRETATION:

Vitamin B_{12} is extrinsic factor. It is only absorbed in the presence of a specific protein substance, intrinsic factor. The site of absorption of vitamin B_{12} is the small intestine, the terminal ileum. The manner of absorption of vitamin B_{12} is uncertain, but is seems probable that the vitamin is bound by intrinsic factor and that the intrinsic factor is bound by receptors in the intestine in the presence of calcium.

Pernicious anemia patients in relapse have low serum levels, below 100 micromicrograms/ml. Patients who have megaloblastic anemia secondary to pregnancy, partial or total gastrectomy, blind loops following surgery, malabsorption syndrome due to various causes, and utilization of anticonvulsants or chemotherapy, also have low serum vitamin B_{12} levels.

Serum vitamin B_{12} is elevated in acute and chronic myelogenous leukemi di Guglielmo syndrome, and liver disease.

Assays of vitamin B_{12} and folic acid blood levels in various disorders are characterized by megaloblastic anemia show that in pernicious anemia in relapse, the serum vitamin B_{12} is low and the serum folic acid is variable. When vitamin B_{12} is injected, a rapid fall of folic acid occurs within two hours. When folic acid is given to pernicious anemia patients in relapse, a decrease in serum vitamin B_{12} occurs.

In nutritional megaloblastic anemia, folic acid serum levels are low. Folic acid levels are low in renal patients on chronic hemodialysis, patients taking anti-folic acid antagonistic chemotherapeutic drugs for cancer, patients on anti-convulsants and oral contraceptives, and hemolytic anemia patients.

The metabolic roles of vitamin B_{12} and folic acid are closely related. As a deficiency of vitamin B_{12} becomes pronounced, the requirement for folic acid may increase.

WESTERGREN SEDIMENTATION RATE

PRINCIPLE: Whole anticoagulated blood is allowed to settle in a tube at room temperature. The amount of settling is noted after one hour. More rapid settling is seen in acute and chronic inflammatory diseases, tissue damage, neoplasia and immunological diseases.

SPECIMEN: Double oxalated whole blood.

EQUIPMENT:

1. Westergren Tube

2. Long Capillary Tube Filler

3. Rack for holding tubes vertical

4. Timer

PROCEDURE:

1. Fill a Westergren tube with double oxalated whole blood being careful to exclude bubbles from the column.

2. Place tube without agitation in rack so that it is held exactly vertical.

3. Set timer for 1 hour.

4. In exactly 1 hour read the distance of RBC from the tip of the tube.

NORMAL VALUES: Males   0 - 15 mm.
                Females   0 - 20 mm.
                Children   0 - 10 mm.

372

Westergren Sedimentation Rate (Continued):

REFERENCES:

1. Gambino, R. S., Dire, J., Monteleone, M., Budd, D.: "The Westergren Sedimentation Rate". Tech. Bull. Regist. Med. Technologists. 35:1, 1965.

2. Davidsohn, I. and Henry, J. B.,Eds.: CLINICAL DIAGNOSIS BY LABORATORY METHODS, W. B. Saunders Co., Phil., pg. 152, 1969.

INTERPRETATION:

The Westergren procedure is considered to be the procedure of choice. Erythrocyte sedimentation occurs in various phases. The first phase is characterized by rouleaux formation following by rapid sedimentation of the conglutinated red blood cells. Erroneous results occur if excessive anticoagulant is present, variability in room temperature, and tilting of the sedimentation tube. The sedimentation rate in the elderly healthy individual is higher than in younger adults.

The major causes for elevation of the sedimentation rate are:

1. Infectious disease
2. Tissue necrosis
3. Immunologic diseases
4. Pregnancy
5. Neoplastic diseases
6. Anemia

A low sedimentation rate occurs where rouleaux formation is difficult, such as in sickle cell and spherocytic anemia.

WINTROBE SEDIMENTATION RATE

PRINCIPLE: Whole anticoagulated blood is allowed to settle in a tube at room temperature. The amount of settling is noted after one hour. More rapid settling is seen in acute and chronic inflammatory disease states than in normal conditions. Increase in sedimentation rate represents a non-specific response to tissue damage, neoplasia, and inflammation.

EQUIPMENT AND REAGENTS:

1. Wintrobe tube
   120 mm. long with an I.D. of 215 mm. and graduated from 0 to 105 mm.

2. Long Capillary Wintrobe Tube Filler

3. Rack
   Used for holding tubes vertical.

4. Timer

PROCEDURE:

1. Fill a Wintrobe tube with versenated whole blood being careful to exclude bubbles from the column.

2. Place tube without agitation in rack so that it is held exactly vertical.

3. Set timer for 1 hour.

4. In exactly 1 hour read the distance of RBC from the top of the tube.

NORMAL VALUES: Males   0 - 10 mm.
                Females   0 - 20 mm.
                Children   0 - 20 mm.

Wintrobe Sedimentation Rate (Continued):

REFERENCES:

1. Gambino, R. S., Dire, J., Monteleone, M., and Budd, D.: "The Westergren Sedimentation Rate". Tech. Bull. Regist. Med. Technologists. 35:1, 1965.

2. Davidsohn, I. and Henry, J. B., Eds.: CLINICAL DIAGNOSIS BY LABORATORY METHODS, 14th. Ed., W. B. Saunders Co., Phil., pg. 152, 1969.

INTERPRETATION:

Two types of procedures are used for the erythrocyte sedimentation rate (ESR), the Westergren Method and the Wintrobe Method. The Westergren procedure is considered to be the procedure of choice; however, when only a small amount of blood can be obtained, the Wintrobe Method is used. It is not a good method if severe anemia other than that caused by acute hemorrhage is present, as there is some evidence that it occasionally gives misleading low results.

The erythrocyte sedimentation occurs in various phases. The first phase is characterized by rouleaux formation followed by a rapid sedimentation of the conglutinated red blood cells. Erroneous results occur if excessive anticoagulant is present, variability in room temperature, and tilting of the sedimentation tube. The sedimentation rate in the elderly healthy individual is higher than in younger adults.

The major causes for elevation of the sedimentation rate are:

1. Infectious disease
2. Tissue necrosis
3. Immunologic diseases
4. Pregnancy
5. Neoplastic diseases
6. Anemia

A low sedimentation rate occurs where rouleaux formation is difficult such as in sickle cell and spherocytic anemia.

WRIGHT'S-GIEMSA STAIN

PRINCIPLE: Wright's stain is a Romanowsky type of stain. It is a compound stain composed of polychrome methylene blue and eosin. The powder stain is made by combining eosin with basic methylene blue and its oxidation products to form a complex dye, thiozine-eosinate, which is neutral in reaction and soluble in absolute methyl alcohol. The staining properties depend on the balance dissociation of the neutral complex; therefore, the pH of the water and buffer is important.

Giemsa's stain uses purified dyes. The azurophilic properties of the polychrome dye is preserved; however, the erythrocytes are poorly stained and the neutrophil granules are pale.

By using the Wright's stain method and then restaining with Giemsa stain the cellular structure appears sharp and clear.

REAGENTS AND EQUIPMENT:

1. Wright's Stain
   Add 6.0 gm. Wright's stain (purchased through Matheson, Coleman, and Bell) to 1 gallon methyl alcohol. Mix and let stand for at least two weeks. Filter fresh each day after the two week period before using.

2. Giordano's Buffer Solution, pH 6.4
   (Purchased commercially through Van Waters and Rogers, Inc.)
   Use fresh daily. Wright's added until sheen on surface.

3. Giemsa's Stain
   a). Stock Solution
      Dissolve 1.52 gm. Giemsa stain in 100 ml. glycerin at 60°C. for 10 minutes. Add 100 ml. methanol, and allow to stand overnight and filter.

   b). Working Solution
      Make fresh daily by using 300 ml. pH 6.4 buffer (Giordan's buffer) and 6.7 ml. Giemsa stock.

COMMENTS ON PROCEDURE:

1. If the stain is too acid, the erythrocytes will be bright red and the nuclei of the leukocytes will be pale blue to colorless.

Wright's-Giemsa Stain (Continued):

2. If the stain is too basic, the erythrocytes will be slate blue.

PROCEDURE:

1. The sequence for staining blood films is as follows:
   a). 30 seconds in methyl alcohol
   b). 2 minutes in Wright's stain
   c). 4 minutes in Wright's buffer
   d). Rinse in water
   e). 4 minutes in Giemsa buffer
   f). Rinse in water

2. The slide is allowed to air dry before microscopic examination.

REFERENCE: Miale, John B.: LABORATORY MEDICINE HEMATOLOGY 4th. Ed.
C. V. Mosby Co., St. Louis, pgs. 1208-1209, 1972.

INTERPRETATION:

This procedure is utilized primarily to stain peripheral blood smears
and bone marrow smears. Smears of peripheral blood are evaluated
for abnormalities of white blood and red blood cells and platelets.

The indications for aspirating bone marrow and preparing smears for
interpretation are numerous. A few of the important indications are:

1. Assessment of anemia
2. Assessment of leukemia
3. Assessment of leukopenia
4. Assessment of thrombocytopenia
5. Identification of bone marrow parasites
6. Diagnosis of lipid storage disease
7. Follow-up of therapy of anemia and leukemia
8. Assessment of hypoplasia or aplasia
9. Assessment of plasmocytic disorders
10. Assessment of metastatic cancer

ATLAS OF ABNORMALITIES
OF MORPHOLOGY IN BONE MARROW
AND PERIPHERAL BLOOD

Bone Marrow Morphology

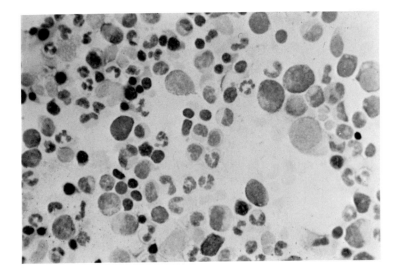

Fig. 1   Bone Marrow Smear demonstrating orderly matura-
tion of myeloid, erythroid and megakaryocytic
cell series and M:E ratio of 4:1.

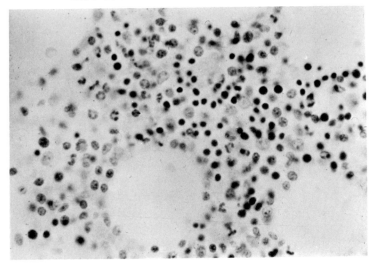

Fig. 2   Section of bone marrow demonstrating orderly mat-
uration of myeloid, erythroid, and megakaryocytic
cell series and M:E ratio of 4:1. The ratio of
bone marrow fat related to nucleated cells is 1:1
which is a normal ratio. Normoblasts have a clear
cytoplasm, myeloid cells a pink cytoplasm, and
histiocytes, lymphocytes, and plasma cells have a
violet cytoplasm in hematoxylin and eosin stained
sections.

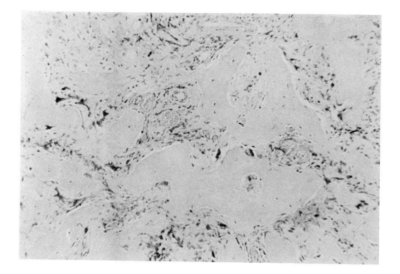

Fig. 3   Section of bone marrow demonstrating extensive
          fibrosis of bone marrow in myelofibrosis. This
          condition will result in myeloid metaplasia and
          peripheral blood leukoerythroblastosis.

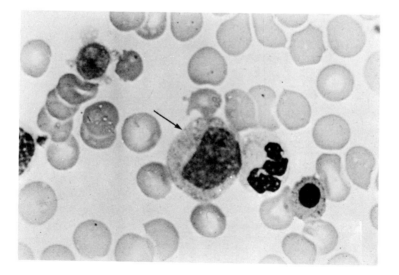

Fig. 4   Peripheral blood smear demonstrating leukoerythro-
          blastosis. Immature myeloid cells (myelocyte-
          arrow) and a normoblast are present indicating
          myelophthsic process due to space-occupying bone
          marrow lesion with myeloid metaplasia.

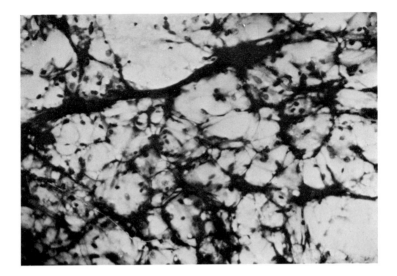

Fig. 5   Bone Marrow section from a patient with aplastic
          anemia. Bone marrow spicule substance and fat
          are present with only a few histiocytes, plasma
          cells, and lymphocytes. No myeloid, normoblasts,
          or megakaryocytes are evident.

Myeloid Maturation

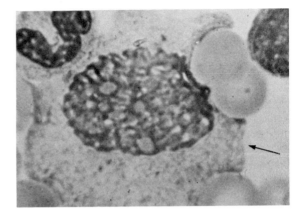

Fig. 6   Ferrata Cell (arrow) which is a hematopoietic reticulum cell or histiocyte, especially seen in the bone marrow in myeloproliferative conditions or hypoplastic bone marrows.

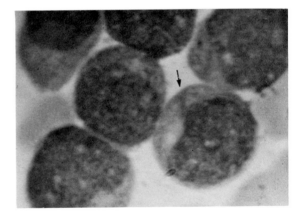

Fig. 7   Myeloblasts in acute myelogenous leukemia with Auer Rod (arrow) with fine nuclear chromatin and multiple nucleoli in bone marrow. Auer rods are not found in non-neoplastic myeloblasts.

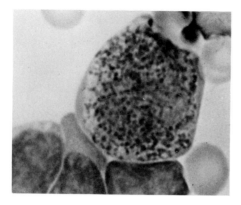

Fig. 8   A promyelocyte with a nucleus consisting of
finely granular chromatin and nucleolus and
prominent azurophilic cytoplasmic granules
in bone marrow.

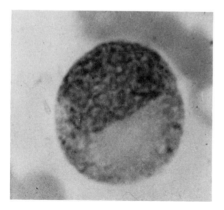

Fig. 9   A myelocyte with eccentric nucleus and neutrophilic substance throughout the cytoplasm in
bone marrow.

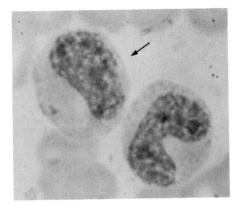

Fig. 10   A metamyelocyte (arrow) and band neutrophilic leukocyte in bone marrow.

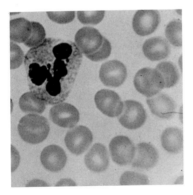

Fig. 11   Polymorphonuclear neutrophilic leukocyte
with nuclear drumsticks which is a nuclear
structure found in females in peripheral
blood.

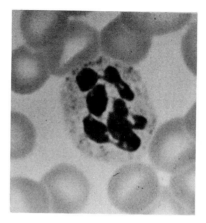

Fig. 12   Hypersegmented polymorphonuclear neutrophil in peripheral blood characteristic of vitamin B_{12} deficiency or folic acid deficiency. Hypersegmentation may also be present on a hereditary basis.

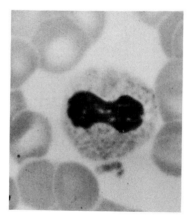

Fig. 13   Neutrophilic band leukocyte with dumbell-shaped nucleus in Pelger-Hüet Anomaly in peripheral blood.

385

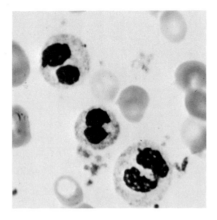

Fig. 14   Pelger-Hüet Anomaly of neutrophilic leukocytes
in which the leukocytes have two lobes in peripheral blood.

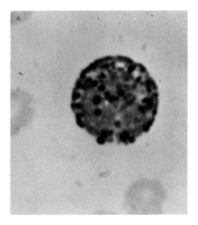

Fig. 15   A basophilic leukocyte in the peripheral blood
containing numerous basophilic granules.

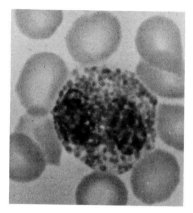

Fig. 16   Normal eosinophil usually containing a bilobed
nucleus in peripheral blood.

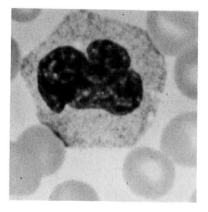

Fig. 17   Normal monocyte in peripheral blood.

Erythroid Maturation

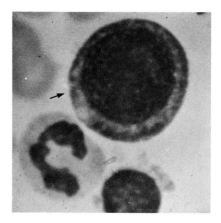

Fig. 18   Bone marrow smear demonstrating a pronormoblast
(arrow) which has a nucleus with fine chromatin
and nucleolus.

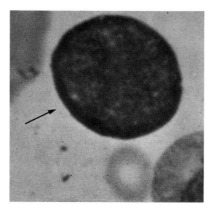

Fig. 19   Bone marrow smear demonstrating a basophilic
normoblast (arrow) which has a nucleus with
a coarser chromatin than the pronormoblast
and a darker blue cytoplasm than the pronormoblast.

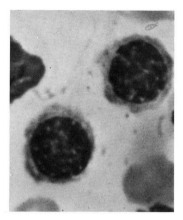

Fig. 20   Bone Marrow Smear demonstrating polychromatophilic
normoblast which has a smaller size than the basophilic normoblast, more pyknotic nucleus with
coarse chromatin and gray cytoplasm.

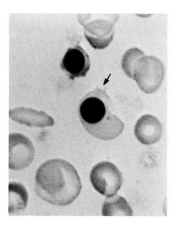

Fig. 21   Orthochromic normoblast with red cytoplasm
(arrow) in peripheral blood.

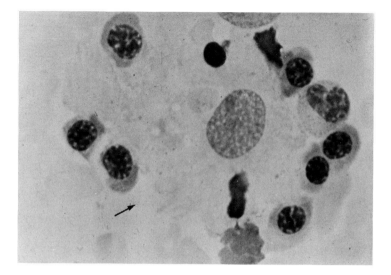

Fig. 22　A "Nurse Cell" (arrow) which is a histiocyte containing iron surrounded by numerous normoblasts in
a bone marrow smear. This is an erythroid island
in which iron is transferred to the normoblasts
from the histiocyte containing iron.

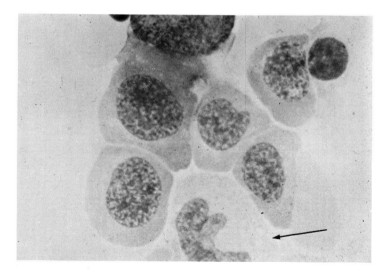

Fig. 23　Bone Marrow Smear demonstrating reversal of M:E
ratio with megaloblastic hyperplasia in pernicious
anemia. The megaloblasts are large and have fine
nuclear chromatin. A giant metamyelocyte is
present (arrow).

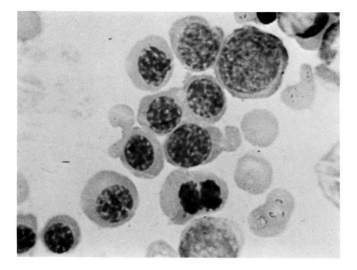

Fig. 24   Normoblastic hyperplasia in bone marrow with
reversal of M:E ratio associated with hemolytic
anemia or acute hemorrhage.

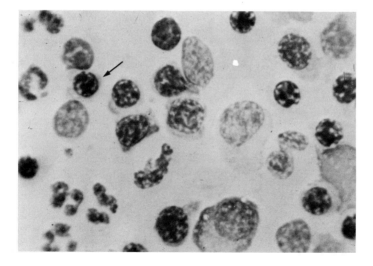

Fig. 25   Bone Marrow Smear demonstrating normoblastic
hyperplasia in iron deficiency anemia or Thalassemia. The normoblasts are small and have deficient serrated cytoplasm (arrow).

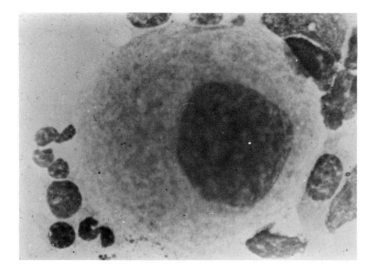

Fig. 26   Normal megakaryocyte with fine granular smooth
            cytoplasm in bone marrow smear.

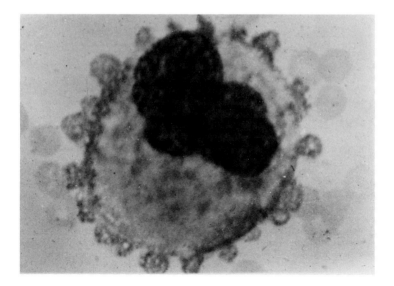

Fig. 27   Immature megakaryocyte in bone marrow smear with
            serrated coarsely granular cytoplasm. Giant blue
            platelets are being produced. This abnormal young
            megakaryocyte is found in conditions in which rapid
            megakaryocytic turnover is present such as in idio-
            pathic thrombocytopenic purpura.

Bone Marrow-Prussian Blue Iron Stain

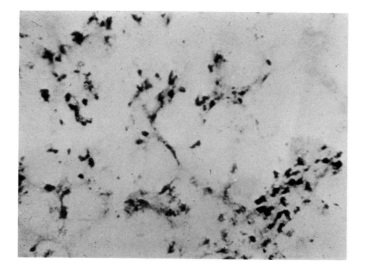

Fig. 28   Prussian Blue Stain of a normal bone marrow smear
demonstrating iron in marrow histiocytes.

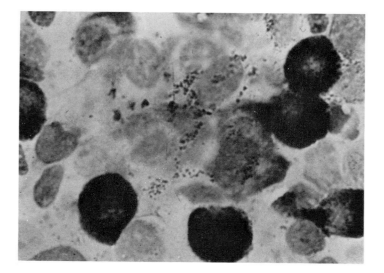

Fig. 29   Prussian Blue Stain of bone marrow demonstrating
marked deposition of iron in histiocytes in
patient with anemia of chronic disease.

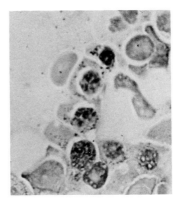

Fig. 30   Prussian Blue Stain of bone marrow demonstrating
presence of many ring sideroblasts found in sideroblastic anemia. The iron is found in ring form
around the nucleus of the normoblast.

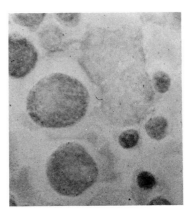

Fig. 31   Prussian Blue Stain of bone marrow demonstrating
lack of iron in histiocytes in patient with iron
deficiency anemia.

Plasma Cell Series

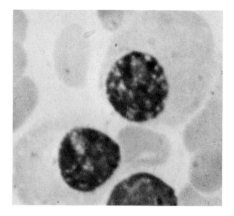

Fig. 32   Plasma cells with eccentric nuclei and coarse
nuclear chromatin in bone marrow.

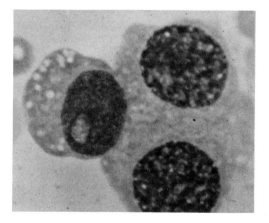

Fig. 33   Plasmablasts in multiple myeloma with eccentric
nuclei, fine nuclear chromatin, and nucleoli in
bone marrow.

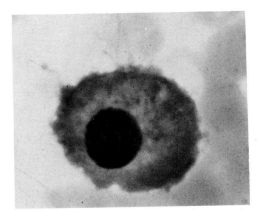

Fig. 34   Flame cell which is a plasma cell associated
with production of IgA immunoglobulin in bone
marrow.

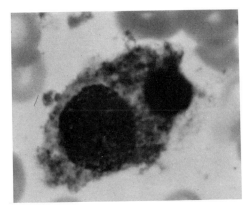

Fig. 35   Plasmablast from smear of multiple myeloma
patient exhibiting phagocytic activity. The
plasmablast is ingesting a lymphocyte.

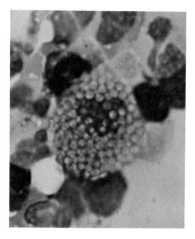

Fig. 36   Bone Marrow Smear demonstrating a Morula cell
          (Mott or Grape cell) due to active production
          of immunoglobulin by a plasmablast in multiple
          myeloma. These cells may also occur in benign
          conditions in which plasma cells actively pro-
          duce immunoglobulin.

Lymphocyte Series

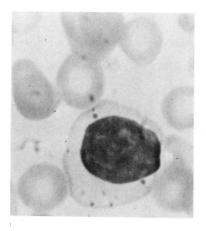

Fig. 37   Normal lymphocyte in peripheral blood.

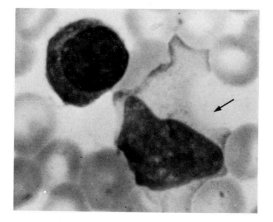

Fig. 38   Two atypical lymphocytes in infectious mononucleosis Downey Type I (arrow) and Downey
Type III plasmacytoid type in peripheral blood.

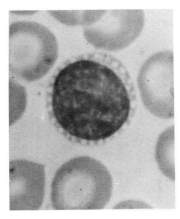

Fig. 39   Sezary syndrome cell in peripheral blood containing numerous vacuoles surrounding the nucleus.
The vacuoles are PAS positive.

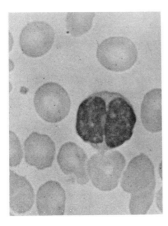

Fig. 40   Peripheral blood demonstrating a lymphocyte with
a deeply clefted immature nucleus, prominent
Rieder Notch ("Buttock Cell"). This type of cell
may be seen in the peripheral blood in Mycosis
Fungoides, Sezary syndrome, or undifferentiated
lymphoma when the neoplastic cells invade the blood
stream.

405

Abnormal Cells in Bone Marrow and Peripheral Blood

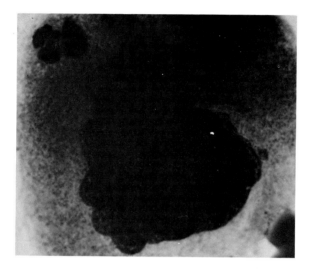

Fig. 41   Bone Marrow Smear demonstrating emperipolesis of
a polymorphonuclear neutrophil in a megakaryocyte
(wandering in and out of PMN's into megakaryocytes)
in various neoplastic, metabolic, inflammatory, or
drug induced diseases affecting megakaryocytes.

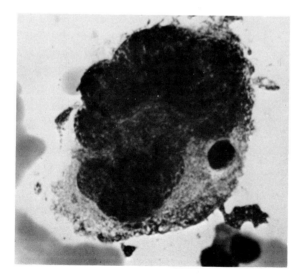

Fig. 42   Bone Marrow Smear demonstrating emperipolesis of a
lymphocyte in a megakaryocyte (wandering in and out
of lymphocytes into megakaryocytes) in various neoplastic, metabolic, inflammatory, or drug induced
diseases affecting megakaryocytes.

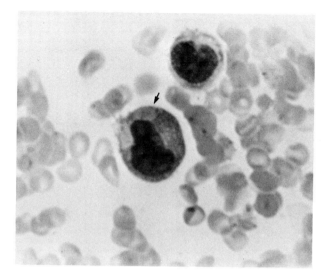

Fig. 43   Bone Marrow Smear demonstrating malignant histiocyte exhibiting phagocytosis of erythrocytes
(arrow). This condition is malignant histiocytosis or histiocytic medullary reticulosis and
results in a hemolytic anemia.

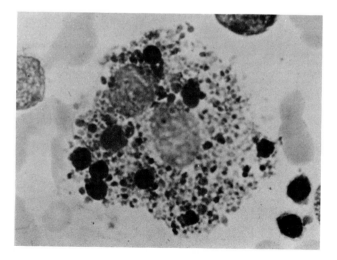

Fig. 44   Bone Marrow Smear demonstrating a histiocyte
which has assumed the function of a macrophage
and is ingesting and removing necrotic cellular
debris.

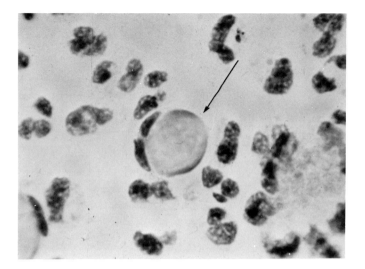

Fig. 45   L. E. cell preparation of peripheral blood demonstrating a lupus erythematosus cell (arrow). The polymorphonuclear neutrophil has ingested a homogenous smooth mass of DNA presumably from a lymphocyte nucleus. The PMN nucleus is eccentric.

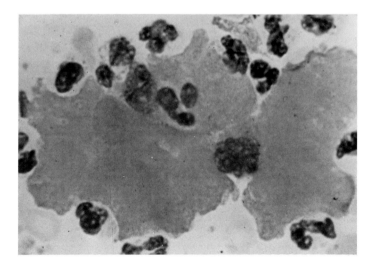

Fig. 46   A L. E. rosette in peripheral blood with numerous polymorphonuclear neutrophils surrounding a large amount of smooth homogeneous DNA substance.

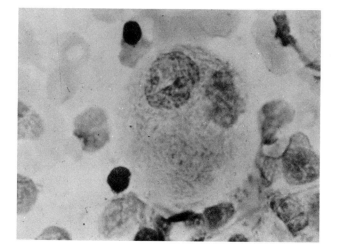

Fig. 47   Bone Marrow Smear demonstrating a Gaucher cell
which is found in Gaucher's disease. The cell
is a histiocyte containing accumulated cerebro-
side due to the deficiency of cerebrosidase in
Gaucher's disease. This type of cell is also
present in bone marrows of chronic myelogenous
leukemia and thalassemia major because of the
large amount of cellular destruction in these
conditions.

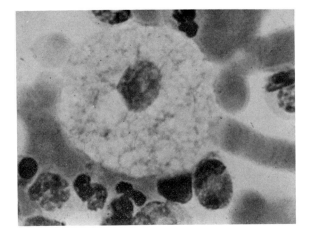

Fig. 48   Bone Marrow Smear demonstrating a phagocyte containing vacuolated cytoplasm. The ingested substance is sphingomyelin. This is a Niemann-Pick
cell.

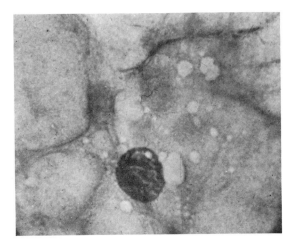

Fig. 49   Bone Marrow Smear demonstrating phagocyte
ingesting amyloid which is located in the
bone marrow in systemic amyloidosis.

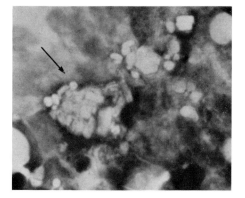

Fig. 50   Macrophages (arrow) in bone marrow con-
          taining cystine crystals in cystinosis
          which is an inherited storage disease.

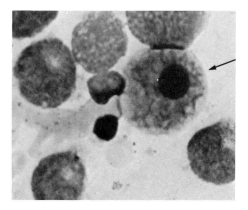

Fig. 51   Sebaceous cell in bone marrow smear which is an
          artefact derived from the sebaceous apparatus
          of skin incurred during bone marrow aspiration.

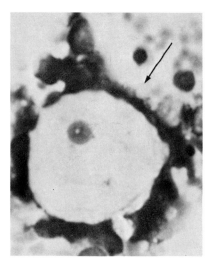

Fig. 52   Macrophage (arrow) in bone marrow smear which
           is filled with lipid from phagocytic activity.

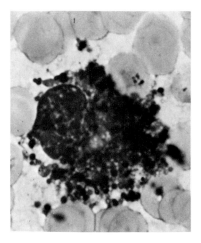

Fig. 53   Bone Marrow Smear demonstrating a
           phagocyte containing mucopolysacchar-
           ide as is found in Hurler's syndrome
           or ceroid in Sea Blue Histiocyte syndrome.

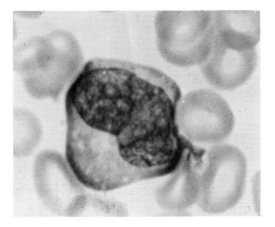

Fig. 54   Reed-Sternberg cell from a bone marrow
           smear obtained from a patient with Hodgkin's
           disease. The patient had IV B disease with
           bone marrow involvement, identified in bone
           marrow aspirate and biopsy section.

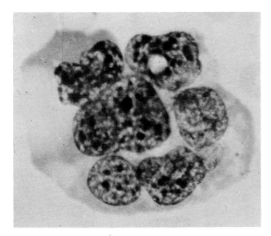

Fig. 55   Bone Marrow Smear demonstrating a multinucleated
           megaloblast. Polyploidy is present with the
           nuclei varying in size and shape. The bone marrow
           was diagnostic of di Guglielmo syndrome. Rarely
           this type of cell may be seen in infectious disease
           affecting the normoblast maturation.

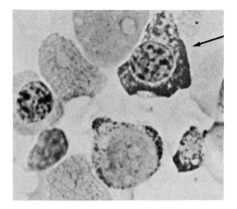

Fig. 56   PAS stain of megaloblastic anemia demonstrating
           PAS positive glycogen in megaloblast in bone
           marrow (arrow) thus, this finding indicates that
           di Guglielmo syndrome is present. PAS positive
           normoblasts are also present in thalassemia and
           not in pernicious anemia.

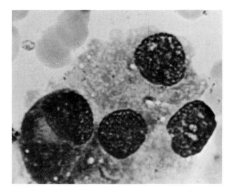

Fig. 57   Osteoblasts in bone marrow with
           eccentric nuclei and fine nuclear
           chromatin resembling plasmablasts.
           Plasmablasts contain cytoplasmic acid
           phosphatase while osteoblasts contain
           alkaline phosphatase.

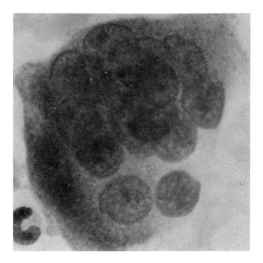

Fig. 58   Bone Marrow Smear demonstrating an
           osteoclast associated with diseases
           in bone and bone marrow in which bone
           destruction is occurring. The cell is
           multinucleated with nuclei equal in size,
           shape, and staining quality.

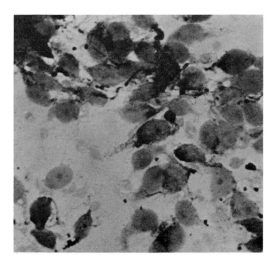

Fig. 59   Bone Marrow Smear demonstrating groups of meta-
           static malignant melanoma cells. The cells are
           spindle shape and contain melanin.

417

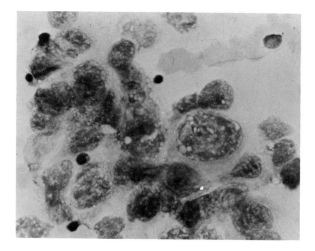

Fig. 60   Bone Marrow Smear demonstrating a collection of
           metastatic malignant epithelial cells from the
           prostate. The cells vary in size, shape, and
           staining quality. Usual primary sites of epith-
           elial malignancies which metastasize to bone
           marrow are prostate, lung, breast, kidney, and
           thyroid.

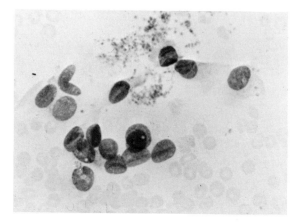

Fig. 61   Peripheral blood smear demonstrating aggregation
           of endothelial cells from vein wall. Blood smear
           was obtained from a venipuncture.

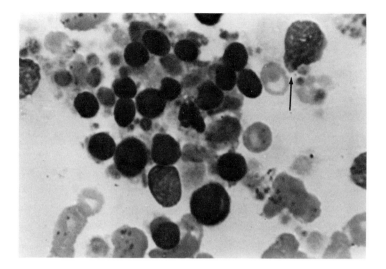

Fig. 62   Megakaryocytic myelosis with portions of nuclei
of megakaryocytes circulating in peripheral blood
associated with numerous platelets and normoblasts.

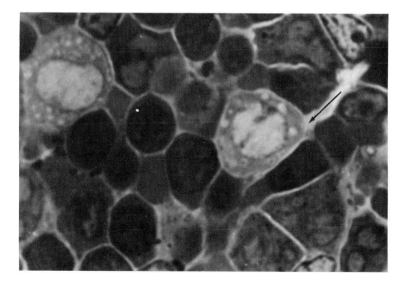

Fig. 63   Bone Marrow Section demonstrating numerous vacuoles
in pronormoblasts.   Vacuoles were caused by Chloramphenicol toxicity.

419

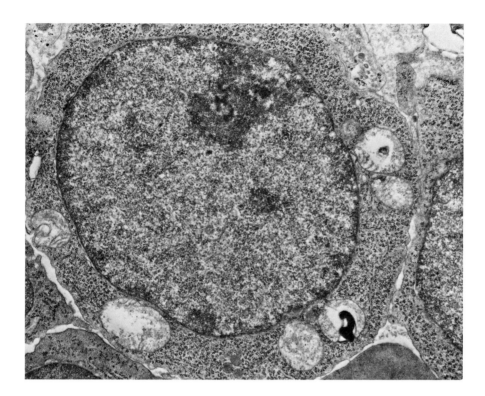

Fig. 64   Electron Microscopic Section of bone marrow pronormoblast demonstrating Chloramphenicol induced
vacuoles in mitochondria surrounding the nucleus.
Electron dense central bodies are present in some
of the vacuoles.

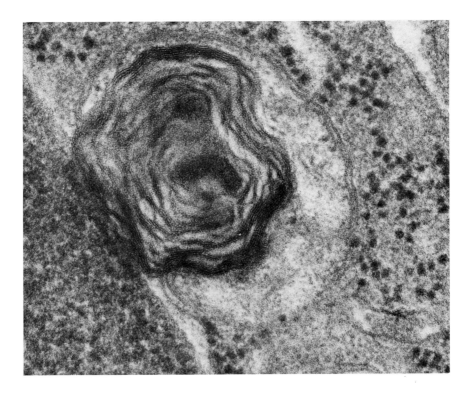

Fig. 65   Electron Microscopic Section of a mitochondrion
           of a pronormoblast with dense bodies in center
           of whorled structure which may be derived from
           outer membranes of mitochondrion. The mitochon-
           drial lesion was induced by Chloramphenicol.

Abnormalities of the Erythrocyte

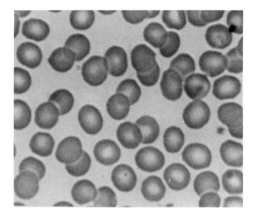

Fig. 66   Normal erythrocytes in peripheral blood. Normal
size and normal chromasia. Normal number of
platelets and normal size.

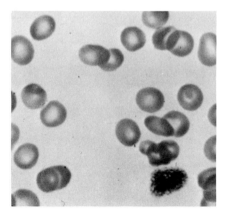

Fig. 67   Giant immature platelet with thrombocytopenia
in peripheral blood.

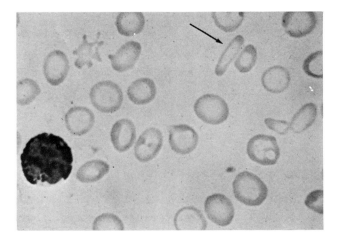

Fig. 68   Microcytic hypochromic anemia with "pencil cells"
(elliptical hypochromic erythrocytes) in peripheral
blood associated with chronic iron deficiency.

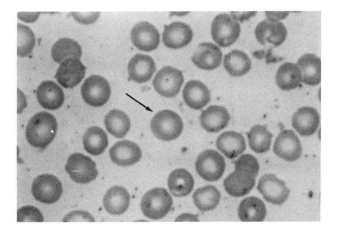

Fig. 69   Round macrocytes (arrow) associated with various
hepatic diseases in contrast to elliptical or
oval macrocytes found in PA in peripheral blood.

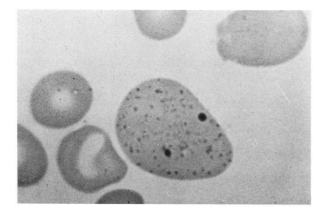

Fig. 70   Elliptical or oval macrocyte of pernicious anemia
in peripheral blood containing numerous basophilic
inclusions which are Prussian Blue positive iron
granules.   Round macrocytes occur in liver disease.

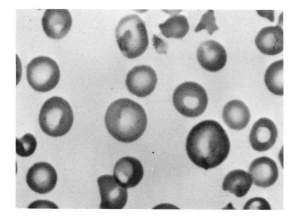

Fig. 71   Peripheral Blood Smear demonstrating normocytic
anemia with fragmented erythrocytes, schistocytes,
or triangle cells found in thrombotic thrombocytopenic purpura.   A marked decrease in platelets has
occurred.

Intracorpuscular Hemolytic Anemia

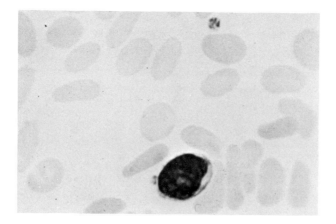

Fig. 72   Numerous elliptocytes found in hereditary ellipto-
           cytosis in peripheral blood.

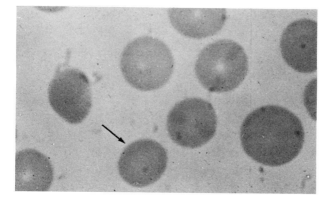

Fig. 73   Peripheral Blood Smear demonstrating spherocytes
           (arrow) which are small and dark erythrocytes
           found in hereditary spherocytosis.

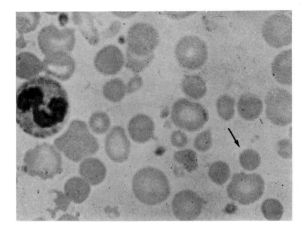

Fig. 74   Numerous spherocytes (arrow) in peripheral blood
caused by acute thermal injury in a patient with
extensive body burn.

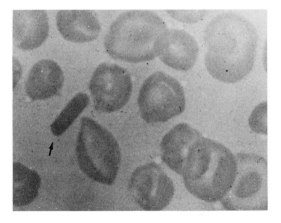

Fig. 75   Hemoglobin C crystal with numerous target cells
(leptocytes) in Hemoglobin C disease in peripheral
blood.

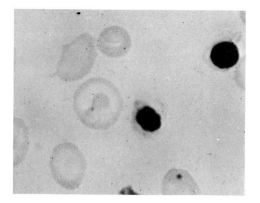

Fig. 76   Peripheral Blood Smear demonstrating hypochromic
microcytic erythrocytes of thalassemia major.
In addition target cells and normoblasts are
frequently present.

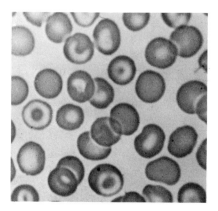

Fig. 77   Target cells present in peripheral blood in patient
who has had a splenectomy. The differential diagnosis is Hemoglobin C disease, thalassemia major,
or obstructive jaundice with liver disease.

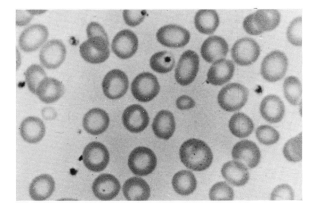

Fig. 78   Peripheral Blood Smear demonstrating microcytic
hypochromic erythrocytes found in thalassemia
minor.

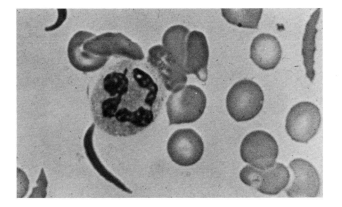

Fig. 79   Sickle cells in peripheral blood in patient with
homozygous Hemoglobin S disease.

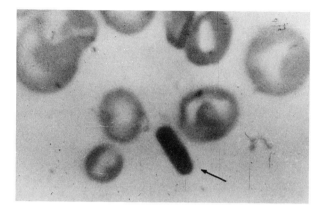

Fig. 80   Hemoglobin S crystal in peripheral blood. A
similar type structure may be a Hemoglobin C
crystal in Hemoglobin C disease.

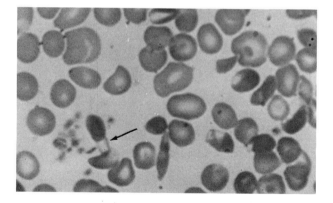

Fig. 81   Peripheral Blood smear demonstrating blister
cell (arrow) associated with pulmonary infarction in homozygous Hemoglobin S or Hemoglobin SC
disease.

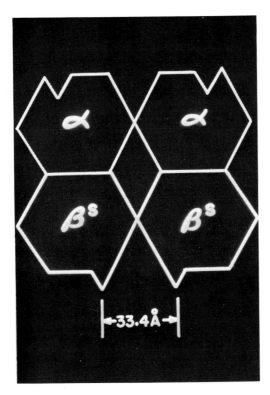

Fig. 82 Oxygenated
Hemoglobin S
Tetramer demon-
strating no
lateral shift
of Beta S
chains.

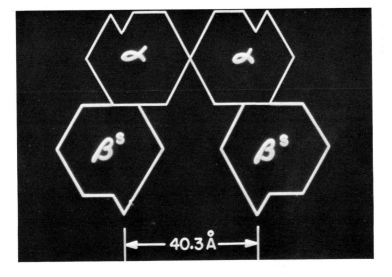

Fig. 83   Deoxygenated Hemoglobin S Tetramer demonstrating
lateral shift of Beta S chains.

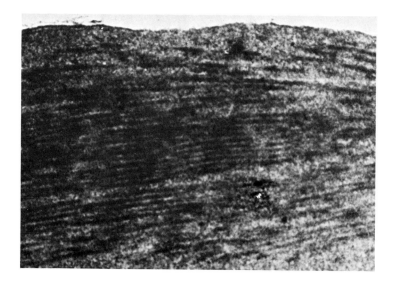

Fig. 84   Electron Microscopic Section of sickle cell
demonstrating microfilaments of Hemoglobin S
crystals at periphery of erythrocyte.

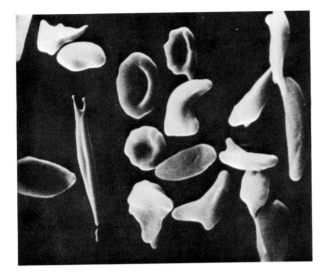

Fig. 85   Scanning Electron Microscopy Photo of
           deoxygenated sickle Hemoglobin erythro-
           cytes. Various shapes of sickled erythro-
           cytes are present.

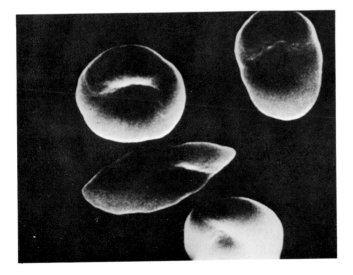

Fig. 86   Scanning Electron Microscopy photo of
           oxygenated sickle Hemoglobin erythrocytes.

Laboratory Tests for
Sickle Cell Disease

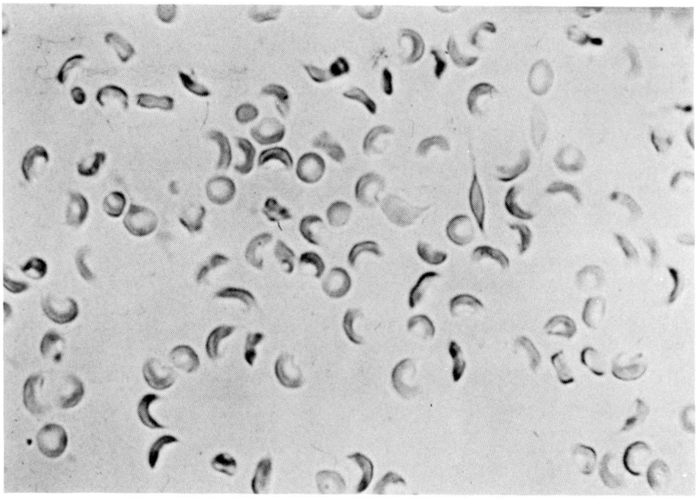

Fig. 87   Positive sickle cell preparation utilizing metabisulfite as the deoxygenating substance with
peripheral blood erythrocytes. This test may
be negative with AS trait.

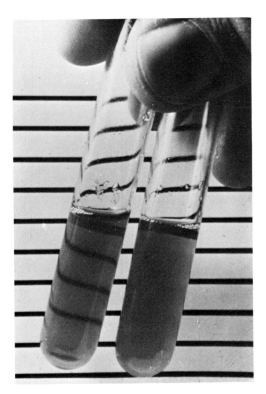

Fig. 88   Dithionite Tube Test demonstrating cloudy
solution of sickling Hemoglobin, right, and
clear solution of non-sickling Hemoglobin,
left (black lines visible through solution).
False positives occur in macroglobulinemia
and in polycythemia.

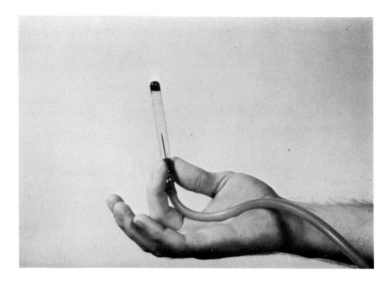

Fig. 89   Murayama Test - Deoxygenated hemolysate of Hemoglobin S which has gelled at 37°C.

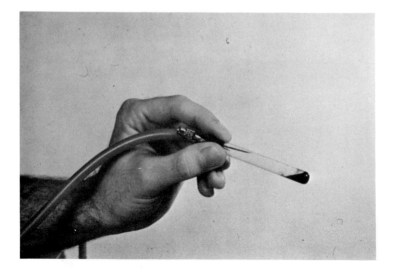

Fig. 90   Murayama Test - Deoxygenated hemolysate of Hemoglobin S which has liquefied when the gel formed
at 37°C. is quickly cooled to 0°C. Hemoglobin C
(Harlem) exhibits similar gel-sol properties.

Extracorpuscular Hemolytic Anemia

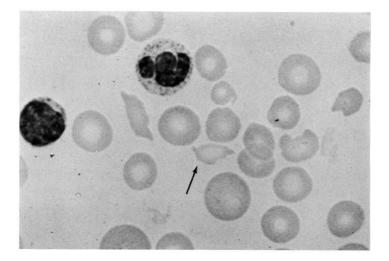

Fig. 91   Fragmented erythrocytes, schistocytes, or triangle cells found in peripheral blood in disseminated intravascular coagulation, heart valve
hemolysis, or hemolytic uremic syndrome. Spherocytes are also present.

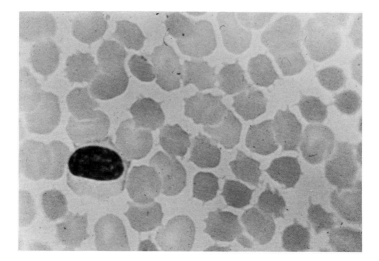

Fig. 92   Peripheral Blood Smear demonstrating acanthrocytes
or Burr cells associated with hemolytic uremic
syndrome or abeta-lipoproteinemia. Spherocytes
are present.

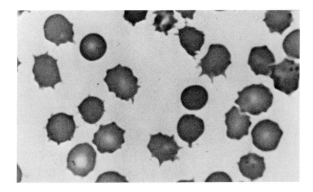

Fig. 93   Spur cells in peripheral blood with more pointed
           spikes than Burr cells.   Spur cells are associated
           with various hepatic diseases.

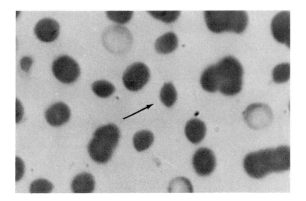

Fig. 94   Peripheral Blood Smear demonstrating the "Torquati"
           sign found in conditions with increased IgM, such as
           Waldenstrom's macroglobulinemia or multiple myeloma.
           The "Torquati" cell (arrow) is heavily coated with
           IgM resulting in an elliptical microspherocytic
           (pseudospherocyte) erythrocyte with a faint halo.

443

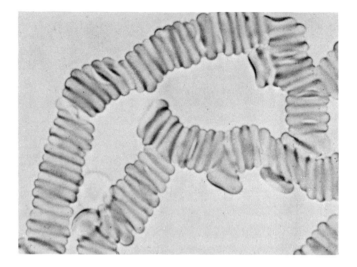

Fig. 95   Peripheral Blood erythrocytes in rouleaux formation secondary to elevated IgM.

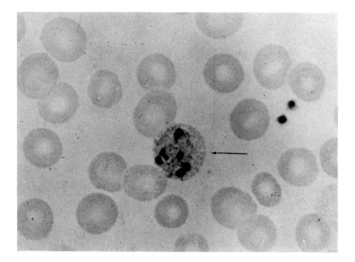

Fig. 96   Peripheral Blood positive for malaria with an organism present within an erythrocyte (arrow).

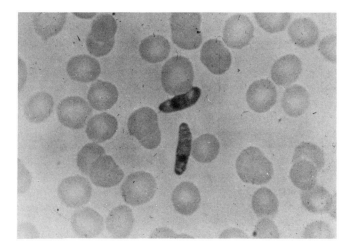

Fig. 97   Peripheral Blood Smear positive for gametocytes
of _Plasmodium_ _falciparum_.

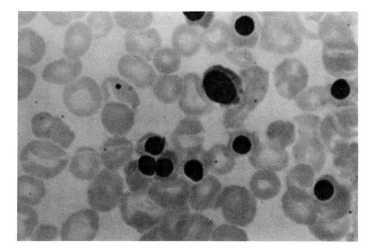

Fig. 98   Numerous normoblasts in peripheral blood of newborn infant with Rh erythroblastosis hemolytic
anemia.   Erythrocytes are macrocytic and many
reticulocytes are present.   ABO erythroblastosis
is associated with spherocytosis.   445

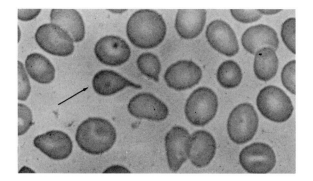

Fig. 99   Tear drop or tadpole cells (arrow) in peripheral
blood associated with myelofibrosis, myeloid
metaplasia with splenomegaly, and splenic disease.

Intraerythrocytic Inclusions

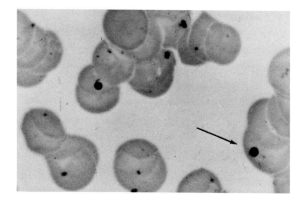

Fig. 100   Peripheral Blood Smear demonstrating Howell-Jolly
Bodies in erythrocytes. These inclusions are portions of the nucleus of the normoblast which should
be "pitted" from the erythrocyte by the spleen.
Thus, the inclusions are present in the erythrocytes
in individuals who have had a splenectomy or have
a diseased non-functional spleen.

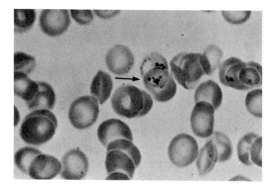

Fig. 101   Peripheral Blood Smear demonstrating siderocytes
(Pappenheimer Bodies) containing iron granules
(arrow). This abnormality in the peripheral blood
indicates that absence of the spleen with loss of
splenic "pitting" function is present. The abnormality may also be found in patients with splenic
disease and functional asplenia.

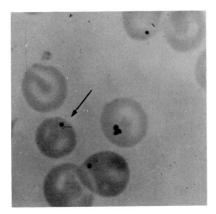

Fig. 102   Prussian Blue Stain of peripheral blood demonstrating erythrocytes with Prussian Blue positive
iron granules in erythrocytes which are designated
Pappenheimer Bodies in siderocytes.

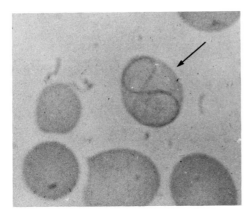

Fig. 103   Cabot ring which represents the rim of the nucleus
of the normoblast in an elliptical macrocytic erythrocyte of pernicious anemia in peripheral blood.

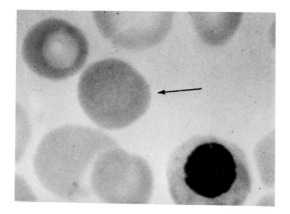

Fig. 104 Polychromatophilic erythrocyte (arrow) which represents a reticulocyte in a Wright-Giemsa Stain of peripheral blood.

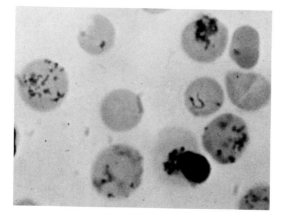

Fig. 105 New Methylene Blue Stain of peripheral blood demonstrating reticulocytes containing stranded and punctate RNA in young erythrocytes.

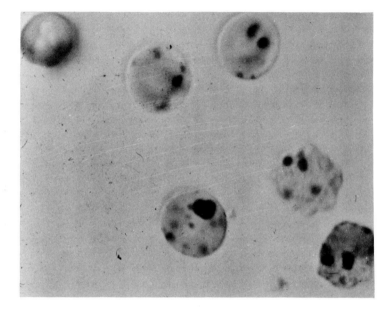

Fig. 106   Heinz Body preparation of peripheral blood demonstrating positive result.   50 percent of the erythrocytes contain 5 or more Heinz-Ehrlich Bodies which
represent precipitated oxidized Hemoglobin in a
patient who has an absence or deficiency of Glucose-
6-Phosphate Dehydrogenase and who received a drug
or had a disease such as diabetic ketoacidosis,
viral hepatitis, or septicemia which caused the
oxidation and precipitation of the Hemoglobin.

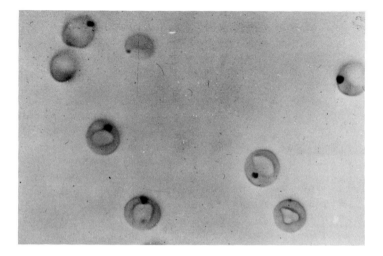

Fig. 107   Heinz Body preparation of peripheral blood demonstrating a negative result.   More than 50 percent
of the erythrocytes have less than 5 Heinz-Ehrlich
Bodies.   See previous photograph.

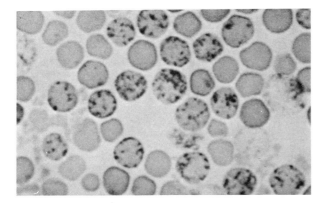

Fig. 108   Intraerythrocytic inclusions of precipitated
hemoglobin in unstable Hemoglobin H disease
in peripheral blood.

Cytoplasmic Inclusions in
White Blood Cells

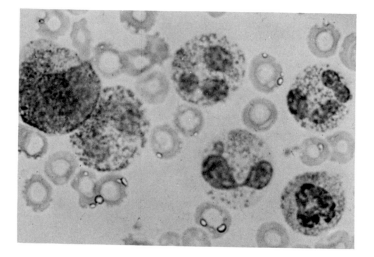

Fig. 109   Peripheral Blood neutrophilic leukocytosis with left shift. Marked toxic granulation of leukocytes is present.

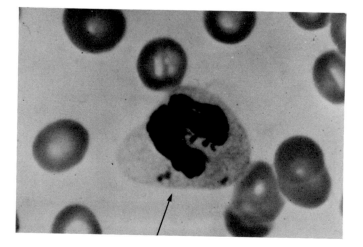

Fig. 110   Peripheral Blood neutrophilic leukocyte containing cytoplasmic Döhle Bodies (arrow) which consist of RNA. This occurs in severe bacterial sepsis, burn patients, malignancy, and pregnancy. It also may be inherited in May-Hegglin anomaly.

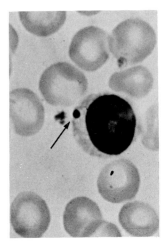

Fig. 111   Peripheral Blood lymphocyte containing
mucopolysaccharide in Alder's anomaly.

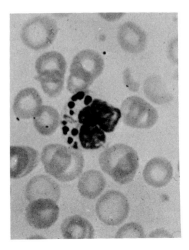

Fig. 112   Peripheral Blood neutrophilic leukocyte
in Chediak-Higashi syndrome containing
cytoplasmic inclusions which are present
in the lysosomes.

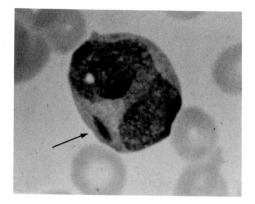

Fig. 113   Peripheral Blood Smear demonstrating monoblast
in acute monocytic leukemia with lysosomal Auer
rod.

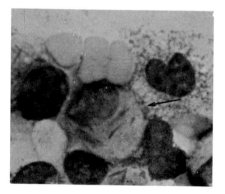

Fig. 114   Auer rods in bone marrow plasmablasts in multiple
myeloma.

Bone Marrow and
Peripheral Blood in Leukemia

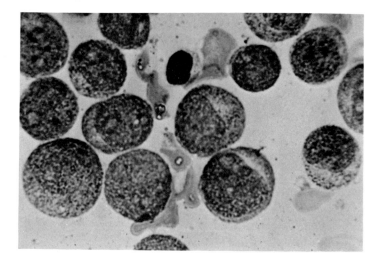

Fig. 115   Bone Marrow Smear demonstrating numerous myeloblasts found in acute myelogenous leukemia. The
M:E ratio is 100:1. The myeloblasts have nuclei
with fine chromatin, numerous nucleoli, fine
nuclear membrane, moderate cytoplasm, and no
vacuoles in cytoplasm.

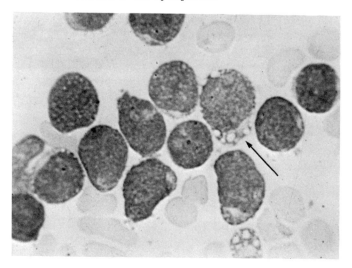

Fig. 116   Lymphoblasts in bone marrow in acute lymphocytic
leukemia containing coarse nuclear chromatin, few
nucleoli, and cytoplasmic vacuoles (arrow).

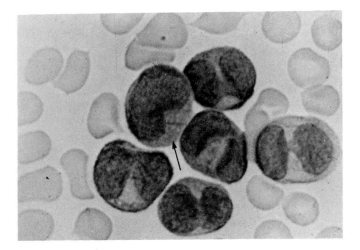

Fig. 117   Monoblasts in the peripheral blood in acute
           monocytic leukemia.   The nuclei are convoluted
           and contain fine chromatin.   An Auer rod is
           present (arrow).

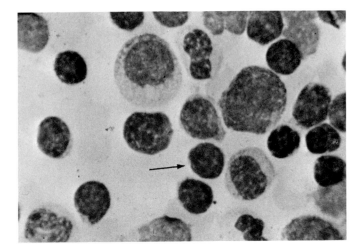

Fig. 118   Bone Marrow Smear demonstrating prominent infil-
           trate of mature lymphocytes found in chronic
           lymphocytic leukemia.

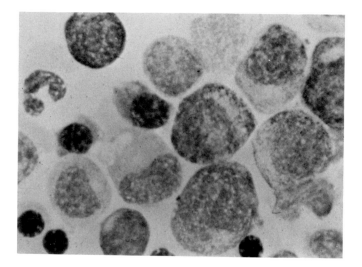

Fig. 119   Bone Marrow Smear from a patient with chronic
myelogenous leukemia. The M:E ratio is 50:1.
All stages of myeloid cellular differentiation
are present with a moderate left shift to
immaturity.

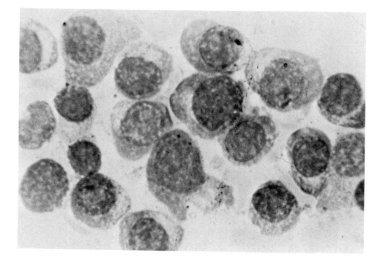

Fig. 120   Prominent proliferation of plasma cells and immuno-
blastic lymphocytes in bone marrow of patient with
Waldenstrom's macroglobulinemia.

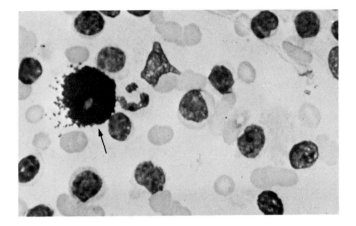

Fig. 121 Mast cell (arrow) present in bone marrow smear
of patient with Waldenstrom's macroglobulinemia.
The presence of mast cells in this disease is
common.

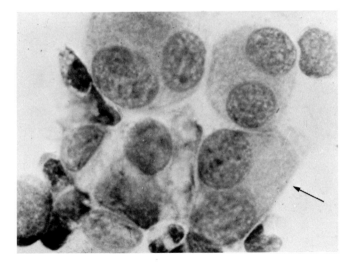

Fig. 122 Bone Marrow Smear demonstrating marked increase
in immature dysplastic megakaryocytes (arrow)
found in megakaryocytic myelosis (a condition
which is present in the myeloproliferative syndrome) or in conditions associated with thrombocytopenia, such as idiopathic thrombocytopenic
purpura.

463

Special Stains

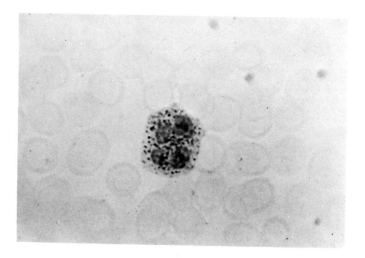

Fig. 123   Alkaline Phosphatase Stain demonstrating neutrophilic leukocyte positive for alkaline phosphatase
in peripheral blood.

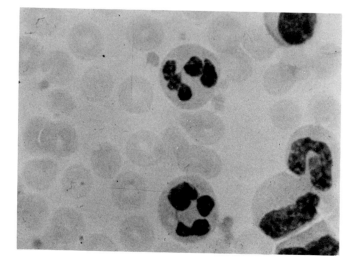

Fig. 124   Alkaline Phosphatase Stain demonstrating neutrophilic leukocytes negative for alkaline phosphatase as is seen in acute or chronic myelogenous
leukemia in peripheral blood.

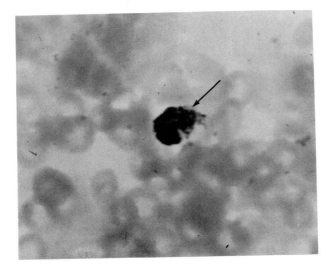

Fig. 125 NBT Stain demonstrating neutrophilic
leukocyte containing formazan granule
(arrow) in peripheral blood.

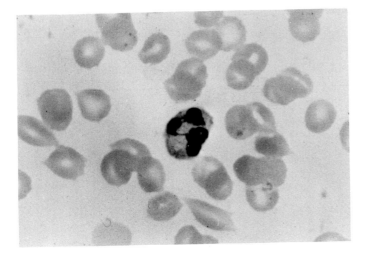

Fig. 126 NBT Stain demonstrating a polymorphonuclear neutrophil in peripheral blood which does not contain a formazan precipitated granule.

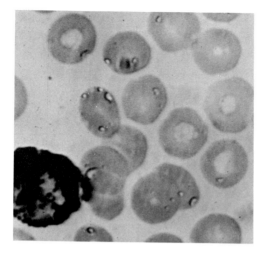

Fig. 127 A Peroxidase Stain of peripheral blood
demonstrating peroxidase positive polymorphonuclear neutrophil. Lymphocytes
are peroxidase negative.